THE Men's Health and Women's BIG BOOK of SEX

GW00994243

RODALE

THE Women'sHealth BIG BOOK of SEX

RODALE

Credits

COVER
Photography by Antoine Verglas
Styling by Karen Shapiro
Hair & Makeup by Donna Fumoso @ Ford Artists

BETTER SEX (His/Hers)
Photography by Antoine Verglas
Wardrobe Styling by Karen Shapiro / Prop Styling by Alistair Turnbull @ Pat Bates
Hair & Makeup by Giovanni Giuntoli @WT Management

OWNER'S MANUAL
Illustrations by Bryan Christie

WHAT MEN/WOMEN WANT; POSITIONS
Illustrations by Byron Gray
Photography by Alex Freund
Wardrobe/Prop Styling by Lisa Mosko
Hair by Tomo Nakajima for Halley Resources / Sally Hershberger Salon
Makeup by Greg Vaughan @ L'Atelier NYC using MAC

FITNESS (His, Hers, Ours)
Photography by Beth Bischoff
Wardrobe Styling by Kathy Kalafut
Hair & Makeup by Kyra Dorman for ArtistsByTimothyPriano.com
Trainers: Dean Graham, Jeff Bell
Clothing Credits - HERS: Top by Lucy, Shorts by Body Wrappers, Shoes by New Balance,
HIS: Shorts by Asics, Shoes by Puma

A-Z of LOVEMAKING (His/Hers)
Photography by Jon Ragel
Wardrobe Styling by Lisa Mosko / Prop Styling by Alistair Turnbull @ Pat Bates
Hair & Makeup by Giovanni Giuntoli @ WT Management

RED HOT MONOGAMY (His/Hers)
Photography by Robert Whitman
Wardrobe/Prop Styling by Lisa Mosko
Hair & Makeup by Chris Newburg @ RJ Bennett

SEX DIET

LIFESTYLE	FOOD
Photography by Robert Whitman	**Photography by Thomas MacDonald**
Wardrobe/Prop Styling by Lisa Mosko	Art Direction and Prop Styling by Tara Long
Hair & Makeup by Chris Newburg @ RJ Bennett	Food Styling by Melissa Reiss

The following excerpts were reprinted with permission: Chapter 5: The Sexual Diagnostic (WH)/page 66 "Sex Repairs" by Leslie Goldman, copyright © by *Women's Health* (July 2007); Chapter 6: The Better Sex Diet/page 100 some recipes adapted with permission of Amy Reiley from *The Love Diet* by Juan-Carlos Cruz & Amy Reiley (Life of Reiley:2010), www.lifeofreiley.com; Chapter 7: Make Lust Last (WH)/page 126 "Your Honey or Your Wife" by Hugh O'Neill, copyright © *Men's Health* (January 1996); Chapter 7: Make Lust Last (WH)/page 142 "Have Amazing Sex All Month Long" by Elise Nersesian, copyright © *Women's Health* (November 2009).

Contents

Index

Boldface page references indicate illustrations. Underscored references indicate boxed text.

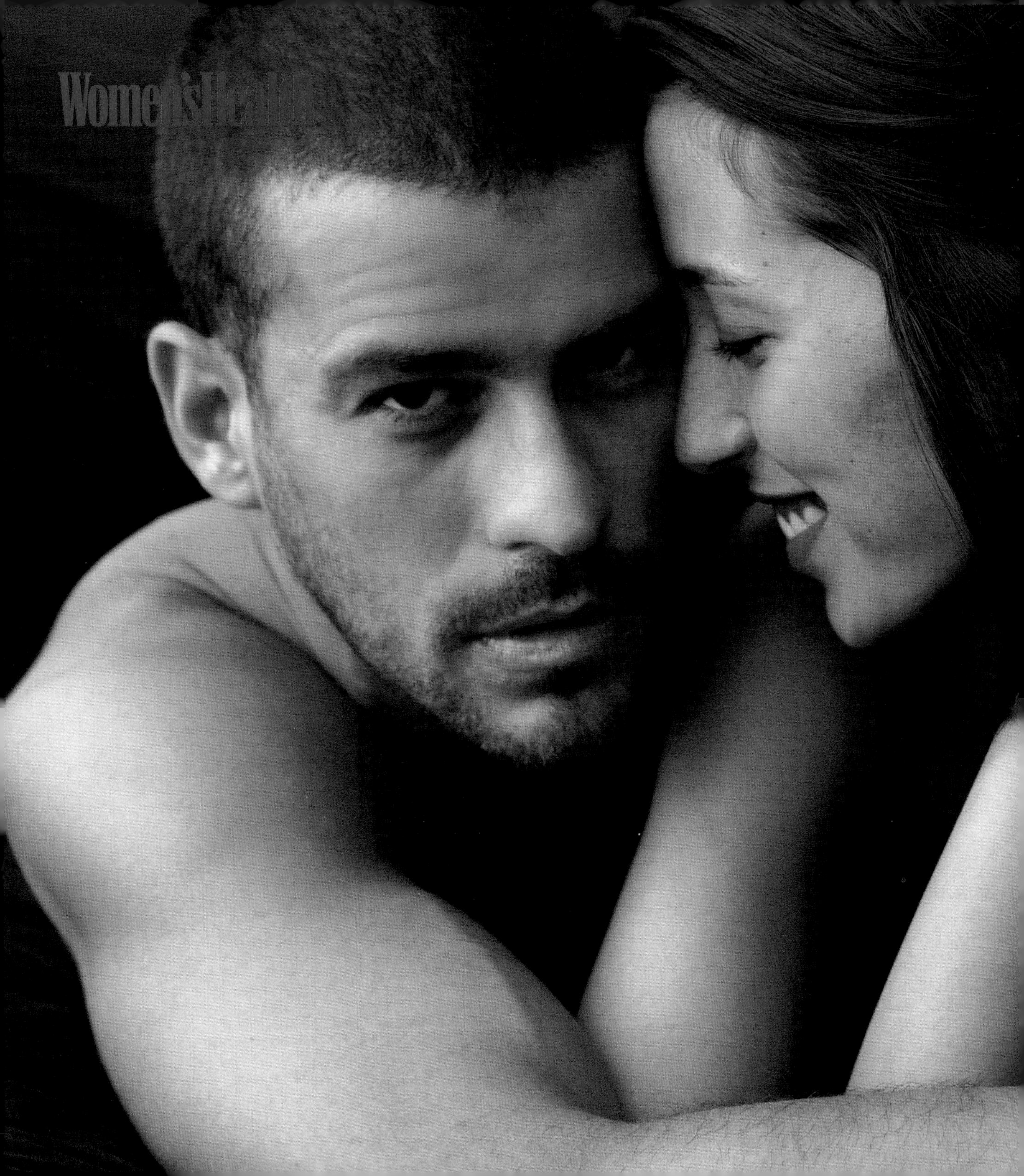

Chapter 1
Better Sex Starts Here

A LEANER, STRONGER, HEALTHIER BODY AND MIND
MEAN MORE—MUCH MORE—PLEASURE FOR YOU

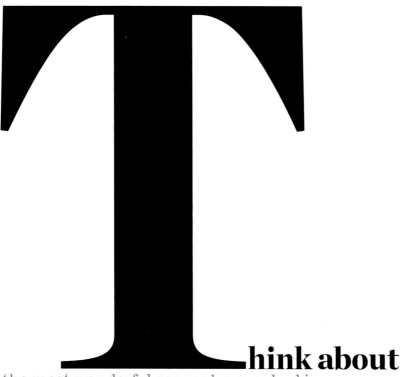hink about

the most wonderful sex you've ever had in your life. Maybe it was last night after Leno, last month on a romantic getaway in Cabo San Lucas, or last year during a quickie with your guy in the laundry room at your friend's cocktail party.

Whenever it was, in all likelihood, more was right with the world than just the sex you were having. Indulge us as we do a little mind-reading: You probably felt great about your relationship. You were totally emotionally connected to your partner or at least sharing the same sexy, carefree vibe. You felt energized. You liked the way your body looked and felt naked. Your partner was attentive and loving. You felt confident, safe, and happy. And probably more than a little naughty in a highly arousing way.

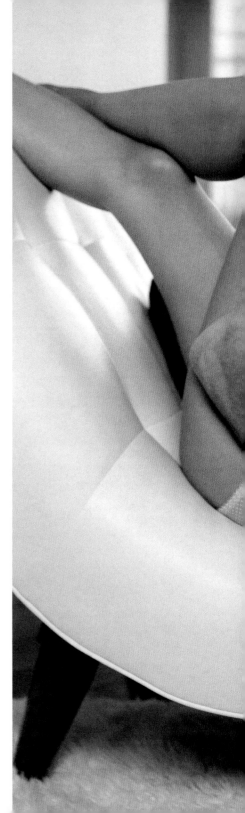

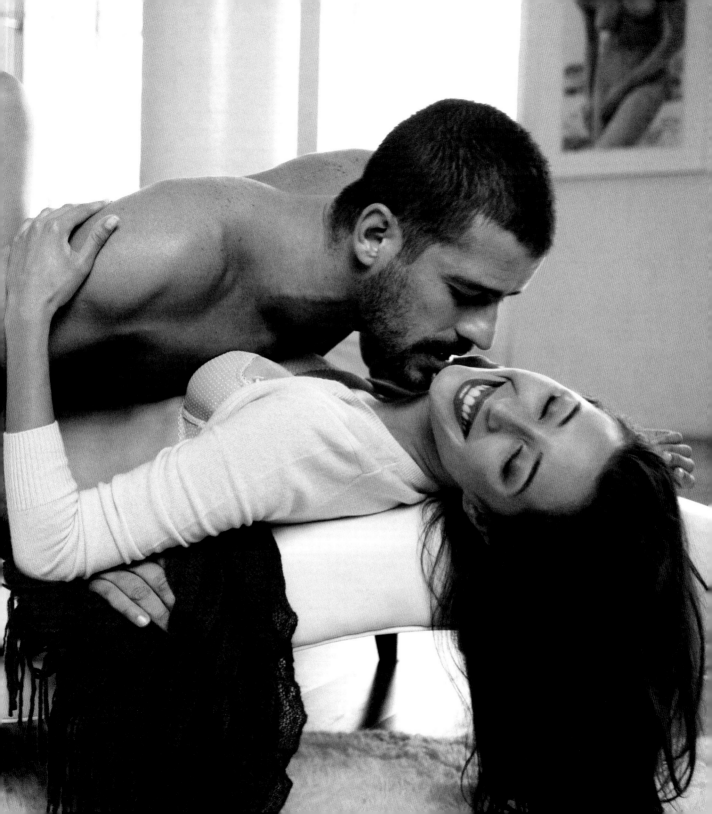

Does that describe your state of mind and body? We'd bet on it because, again and again, women like you have told us that those are the key ingredients of great sex.

That's the kind of sex we hope you'll have after you've read *The Women's Health/Men's Health Big Book of Sex*. We want to provide you (and your partner) with the tools you'll need to achieve a healthy intimacy where great sex with fabulous orgasms is not the only goal, but just one important, exciting, and pleasurable component of a dynamic relationship. (No worries: the multiple-orgasm-achieving tips figure heavily in later chapters.)

First, let's put aside some common notions about sexuality, notions that might be keeping you from reaching that healthy intimacy:

- Everyone else must be enjoying frequent, bed-quaking orgasms but me.

- Men always feel like having sex and, for them, even bad sex is pretty good.

- Because I don't desire intercourse as strongly as my guy, something must be wrong with me or our relationship.

- I feel kind of slutty when I initiate sex or ask for something out of the ordinary.

- When he kisses me or pats my butt, I think he just wants sex.

- A new position, lube, pill, toy, or technique will be "the answer."

- Our sex resembles nothing I see in movies.

- Do I look fat out of these jeans?

All of those thoughts are common, natural, and understandable given our cultural influences and the media's pervasive portrayal of how sex should look, sound, and feel. But what they really point to is the need for you to find out what makes you feel confident enough in body and mind to enjoy the pleasures of sex.

Getting back to the greatest sex you ever had: Where did it go? Back to Cabo San Lucas? Maybe you don't even miss it because well, lately, your libido has gone AWOL. Don't worry. You're not alone. A recent study published in the journal *Archives of Internal Medicine* reports that more than one in three American women experience low sexual desire.

But there's good news: According to sexual health experts we spoke with, reclaiming pleasure is a matter of taking certain proactive steps—practice, if you will—to create a positive atmosphere of emotional comfort and physical health. This book is designed to help you accomplish just that with exercise and diet tips, health advice, stress reduction tricks, and relationship-strengthening exercises—and, of course, some secret saucy moves that'll rock his world and yours!

We can promise you a better sex life long before you reach the simple trick that'll triple your pleasure in Chapter 8.

The Big Book of Sex Will Make You Fit for Sex

Have you ever jumped your man's bones after a workout at the gym?

61

Percentage of women who say they have felt distracted during sex because they were thinking about how their body looked to him.

Can't figure out just what came over you? Well, we know.

Exercise may spark the libido better than a romantic dinner thanks to your sympathetic nervous system. Huh? Let us explain. During research done at the Meston Sexual Psychophysiology Laboratory at the University of Texas in Austin, a group of women was asked to visit the lab on two different days. One day, they watched a travel documentary followed by an erotic film. Another day, they were instructed to exercise for 20 minutes on a stationary cycle at a fairly intense clip, 70 percent of their maximum heart rate. When they finished the workout, they watched an erotic video. On both days, sexual arousal was measured using a probe called a photo-plethsymograph that gauges flow of blood to the vagina and subsequent lubrication. (It doesn't sound fun to us either, but it was for the good of science and better sex!) The result: On the day they exercised, the women became much more aroused—a whopping 150 percent more—while watching the erotic film than they did on a non-exercise day.

So what's the connection? Exercise activated the sympathetic nervous system, which prepared the body for sexual arousal, explains Cindy M. Meston, PhD, director of the lab. "When put in a sexual situation, women's bodies responded more quickly and intensely than when they hadn't exercised."

So, if you're not feeling particularly frisky, trigger your sympathetic nervous system by doing something energizing

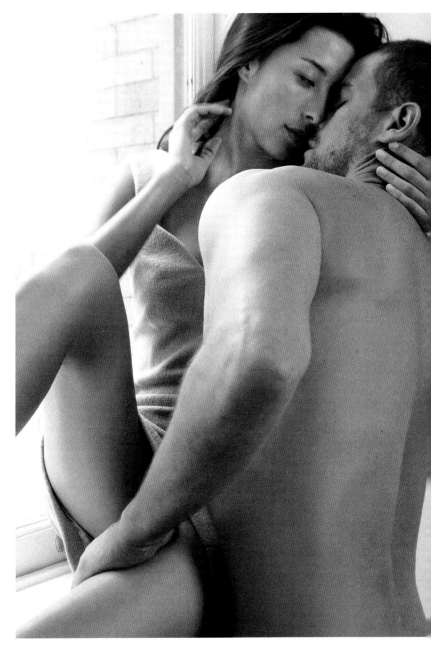

Better Sex Starts Here

BELLY-BLOATING HABITS TO BREAK

Researchers at the University of Massachusetts analyzed the eating habits of 500 people and identified common behaviors that contributed to their becoming dangerously overweight. Here's how much these habits increase your chances of becoming obese:

43% Waiting more than 3 hours after waking up to eat breakfast

69% Eating out for more than a third of your meals

101% Going to bed on an empty stomach

137% Eating out for breakfast regularly

450% Not eating anything for breakfast at all

like taking a spin class, playing tennis, going bowling, or challenging your boyfriend in a game of … handball. Turkish researchers using Doppler ultrasonography measured significantly greater clitoral blood flow in 25 female handball players than in a similar group of 25 non-athletic Turkish women, according to a a study reported in the *Journal of Sexual Medicine*. The handball players also scored higher on questionnaires that measured sexual satisfaction. Both results, the researchers say, suggests that good fitness correlates with better sex.

Need more incentive to get moving? Here are more reasons exercise can wake up your libido.

You'll be happier. Exercise is a terrific mood and libido booster. Going for a run on a beautiful day triggers your brain to release endorphins, feel-good neurochemicals that elevate mood and take your mind off work so you can focus on more pleasurable pursuits. Numerous studies show that exercise can even fight clinical depression, which is a prime destroyer of sexual desire and performance. Psychiatrists at the University of Texas Southwestern's Mood Disorders Research Program and Clinic found that patients suffering from depression who did moderately intense aerobics for 35 minutes a day experienced a nearly 50 percent decline in depression symptoms, which is comparable to the effect of antidepressant medication like Prozac or Zoloft, but without the negative sexual

side effects. Exercise also provides opportunities for more social interaction, which helps with self-esteem and self-image.

You'll want to do it more. A Harvard University study of 160 male and female swimmers in their 40s and 60s showed a positive relationship between regular physical activity and the frequency and enjoyment of sexual intercourse. The research showed that swimmers in their 60s reported sex lives comparable to people in the general population who were 20 years younger.

You'll have healthier arteries. LDL, commonly known as the "bad" cholesterol is the waxy stuff that clogs arteries and, more critically, causes the arterial inflammation that leads to most heart attacks. It doesn't just gunk up the heart arteries; cholesterol deposits can choke the tiny arteries leading to and within the vagina and block blood flow like a jack-knifed tractor trailer blocks traffic. Unfortunately, exercise may not reduce LDL cholesterol levels directly, but evidence does prove that it raises the good HDL cholesterol. HDL acts like arterial drain cleaner, picking up excess cholesterol from artery walls and carting it to the liver for removal from the body. Moderate to intense aerobic exercise has been shown to have a clear effect on raising HDL levels. Studies at Auburn University show that 30 to 45 minutes of vigorous exercise for four consecutive days can raise HDL levels by four to six points. What's more, exercise reduces triglycerides, another dangerous form of blood fat that contributes to cardiovascular disease in men and women.

You'll look sexier, which means you'll feel sexier. Exercise tones, tightens, and keeps the weight off—and we all know how good we feel after a workout. All of that leads to a better body—and a better body image—which then leads to more time in the sack. Studies show that women with a negative body image have lower sex drives, more trouble becoming lubricated, and less frequent orgasms. One study at Meston's lab involved 85 college women who filled out body image questionnaires and then were sent to private rooms, given erotic reading material, and asked to rate how turned-on the story made them feel. Those women who felt good about their bodies reported much greater arousal and desire from the reading than the women who felt bad about their bodies.

You'll sleep sounder and have erotic dreams. Exhausting your muscles will help you get to sleep faster and sleep deeper, according to National Sleep Foundation scientists. One study found that sleep-lab patients who exercised three times a week for 8 weeks improved their quality of sleep by nearly 25 percent. Deep, restful sleep is important to good sexual function. When you have rejuvenating sleep, you produce norepinephrine and dopamine, two neurotransmitters that play a role in desire and arousal. A full night's sleep, 7 to 8 hours, ensures

that you'll experience rejuvenating REM—meaning you'll be totally rested and ready to have fun in bed instead of fall dead asleep as soon as you hit the pillow.

The Big Book of Sex Will Help You Lose Weight

Being overweight can depress anyone's sex life. A survey of 1,210 people of different weights and sizes conducted by researchers at Duke University Medical Center showed that obese people were 25 times as likely to report dissatisfaction with sex as normal weight people. The fantastic news is that good sex can be achieved without a substantial change in body composition. Several studies have shown that people report much greater enjoyment of sexual activity following just a 10 percent weight loss, says Martin Binks, PhD, clinical director of Binks Behavioral Health and an assistant consulting professor at Duke University Medical Center. "It's important to realize that these folks did not get to some ideal weight, but rather that just moderate improvements that we know benefit overall health also helped in the bedroom," he says.

Some other ways taking off pounds can lift your love life:

You'll boost testosterone. The male hormone testosterone (which women produce, too, except in much smaller quantities) is associated with sex drive. In fact, women with low libido can receive a prescription for testosterone

32

Percentage of women in one survey who said they masturbated in the previous 3 months to help themselves fall asleep.

to jumpstart their desire. But there are natural ways to elevate your T levels. Physical, competitive sports and endurance exercise, for example. Since women have far less of the hormone to start with, they actually get a bigger lift from competition than men do. Beach volleyball, anyone?

You'll avoid the big sex killer: diabetes.
Studies show that people with diabetes are more likely to suffer from sexual dysfunction than healthy people are. What's more, sexual health problems start showing up as much as a decade earlier in these people. Type 2 diabetes, or adult-onset diabetes, occurs when the body becomes resistant to insulin over time because it has been flooded with massive amounts of glucose. When your pancreas doesn't produce enough insulin to effectively do its job, the glucose starts to do damage, including to your sex life. Over time high blood sugar causes damage to nerves and blood vessels, which affects blood flow to the genitals, and reduces testosterone. But by losing belly fat through diet and exercise, you can improve your sensitivity to the insulin hormone and actually reverse type 2 diabetes. In one Austrian study, people with type 2 diabetes on a 4-month-long strength training program significantly lowered their blood sugar levels and vastly improved control over their diabetes.

You may increase your sex drive.
High-fat meats, other saturated fats, and trans fats in processed foods decrease testosterone levels and lower libido. By replacing the fatty-foods in your diet with fresh vegetables, fruits, whole grains, and lean proteins you may increase your desire to have sex as well as your stamina.

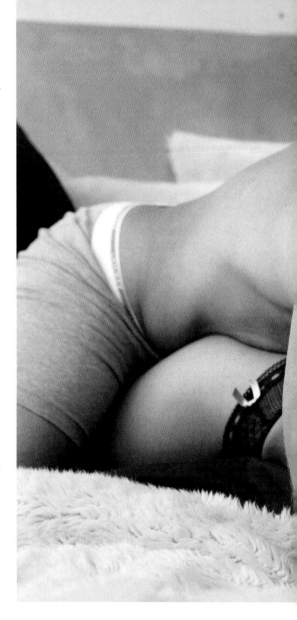

FLEX FOR SEX

Women who practice yoga regularly report a boost in sex drive, according to *The Journal of Sexual Medicine.*

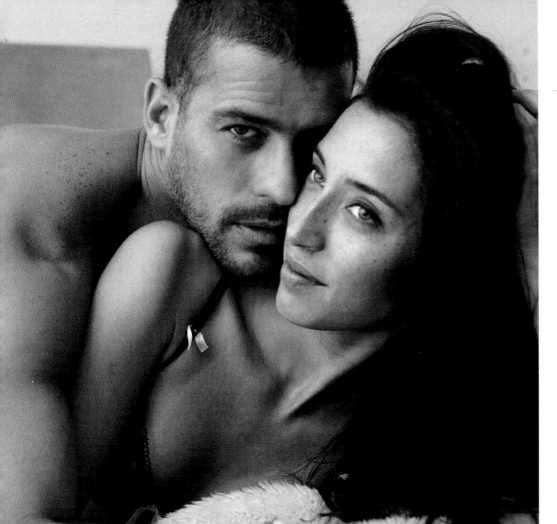

50

Percent decrease in pain sensitivity due to stimulation of the clitoris and vaginal walls, according to studies at Rutgers University. Similar research shows that arousal can reduce migraine and lower back pain.

You'll pave the way to greater arousal. As we mentioned, high cholesterol disrupts the pathways that feed blood to the genitals. Studies have shown a direct correlation between blood cholesterol levels and blood flow problems. But you can significantly improve your cholesterol profile with medication—or naturally. Boosting your dietary fiber intake is one way. Eating oatmeal, beans, and other foods high in soluble fiber can open the floodgates to blood flow to the vagina. Better blood flow equals easier arousal leading to greater desire.

More Sex = Better Health

IF YOU NEED ANY MOTIVATION TO PUT MORE EFFORT INTO HAVING MORE SEX, CONSIDER THIS: SCIENTISTS SAY SEX IS GOOD FOR YOUR BRAIN.

A 2010 study at the Neuroscience Institute of Princeton University suggests that having a lot of sex may actually boost brainpower. Well, at least it works for animals. Researchers found that rats that had a once-a-day sexual encounter increased the number of new neurons in the hippocampus, the area of the brain responsible for long-term memory and attention, when compared with rats that had little or no sex. What's more, regular sex appeared to stimulate the growth of dendritic spines—branches of neurons that conduct electrical signals.

Human studies, too, show the brain benefits of good sex. Researchers at the University of West Scotland found that sex, like exercise, releases anxiety, lowers stress hormones, and can help people ease mental pressure for at least a week. In the study 46 women and men were put in a stressful situation involving speaking and working with math problems in front of an audience. Participants were also asked to keep a diary of their sexual activity for 2 weeks prior to the test. It turned out that those who had sex were the least stressed out, and their blood pressures returned to normal faster after the public speaking test than it did for the participants who abstained from sex. "People who had penile-vaginal intercourse did twice as well as people who only masturbated or had no sex at all," says psychologist and lead researcher Stuart Brody.

A roll in the hay keeps the doctor away.

Take two and call us at the end of the week. People who have sex once or twice weekly have stronger immune systems than people who have sex less than once a week, according to a study at Wilkes University in Pennsylvania by psychologists Carl Charnetski, PhD, and Francis Brennan Jr., PhD. In their book, *Feeling Good is Good for You: How Pleasure Can Boost Your Immune System and Lengthen Your Life,* the researchers described a study in which they took saliva samples from 111 college students and surveyed them on their frequency of partner sex over the course of a month. Analysis showed that the saliva of the students who had sex once or twice a week had 30 percent more of the antigen immunoglobulin A (IgA) than students who had sex less often. "IgA is the body's first line of defense against colds and flu," says Charnetski. Other studies show that happy relationships are good for health. In one experiment reported in the *New England Journal of Medicine,* University of Pittsburgh scientists shot live rhinovirus up the noses of volunteers. Those who reported having strong ties with lovers, friends, and family were the least likely to catch a cold.

Good lovin' is better than a bandage.

Love helps bodies heal faster. Researchers at Ohio State University Medical Center inflicted minor blister wounds on the arms of 45 married couples during 24-hour visits on two different occasions. On the first visit, the couples were prompted to have a supportive, positive discussion. Two months later, after new wounds were administered, the couples were prompted to argue. Results showed that wounds healed nearly twice as fast after the warm and positive interaction than after the argument.

More sex may turn back the clock.

Can having sex keep wrinkles away? British neuropsychologist David Weeks of Royal Edinburgh Hospital believes so. In a 10-year-long study, he interviewed 3,500 adults in England and the United States and found that people who reported having sex four times a week looked about 10 years younger than they actually were. Pleasure derived from having loving sex releases hormones, including human growth hormone, that are crucial in preserving youth, he says.

Frequent orgasms may protect against cancer.

A French study in *The Journal of Clinical Epidemiology* found a correlation between lack of vaginal intercourse and increased risk of breast cancer. Some scientists theorize that sperm may contain antigens. Others believe hormones like oxytocin and DHEA that increase during arousal may provide some protective effect.

Love longer, keep him around longer.

It's no secret that women typically outlive men. But having regular sex may help women protect their husbands' health. An Irish study published in the *British Medical Journal* tracked the mortality of 1,000 middle-age men over the course of a decade and concluded that sexual activity may have a protective effect on middle-age health. By comparing men according to age and health, researchers found that men who had the highest frequency of orgasms had a death rate 50-percent lower than men who did not ejaculate frequently.

Couples who have more sex are happier!

An Australian survey of 5,000 people showed that married men and women are significantly more likely to report being happy than their single counterparts. Could it have something to do with the fact that sex is easier for cohabiting couples? According to a national sex survey conducted by the University of Chicago, sexual activity is 25 percent to 300 percent greater for married couples compared to non-married people, depending on age.

Doing it burns calories.

Due to its brevity, having an orgasm fries only two or three calories. But the prelude can burn quite a bit more. Depending on your weight and vigor of the lovemaking session, you'll likely churn through 50 to 200 calories.

Women'sHealth

Chapter 2
The Vagina:
An Owner's Manual

BECOME BETTER ACQUAINTED WITH

YOUR PRIVATE PARTS FOR

GOOD HEALTH AND STEAMIER SEX

Humor

us for a sec: If the average woman had a Facebook page for her private parts (we know, shut up), odds are that her relationship status would be "it's complicated" and she'd desperately need to post a profile picture. After all, new research from the Center for Sexual Health Promotion at Indiana University-Bloomington suggests that she hasn't checked herself out much—only 26 percent of women look closely at their vaginas on a regular basis. There's a logical reason for this. Guys have it easier. Their junk is dangling there, just waiting to be, um, adjusted. Female parts are internal, so it's more difficult to see what you are working with. But there's more to it than that. As children, we were often taught not to explore our private parts. Mom probably had the menstruation and sex talk but went nowhere near detailing the clitoris.

The Vagina: An Owner's Manual

"Many women never connect with their sexual anatomy because of our society's 'keep away' attitude toward the vagina and vulva," says Elizabeth G. Stewart, MD, author of *The V Book*. Well, here's some incentive to change all that: The more you make your vagina your business, the more sexual pleasure you'll experience.

In a study published in the *International Journal of Sexual Health*, scientists found that females who have a positive view of their genitals are more comfortable in their skin, more apt to orgasm, and more likely to experiment in bed. In fact, just looking at your vagina can be a turn-on. "Research shows that seeing signs of sex helps inspire arousal and lubrication," says Debby Herbenick, PhD, research scientist at Indiana University and author of *Because It Feels Good* and a *Men's Health* contributor. So allow us to scroll down there, if you will, for a better view.

To start, let's clear up one of the biggest misconceptions about the vagina. It's not the entire genital area. If you're standing naked in front of a full-length mirror, you're actually looking at the vulva, the exterior portion of your privates.

If you think of your privates as an ensemble, there are the supporting actors (like the vulva) and the marquee stars (the clitoris and G-spot). Every part is there to entertain your sexual needs, but to milk the best performance out of each one, you've got to show them some love. So lock the bedroom door, prop a few pillows up on the bed, grab a hand mirror, and join us for a very personal tour.

On the Mound

As we mentioned earlier, on the outside you'll see your vulva, including the mons pubis and two folds of skin called the labia majora (the "outer lips"). Both contain layers of fatty tissue that protect your clitoris and vagina. As for the hair, scientists believe it is there to trap pheromone-containing secretions that attract males. While pleasure reception is typically weak in this area, manual play can help increase the signal. "Rubbing the pubic mound and outer lips readies the clitoris for stimulation," says Herbenick.

The outer lips come in all shapes, colors, and sizes. They're wrinkled in some women, smooth in others, and both are normal. Just as a male's erectile tissue fills with blood during stimulation, so will these female tissues swell. Now, if you gently push apart the outer lips, you'll reveal a thinner set of lips called the labia minora. These hairless flaps are loaded with blood vessels, nerve endings, and secreting glands. "To the naked eye, the glands look like tiny bumps," says Diana Hoppe, MD, and author of *Healthy Sex Drive, Healthy You: What Your Libido Reveals About Your Life*. "They release secretions that actually help to separate your lips for easier penetration."

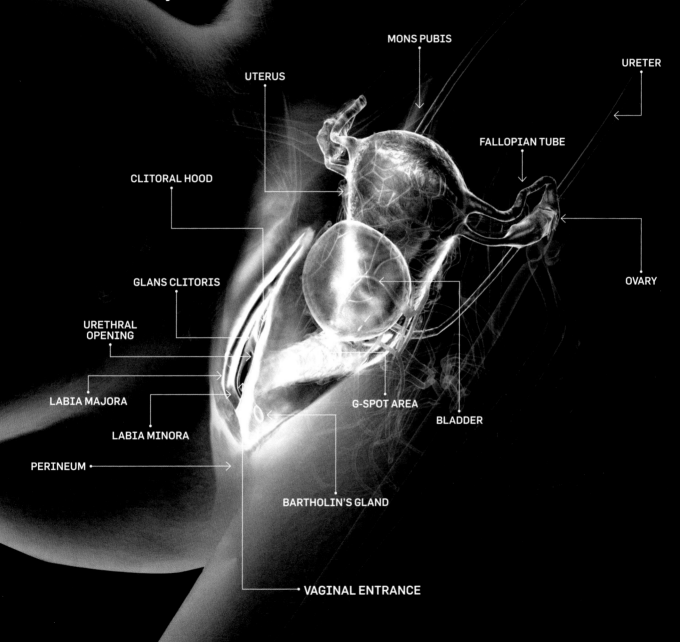

Your Sexual Anatomy

MONS PUBIS

UTERUS

URETER

CLITORAL HOOD

FALLOPIAN TUBE

GLANS CLITORIS

OVARY

URETHRAL OPENING

LABIA MAJORA

G-SPOT AREA

LABIA MINORA

BLADDER

PERINEUM

BARTHOLIN'S GLAND

VAGINAL ENTRANCE

They're not the only things lubing up your nether regions. There are Bartholin's glands (although because they're microscopic, you can't actually see them) on either side of your vaginal opening. As you get aroused, these glands lubricate the vaginal canal, from the opening right down to the cervix, where the canal ends. They typically release only about two drops, which is why many women still need plenty of foreplay and lubrication to stay wet.

Press Here for Pleasure

The clitoris is that proud little pink button roughly the size of a pencil eraser, and she's there for sexual pleasure only. The girl's got some nerve—8,000 nerve endings to be exact, the largest number found in any one place in the entire body and double the amount found in a man's penis. (Guys, if you're reading this, remember that. It's tons more sensitive than your penis, so stimulating it the way you do yourself can be too much—to the point of hurting. It's always best to ask how she likes to be touched.)

Now, what you may not know about your clitoris is that it's larger than it seems, and it's got legs. Literally. "We only see the head of the clitoris," says Herbenick. But it has a body that's shaped like a wishbone, with two legs (also known as crura) that reach three-inches deep into the vagina, just under the pubic mound and straight

"You Can Lose Stuff In It" & Other Myths About Your Vagina

Myth 1. Where did my tampon go?
It's not in there. Nor is that missing universal remote. The vagina is like a sock, no longer than 7 inches, and it ends at a microscopic hole that only sperm can slip through.

Myth 2. It smells like low tide.
Of all the myths, this is the one that angers experts the most—especially because it keeps women from accepting and enjoying oral sex, the prime gateway to orgasm. Experts chalk it up to years of douching advertising, and the perception that vaginas should smell like rosewater. Um, they don't. Every woman has her own unique scent, a version of musk that men are biologically wired to be attracted to. Know your normal scent. If it's much different than usual, that could be the sign of an infection.

Myth 3. Some are too tight; others too loose.
Unless a woman is a virgin or she's had a traumatic birthing experience with multiple children, there aren't big anatomical differences in the vaginal canal. Usually, feeling too tight or loose is a matter of lubrication—too much and there's not enough friction, or not enough and every penis feels Magnum-size. Always have a tube of lube within reach if you tend to be dry, or keep a hand towel nearby and pat your genitals off if you're sopping wet. Kegels (See "Squeeze Play," page 21) can easily help strengthen the pelvic floor and the muscles around the vagina.

into G-spot territory (but more on that later). That gives the clitoris incredible sexual reach and depth. "It's the beginning and end of the orgasm, the powerhouse of the orgasm," says Ian Kerner, PhD, author of *She Comes First: The Thinking Man's Guide to Pleasuring a Woman.* "It connects with every single structure in the genitals."

The best way to make the clitoris happy is through direct, consistent yet gentle oral and manual stimulation. But it's also quite responsive during woman-on-top and a twist on mission-ary called Coital Alignment Technique (CAT). In this position, your guy enters you as he normally would during missionary with two simple tweaks: he inches his body up, until his shoulders rest above yours and the base of his penis directly hits your clitoris, and then he grinds in a circular motion instead of thrusting, which creates more friction against the clitoris. See Chapter 8—"The Big Book of Sex Positions Sampler"—for the juicy details.

Friction can feel fabulous, but sometimes the little starlet can be a touch overexposed. As you head toward climax, the clitoris swells in size, which can make sex painful. Some women report that clitoral stimulation at this point can feel like an irritating tickle, and in some cases, like a really sharp shock. To protect itself, the clitoris retreats under the protective awning of the clitoral hood. Often, lightening up the stimulation a bit will make it feel good again.

An overly sensitive clitoris is kind of your body's way of saying "let the vagina soak up some of the sexual spotlight, please!" The 4- to 7-inch canal (depending on the woman) holds very sensitive nerve endings, mostly in the first 2 to 3 inches of the vagina. That's why when a woman is giving birth and the baby is crowning they call it the ring of fire. To stimulate these first few inches of the vaginal canal, try shorter, shallower thrusting during sex.

What Lies Beneath

Right under the clitoris, you'll see the urethral opening, the end of a short vessel that carries urine from the bladder out of the body. Just below the urethra is the opening of the vagina, called the introitus. Because the two are so close to one another, the thrust-ing of a penis can cause you to feel as if you have to urinate. Sometimes swelling can cause pain.

The vagina is a remarkable, dynamic organ. (Gentlemen, if you think your erection is impressive, consider what this baby can do.) It measures about $4\frac{1}{2}$ inches in length and 2 inches wide. When not aroused, the walls collapse in on one another. The walls are made up of membranes that lubricate the vagina during sex, tissues that are loaded with blood vessels that become engorged during arousal, and highly elastic muscle that allows it to expand deeper and wider for intercourse and childbirth.

DOWNTOWN DICTIONARY

What do you call your Aunt Vagina? Here are some popular terms of endearment:

- **Purse**
- **Lady Bug**
- **Hot Pocket**
- **Cookie Jar**
- **Catcher's Mitt**
- **Jewelry Box**
- **South Beach**
- **Miss Kittty**
- **Hoo Ha**
- **Little Miss Muffet**
- **Love Nest**
- **Muffin**
- **Pink Taco**
- **Twinkie**
- **The Notorious V.A.G.**
- **Whoopie Cushion**
- **Vajayjay (Actually, only Oprah calls it that.)**

That Special Place

Deeper into the vaginal walls is where you'll find one of the vagina's trickiest trump cards: the G-spot. If the clitoris is famous, the G-spot is infamous. Not every woman can tap into its potential, but when she does, the rewards are pretty phenomenal.

The G-spot is a spongy area located an inch or two into the anterior wall of the vagina, just under the pubic mound and right behind the urethra. You've got to feel it to believe it: it has bumpy, knotty striations similar to a walnut. In a study of more than 400 women, Rutgers University sex researcher Beverly Whipple, PhD, and two colleagues found that when this area was stimulated after a woman was already sexually aroused, a dime-size bump of tissue appeared and could sometimes trigger an orgasm. Whipple named the area the G-spot after Ernst Grafenberg, the German doctor who first documented it in 1950. Further examination of this tissue found it identical to that of the male prostate gland, a well-established pleasure zone. Because of this, some doctors believe the G-spot should be renamed the female prostate. Supporting that belief is a study showing the similarity between the fluid expelled by a very small percentage of women through their urethra during a G-spot orgasm (a.k.a. female ejaculation) and that produced by the male prostate.

When searching for the G-spot, you need *a lot* of foreplay first—the tissue doesn't swell and make itself known until you're already *really* turned on. "The G-spot's nerves are contained in fattier tissue, so you have to provide a deeper, firmer pressure to stimulate it," says Kerner. G-spot stimulation also calls for a tag-team approach. You can hit it by having your guy enter you from behind, but your best bet is to have him go down on you with his tongue and fingers. "His mouth should be on your clitoris, and then have him use his fingers in a come-hither motion to apply a firm, rhythmic pressure to the G-spot," says Kerner.

What if you've never found your G-spot, much less ejaculated? Don't sweat it. (For the record, orgasms that originate in this zone generally feel expansive and deep, while orgasms that start in the clitoris often feel more acute and intense.) "Many women say the G-spot enhances their orgasm," says Kerner. "They wouldn't isolate it and say, 'Wow, I just had a G-spot orgasm.' It's more like, 'I just had an orgasm and what he was doing felt really good.' That's why most vibrators come with a clitoral stimulator and a G-spot stimulator. They work in tandem to create what's commonly referred to as a blended orgasm." And while you can have a clitoral orgasm without G-spot stimulation, it's difficult to pull off the reverse. But at the end of the day, it doesn't really matter where it's coming from—an orgasm is an orgasm. And they all feel amazing.

Anatomy of Your Orgasm

The big, Big O can be an elusive thing. These bliss-inducing muscle contractions can explode spontaneously during one sexual encounter, but at other times they require a super-specific setting (soft music, dimmed lights), body position (perhaps the sexy scissors move), and technique (clockwise clitoral stimulation, please) to set them off. And hitting the height of pleasure is no guarantee. In fact, only 24 percent of women climax every time during sex with a partner, according to several major surveys. The rest either hit—or miss—depending on the night, or never orgasm during intercourse at all.

That may be little consolation if what's happening in the bedroom with your partner isn't working for you. When all the right moves don't produce an orgasm, many women wonder if something is wrong with them. A seeming lack of desire complicates things. If you don't want sex as often as your man, you may experience self-doubt. After all, everyone else (especially on TV and in the movies) seems to be so turned on and having a rollicking good time in bed.

Well, rest assured, you are not alone if you notice that your drive is different from your guy's or that orgasms are challenging to achieve. Pharmaceutical companies have tried to pathologize these tendencies as "female sexual dysfunction," but sex researchers now understand they are really quite the normal.

One of the most helpful advances by sex researchers in recent decades has been in recognizing what truly is a typical sexual response in women and how it differs in men. Recent research suggests that for at least one-third of all women, wanting to have sex doesn't necessarily begin with desire but with some sort of cognitive motivation. There needs to be a reason to get sexual, and only after physical arousal is well established does desire kick in. That may be one reason why plenty of foreplay is so crucial to achieving orgasm. During all that groping, kissing, and caressing, your nervous system starts taking notes and fires feel-good messages through the web of nerves that weave their way through your pelvis and up to your brain. This early stage is where a lot of women get tripped up because they can't silence the voices in their heads long enough to focus on the sensations. (When was the last time I had a bikini wax? I hope the kids don't hear us. Am I prepared for that 8 o'clock meeting? Does he think my thighs look huge?) Research by uroneurologists at the University of Groningen in the

THE "COREGASM"
Abs with Benefits

Some *Women's Health* readers have reported finding a hidden gem in their quest for tight abs—secret, solo, hands-free orgasms in the gym. Women say the abs exercises most likely to cause these "coregasms" are hanging leg raises, leg-lowering drills, Roman chair knee raises, and leg exercises on an abductor/adductor machine. Sex researcher Debby Herbenick, PhD, believes the clitoral vibes may be triggered when women bear down on their pelvic muscles while simultaneously squeezing their thighs together and raising their legs. "I don't care why it happens, but I am just happy it does," wrote one satisfied exerciser.

Netherlands shows that the brain's amygdala and prefrontal cortex, which process fear and anxiety, need to be less active during sex in order for women to climax. Once you are relaxed and comfortable, absent of worry, your brain gets the green light to orgasm.

Tip: To keep your mind from wandering out of the bedroom, zero in on one of your senses. Focus on the smell of his skin, relish the feeling of his hands on your body, concentrate on how he tastes while you're kissing. "It sounds counterintuitive, but studies show that lapsing into a sexual fantasy can help a woman become and stay aroused," says Herbenick. "Switching to a sexual mind-set makes you more physically responsive."

Once you are turned on, your nerves communicate to your brain that it's time to increase blood flow. The result: Your genitals become engorged with blood, your breasts swell, and nipples harden. Around this time, the walls of the vagina start to secrete beads of lubrication that eventually get bigger and flow together. The more engorged you are, the more sensitive you become to his touch, causing the nerves to fire back to the brain to pump more blood, creating an increasingly pleasurable loop, says Barry R. Komisaruk, PhD, an adjunct psychology professor at Rutgers University and coauthor of *Orgasm Answer Guide*.

Here's the catch: Keeping that loop going requires patience—yours and his. The average female requires 10 to 20 minutes of rhythmic manual or oral pressure to reach peak arousal. Women often speed up the process before they're properly warmed up because they're worried about taking too long. But don't worry about that: The truth is guys get off on pleasing their mates. Seeing a woman enjoying what he's doing boosts his testosterone levels, turning him on even more.

When you've been sufficiently primed for intercourse, you'll feel a throbbing sensation in your genitals or an intense pressure building on either side of the vaginal wall. This is the ideal time to transition to a sexual position that provides clitoral contact. The CAT positioning mentioned earlier—where the base of his penis aligns with your clitoris—is perfect. Or try a rear-entry or woman-on-top position where he can stimulate your clitoris with his fingers—or you can do it yourself.

Groundbreaking research by Australian urologist Helen O'Connell, PhD, found that the clitoris actually extends way back into the pelvis and plays a significant role in both vaginal and G-spot orgasms. Her research suggests that every climax is actually a blended orgasm involving the clitoris, G-spot, and vagina.

During intercourse the lower part of the vagina narrows in order to grip the penis while the upper part expands to give it someplace to go. Nerve and muscle tension builds up in the genitals, pelvis, buttocks, and thighs. When orgasm occurs, an area of the brain called the paraventricular nucleus spills a wave of oxytocin into your bloodstream. As this neurohormone washes through your pelvic muscles, it causes a series of rhythmic contractions in the uterus, vagina, and anus, at intervals of every .08 seconds. Meanwhile, your heart starts pumping extra oxygen to the pulsating parts to keep them humming along. These contractions will be even stronger if you do Kegel exercises (see below).

While your body is pumping out waves of tingly goodness, your mind falls into a contented trance. The nucleus accumbens, where the brain produces pleasurable feelings (including addictive ones like those you can get from nicotine or drugs), is activated, according to Komisaruk. That's why

you may feel as if you can't get enough of your partner—even one you're lukewarm about—during pleasure.

Soon after an orgasm, your blood pressure and pulse settle down. While blood drains from his penis rather quickly, it stays longer around your vagina, keeping you aroused, and allowing you to achieve multiple orgasms. Psst: Take advantage of this. Wait a minute until your clitoris becomes less sensitive then have him stimulate you with his fingers or tongue to start building to another peak.

Once you've filled your pleasure quota, you'll probably fall into cuddle mode, because there's still leftover oxytocin (the bonding hormone) floating around from your orgasm(s), making you feel especially attached to the person who brought you all that glory.

Squeeze Play AN EXERCISE FOR BETTER ORGASMS

Kegels are named after gynecologist Arnold Kegel who, in the 1940s, prescribed the pelvic floor strengthening exercises to patients to remedy incontinence following childbirth. Now Kegels are considered tried and true orgasm boosters, according to *Women's Health* advisor Laura Berman, PhD, the president and director of Chicago's Berman

Center, which specializes in women's health. "Strengthening your pelvic floor muscles and your transverse abdominals brings more blood to your pelvic region, increases the amount of friction you can generate, and intensifies contractions during orgasm," she says. You can do them inconspicuously anywhere— watching TV, driving, in meetings. Or try this

variation, recommended by Berman, which works the transverse abdominals as well: Lie on your back with knees bent and feet flat on the floor. Place a yoga block or similarly sized object between your thighs. Extend your arms straight alongside your body. Without using your butt muscles, do a Kegel and lift your legs into the air while

simultaneously lifting your shoulders slightly off the ground. Your pelvis and lower back should remain touching the floor, and arms should be straight and slightly higher than your torso, pulling toward the wall in front of you. Hold for 5 to 10 seconds, then release. Do five to ten twice a day, increasing the number as they get easier.

How to Keep Your Private Parts Healthy

Smart lifestyle choices and proper hygiene can do wonders for your body, your self-esteem, and your sex life. Here are some of the good things you should be doing for your breasts and vagina.

Stay at a healthy weight.

By eating a healthy diet and exercising regularly, you'll reduce your risk of obesity, diabetes, and heart disease, all of which are known sexual health destroyers. In addition, being heavy can increase your risk of breast cancer as well as reduce your risk of surviving it, according to Harold P. Freeman, MD, president and founder of the Ralph Lauren Center for Cancer Care and Prevention in Harlem. A low-fat diet can reduce your risk of cancer. Eat cruciferous vegetables, such as broccoli and kale, which contain sulforaphane, a chemical that is believed to prevent cancer cells from multiplying.

Lose the tummy.

Abdominal fat is a bad marker for overall health—including your sexual health—and it can hurt your body image, a significant contributor to low libido. Also an unhealthy diet can lead to arterial plaque buildup, which reduces blood flow to the genitals. (Smoking does similar damage. Nicotine hampers blood flow by constricting blood vessels.)

Cop a feel.

Do a breast self-exam monthly, right after your period when your breasts are not tender or swollen.
1. Lie on a bed and put a pillow under your shoulder for support and lift that arm behind your head. Using the three middle fingers of your other hand, press firmly around the bottom breast, feeling for lumps or thickening.
2. Move around the breast in a circle or up and down, but do it the same way every month so you become familiar with how your breast feels most of the time. Note that a firm ridge in the lower curve of the breast is normal.
3. After examining the entire breast, place the pillow under the other shoulder and repeat the self-exam on the other breast.
4. Finally, check both breasts while standing, with one arm behind your head to examine the upper and outer parts of the breasts near the armpit. It may help to do this while in a warm shower. Lumps may be easier to feel when your skin is soapy and wet. If you feel any lumps or other abnormalities, see your doctor.

Check under the hood.

Examine your vagina once a month at the same time you check your breasts. Making it a habit will help you recognize anything that looks abnormal and may help you catch infections or early warning signs of cancer. Sit on a chair in front of a light. Unless you're extremely flexible, you'll need a hand mirror. Check the whole kit and caboodle from mons to anus. Spread your labia with your fingers and pull back the hood of the clitoris. If you see bumps, warts, or other growths, moles that have changed shape or color, or abnormal discharge or swelling, see your doctor.

Do nothing.

Your private parts have a remarkable built-in self-cleaning system. The vulva and vagina produce an average of one-quarter to a half teaspoon of vaginal discharge every 8 hours, which is why panties carry that helpful strip of cotton fabric. Most of the vaginal secretion is cervical mucous, which effectively neutralizes bacteria and helps maintain a proper acid balance in the vagina that keeps bad bacteria from flourishing. Don't douche, which was popular many years ago, or use over-the-counter feminine products. Both can disrupt the protective bacterial balance, according to Berman. Instead, wash with water and a pH-balanced soap, never colored or perfumed soaps. Pull the hood of your clitoris back and use warm water and a gentle washcloth to wipe away oils and skin particles.

Eat a cup of yogurt every day.

Lactobacillus is a beneficial bacterium that keeps nastier bacteria in check in the vagina. When the number of *Lactobacillus* drops, yeast

spores and bacterial bad boys like *E. coli* can grow, causing an itchy infection. But eating probiotic yogurt, containing the live helpful bacterial, will support the delicate chemical balance in your vagina.

Go commando at night.

Sleeping in boxers or jammies without wearing panties allows the skin to breathe, lowers the temperature of the vulva, and prevents sweating. All help reduce chances of infection.

Inspect his fingers.

Don't let hands—anyone's, including yours—touch your vagina unless they are clean and don't have long or jagged fingernails.

Tread lightly with tampons.

As tender as the vagina may seem, it's actually a pretty tough cookie. When it sustains small scrapes from, say, enthusiastic sex, the vaginal lining can heal surprisingly fast. Another way it gets beat up is improper use of super-absorbent tampons. This is different from scary toxic shock syndrome, a rare, dangerous condition (odds of getting it are about 1 in 100,000) that results from an overgrowth of *Staphylococcus aureus* bacteria. The staph bug can be exacerbated by wearing the same tampon for longer than 8 hours —but is not actually caused by tampons themselves. What tampons can give you are vagi-

nal ulcers that don't cause any discomfort but do make you more vulnerable to sexually transmitted infections. Using a high-absorbency tampon during light flow days or when spotting can draw too much fluid out of the vagina, damaging cells and causing them to erode. The good news is that the vaginal lining is quick to produce new cells, allowing ulcers to heal completely in as little as 48 hours. To prevent vaginal stress, avoid superabsorbency tampons on all but your heaviest days and don't use them at all between periods.

Go to bed earlier.

Irregular sleep patterns or getting fewer than 7 hours of sleep can affect the quality of your sleep and your sexual health. What's more, poor sleep is associated with many health issues that contribute to sexual problems, high blood pressure, obesity, sleep apnea, heart disease, and diabetes.

Keep it to one or two drinks.

A glass of chardonnay may relax you and put you in the mood, but as Shakespeare warned in *Macbeth*, "drink provokes desire, but it takes away performance." Clinical studies have shown that alcohol acts as a depressant in the brain's cerebral cortex, dulling anxiety and inhibitions about sex, but larger amounts can have the opposite effect, messing with your ability to become aroused.

Sextistics

8,000

Number of nerve endings on the visible nub of the clitoris— twice as many as the penis

50

Percentage of women who say they cannot reach orgasm through intercourse alone

46

Percentage of *Women's Health* readers who own a vibrator or other sex toy

51

Percentage of women who say they've faked an orgasm

23

Percentage of women who always climax on top

42

Percentage of women who climax during oral sex

Nearly 1 in 2

Number of women who think orgasm synchronicity makes for better sex

Nearly 90

Percentage of women who say they would like to experience sex outdoors

62

Percentage of women who say they have felt distracted during sex due to worrying about how their body looks

25

Percentage increase in size breast can become when kissed or stroked

50

Percent increase in size of clitoral tissue when erect

27

Minutes it takes the average woman to reach orgasm

14

Percentage of men who stress about timing a simultaneous orgasm

Saturday, 10:34 p.m.

Day and time when you're most likely to have an orgasm

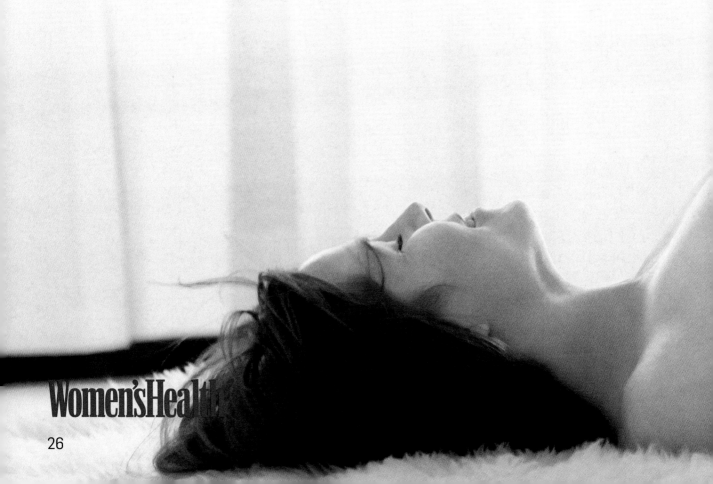

Chapter 3
What Every Man Wants

WANT TO KNOW WHAT'S GOING THROUGH
A GUY'S HEAD AS YOU CRAWL INTO BED?
THE MALE BRAIN'S NEEDS, FEARS,
AND SECRET DESIRES WILL SURPRISE YOU

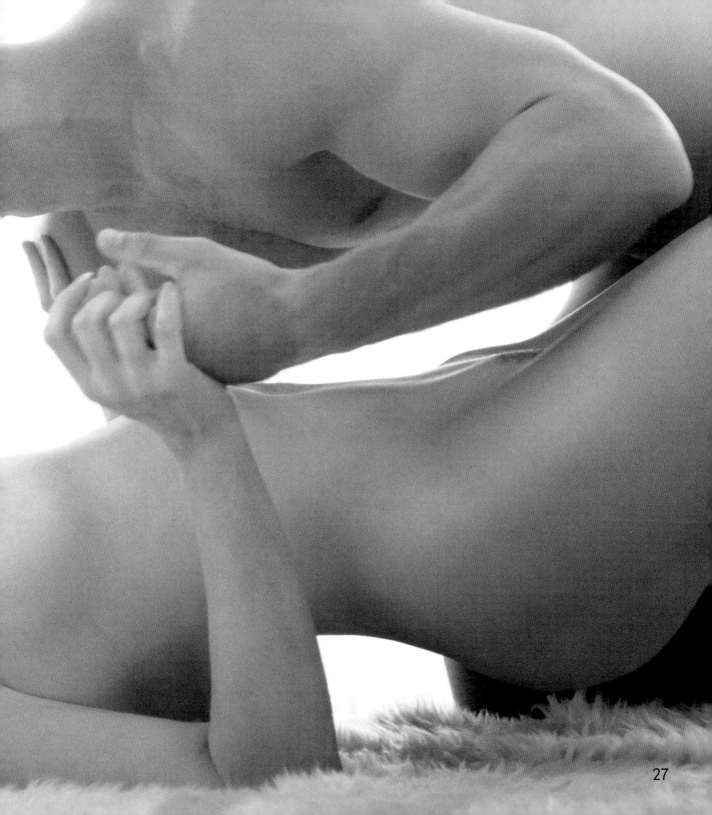

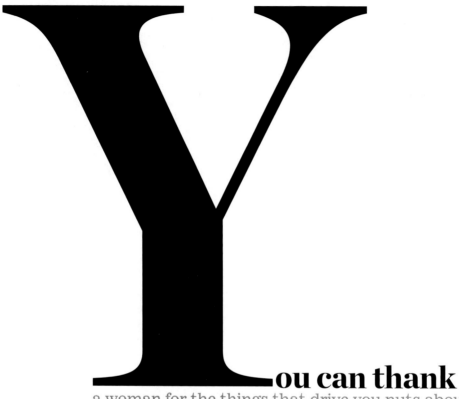

Y

ou can thank a woman for the things that drive you nuts about men. Her name is Mother Nature. She created a male brain that is very different from yours both in structure and behavior. With major direction and influence from hormones, especially testosterone, the male brain develops into "a lean, mean, problem-solving machine," says Louann Brizendine, MD, a professor of clinical psychiatry at the University of California.

That distinction is at the crux of what frustrates women about men—and it continues to fuel the conflict between the sexes. Here's an example: Let's say your boyfriend's or husband's mother says something to tick you off. When he comes home from work,

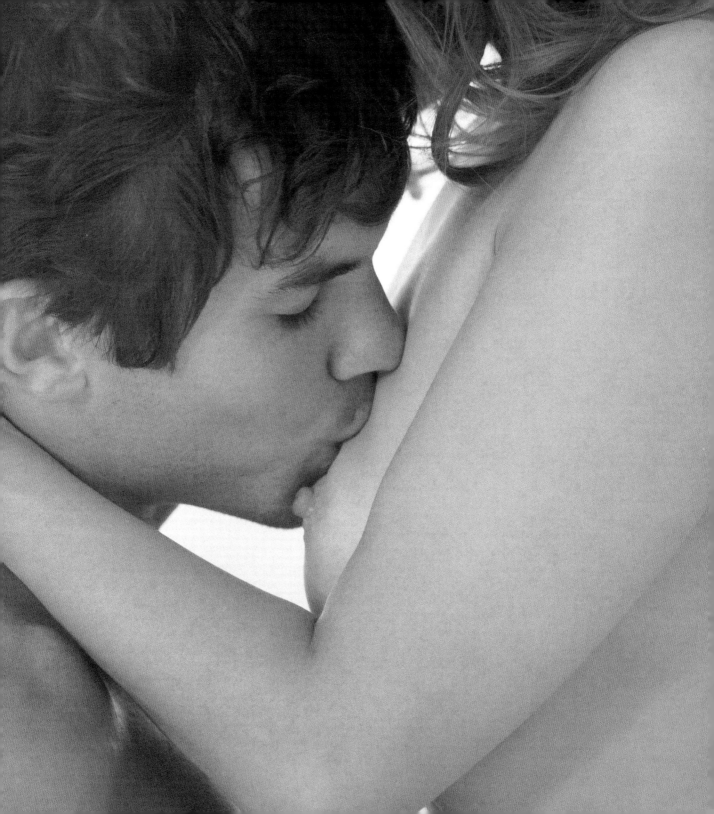

you want to vent, so you sit down and describe what happened, in excruciating (for him) detail, for 20 minutes. Your female brain considers this therapeutic, because your gray matter is much more adept at interpersonal sensitivity than his brain is. Your brain is looking for signals of understanding, commiseration, and support from him. His emotional brain, by contrast, is hard-wired to search and destroy the problem at hand. He's looking to act and to fix the disturbance fast and move on, not to give you what you really opened up for, which is simply a sympathetic ear.

Do you see the difference? Your brain is wired for social communication, his for pursuit and targeted action. The distinction is even clearer when it comes to courtship and sex. Scientists know that male brains contain two and a half times more real estate devoted to sexual pursuit than female brains do. This sexual staging zone is found deep in the brain's core in the medial preoptic area of the hypothalamus.

"Sexual thoughts flicker in the background of a man's visual cortex all day and night, making him always at the ready for seizing sexual opportunity," writes neuropsychiatrist Brizendine in her book *The Male Brain: A Breakthrough Understanding of How Men and Boys Think.*

So, on the most elemental level, a guy is like a big-eyed dog drooling over every female who walks by as if she was a juicy pork chop with breasts. His eyes immediately focus on the female body

THE BIKINI EFFECT

Thinking about sex can impair a man's judgment. Research in *The Journal of Consumer Research* reports that sexual urges make men crave quick rewards when they make decisions about money or food. In the study, men who were given lingerie to fondle or shown videos of women running in bikinis tended to be content with small immediate monetary rewards instead of bigger ones that involved waiting. Sexual stimuli snap men's minds into the present, researchers speculate, making fast rewards more appealing.

form. Although he's not aware of it, instinctively his brain is driving him to ejaculate his DNA into the next generation by having sex with as many females as he can.

But keep in mind that Mother Nature designed your brain specifically to deal with this kind of primal male behavior and use it to your advantage. Because pregnancy and nursing are such dangerous, painful, and time-consuming undertakings, women have evolved to be far more thoughtful and selective about whom they have sex with. The area of your brain that analyzes risk, the anterior cingulate cortex, or ACC, is much larger than it is in a man's brain. You use it to determine whether a potential mate has the brains and the balls to be both a provider and protector for you and your expected offspring. And you do that by sizing up the opposite sex in a far different way than men do—by talking, getting to know him, and assessing his trustworthiness, slowly, consciously, before taking the next step.

In essence, you need to feel safe, comfortable, and intimately connected with a man in order to desire sex with him, while he needs sex in order to feel intimacy. For him, frequent sex is as essential to a satisfying relationship as having frequent intimate talks is for you. When you can recognize these cerebral differences, you may start to see men from a different perspective and form a deeper understanding about what drives them, frightens them, and turns them on. This knowledge will be invaluable to you in your relationships with men, not only with your main guy, but with brothers, father, sons, and friends. But for this book, we'll focus on the male brains you go to bed with—both of them. Give them what they want, and you'll enjoy men more.

Talk more like a man.

We don't mean to clear your throat, speak in deeper tones, and scratch your privates between declaratives. Just get to the point quicker. As much as men love the sound of your voice and really love to help you out, their attention spans are short. Their minds will wander if they don't see a climax and conclusion on your story's horizon. So, as you are sharing the details of today's run-in with Brenda from Business Affairs, skip the transcript of the exchange and create a highlight reel. He'll get the gist if you keep it short and just say what's on your mind—like most men talk when talking with other guys. But, remember, he's not hearing the story for story's sake. He's looking for a problem to fix for you. So, if there isn't one or you're not really looking for solutions, broadcast that to him in black and white: "I'm not looking for you to fix anything; I feel better just having you understand how I'm feeling." Say it your way. Suddenly, you will have given him the reward he was looking for—the satisfaction of having provided something of value to you, the woman he cares about.

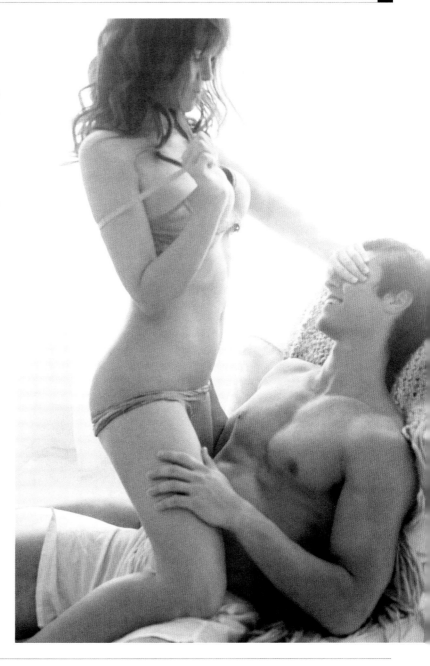

What Every Man Wants

Grab hold of his hand.

Many women think that men don't like cuddling, handholding, and other non-sexual forms of closeness; they're wrong. Men enjoy it as much as you do, but they are conditioned to hide these deep desires to avoid the appearance of weakness—"non-maleness"—in front of other men and even from you. When you display your love in public by grabbing his hand, planting a brief but passionate kiss, touching his thigh with your hand, or grazing his arm with your breasts on purpose, you demonstrate confidence in your sexuality, which men find irresistible.

Give him props.

Remember how hard you worked on those show-and-tell projects in kindergarten, and how good you felt when the class clapped and, at home, dad said "attagirl"? Men are, in many ways, kindergarteners who want nothing more desperately than your appreciation and respect for their hard work. Because that recognition rarely comes from their bosses, it's even more critical that you give it to them on occasion at home when they do something particularly thoughtful or skillful. Men grow up with cultural expectations to be strong and brave, to suppress their emotions, fears, and hurts, so it may be very difficult to detect this need beneath their stoic armor. But, rest assured, it's there; men can be insecure. One of the most effective ways to show your love for

him is to fulfill his need to feel valued and needed as provider and protector. In a poll of *Men's Health* readers, 66 percent said they want women to compliment them on an intangible yet specific quality, something they uniquely possess. Be sincere: "I love how you always can make me feel better" is much more effective than "You're wonderful" because it reinforces his efforts to care for you.

Laugh with and at him.

After her body, her sense of humor is the most attractive thing about women for men who responded to *The Big Book of Sex* survey. But that doesn't mean you have to be quick with jokes and witty one-liners. Simply being able to laugh with him, at him, and at yourself is a sign of intellectual compatibility, says Billy Goldberg, MD, coauthor of *Why Do Men Fall Asleep After Sex?* "Men want a woman who is as comfortable relating her own ridiculous anecdote as she is listening to ours."

Ask for what you want in bed.

Men aren't the best mind readers. But they understand coaching, having spent years playing organized sports. So most of them respond well to feedback and direction. In fact, they would very much enjoy hearing what you'd like them to do to you in bed. If you're not really comfortable asking for specifics, take the pressure off by talking in

73

Percentage of men who are satisfied with their partner's breast size.

generalities when you're not in bed. Once you're between the sheets, "turn requests into erotic expressions, not instructions," says Joy Davidson, PhD, a sex therapist in New York and author of *Fearless Sex*. "Saying 'Oh, do that slower,' isn't an order, it's sexy."

Seduce him with subtlety.

Skip the Lady Gaga impersonation. "With so much explicit imagery in the media, too much exposure isn't seductive," says Robert W. Birch, PhD, a sex therapist. Instead, play a little hide-and-seek. Let your shirt fall from your shoulder, undo one more button, or wear a fitted blouse over a lacy bra and watch him ogle you all night long. "Allow the peep to appear unintentional," Birch says.

Be more assertive.

As much as a man likes to be in control, the bedroom is one place where he would like to see you take more control—and we don't mean by grabbing the TV remote. Be the one to initiate sex. When you take charge, you affirm your desire for him, something he needs both in and out of the bedroom. Take advantage of his notorious propensity for visual cues. Outside of the bedroom, wear strapless dresses that flash a bit of flesh. Wear his boxers around the house. Leaving something to be imagined will drive him wild as men get turned on even more by what they can't see. Slip into the shower with him and soap him

up. At a fancy dinner at a restaurant, clue him in to the fact that you're not wearing any underwear, and see how fast he finishes his crème brulee. When you are shifting from one sex position to another, take him into your mouth and look up at him for a few seconds, then turn around and offer him rear entry. These are just some secret desires we've heard from guys. We're sure you can think of many more.

Watch porn with him.

According to a study at Brigham Young University, 87 percent of men have looked at some form of porn in the past year, and one in five checks out X-rated fare daily. That's probably not surprising to anyone, but what is shocking is how quickly men can become dependent on regular doses of erotic images. The arousal hormones the visuals trigger can become addictive. If you feel erotic material is interfering with your relationship or he's using it to avoid something, you should confront the problem, says sex therapist Sandor Gardos, PhD. One tactic is to suggest watching erotica together. "It becomes compulsive when he feels like he has to hide it," says Gardos. But willingness to share his interest takes the compulsion out of the question. Viewing erotic images together may even enhance your sex life, say sex experts. Focus on genres that you prefer, which are likely to be films containing more storytelling and romance versus raw humping.

HIS TOP 5 REASONS FOR ACCEPTING A BOOTY CALL

1. **I want sexual contact**

2. **She's physically attractive**

3. **Good timing**

4. **She's interested and available**

5. **She's promiscuous**

Keep the lights on.

There's nothing sexier than a woman who lets her guard down in bed. "He loves when he can see and feel your body, and the biggest turnoff for him is your acting embarrassed," says Pepper Schwartz, PhD, a relationships advisor for Perfectmatch.com and author of *Prime: Adventures and Advice on Sex, Love, and the Sensual Years.* So create an environment where you can enjoy yourself—candles, lingerie, whatever you need to relax and feel beautiful. Trust us; he doesn't see the imperfections that women tend to zone in on—all he knows is that he loves your body.

He wants more foreplay.

You think we're kidding. Well, the vast majority of men responding to *The Big Book of Sex* survey said they expect foreplay to last 15 minutes or longer, on par with what the women respondents think. Slow-burning sex isn't better only for you. "Longer foreplay helps men synchronize with their partners, giving them confidence and, as a result, better control over ejaculation," says San Francisco sex therapist Seth Prosterman, PhD. Men know that it takes women longer to become aroused. So, relax and take your time, and put some of your own effort into getting in a sexual mood, suggests Gardos. Fantasize the way you do when you are masturbating alone. Grab your vibrator or use your fingers to start to rev things up. He'll love watching you. When he stimulates you with his hand,

guide him to show him how you like to be touched. Your magic phrase? "Like this." That's all—he'll get the picture. Slip one hand down his backside and pull his pelvis toward you, showing him the motion that turns you on. Don't forget your line: "Like this." During sex,

CHEER HIM UP

Even if his jokes are lame, laugh. Studies at McMaster University in Ontario show that men place a great deal of importance on humor and need affirmation that they are funny.

34

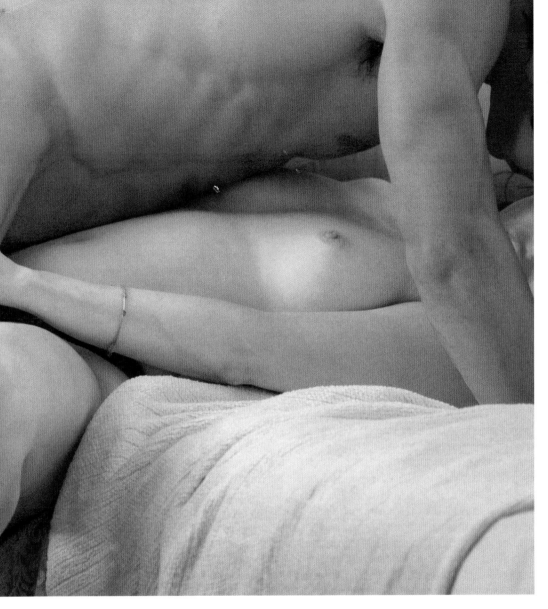

44

Percentage of
men who say they
sleep naked and not
just in summer.

switch positions—you on top. Slowly
kiss him along his neck and collarbone.
Linger by his belt line, looking up at
him as you kiss his abdomen. Then go
down on him slowly, looking up at him
as you take him into your mouth—which
men find to be an incredible turn on.

The double-handed butt grab.

Wrapping your hands around his derriere
will make him feel wanted, which will turn
him on more than any Victoria's Secret
undergarment. Don't be shy about squeezing hard. It's plenty padded back there.

What Every Man Wants | HERS

TENDERIZE HIM

Press here for more emotion. In a study published in *The Journal of Neuroscience,* researchers showed two groups of men emotionally loaded photos, such as a crying child. Beforehand, one group inhaled a nasal spray containing oxytocin, the so-called "cuddle hormone." Those who sniffed oxytocin showed a 30 percent increase in emotional empathy, according to researchers from Babraham Institute in England where the study was conducted. Sorry, you can't buy oxytocin perfume, but you can give your guy a back rub. Regular massages can release the hormone that turns macho men into mushballs.

To find out what he likes, ask.

Guys can be shy about telling you what really turns them on and how they like to be touched down there. So, ask. Your permission to be open will create a safe, comfortable atmosphere that can turn into some really hot sex. Ask him to demonstrate how he masturbates while thinking of you. Note the way he grips his shaft and mimic it. Also, become familiar with his frenulum, one of the most sensitive areas of the penis, which is on the underside of the head. Playful licks and light pressure to the frenulum often coax more blood into the penis for even harder erections. When stimulating him manually, wrap your hand around his penis so that the fleshy pads of your fingers, not the fingertips, rub over the frenulum. Try using a lube—it will make the experience more pleasurable for both of you. Place his hand over yours so he can guide you up and down just the way he likes it. To double his pleasure, stimulate another erogenous zone while playing with his penis—his anus, his testicles, his nipples. Lick the nerve-rich seam running down the middle of his scrotum, then gently push up against the base of his testicles with your hand. That's a way to arouse his prostate, the sensitive gland known as the male G-spot, without having to insert a finger in his anus, according to author Ian Kerner.

He digs it doggy style.

Doing it like the lions on the Discovery Channel is arguably the most popular and arousing position for men. Men love the primal element and find the fantasy submissiveness highly erotic. No wonder it's also the most difficult position for men to hold off orgasm.

The biggest secret sexual turn on for men.

It's not oral sex or the downward dog position, a new sex toy or lube—not even the prospect of a threesome. It's your unbridled enthusiasm and confidence in bed. Remember that men are action- and accomplishment-oriented. So it is exciting for him to know that he is pleasing you, that you want him and are enjoying him as much as he's enjoying you. The more interactive sex is, the better sex is for him and for you. Eighty-seven percent of men say "just lying there" is a serious turnoff, and 57 percent say that silence is a sexual downer. That doesn't mean that you need to have an orgasm to make him feel whole. Don't put that kind of pressure on yourself or him. But you'll satisfy him by letting him know what feels good to you and what he's doing right. Grip the sheets. Grab the headboard. Moan into his ear and talk dirty. Plead. Demand. Direct. "All great sexual encounters deliver a sense of validation that you really have something special," says Prosterman. And your over-the-top passion can help a man feel closer to you emotionally—something guys say is one of the most important elements of unforgettable sex.

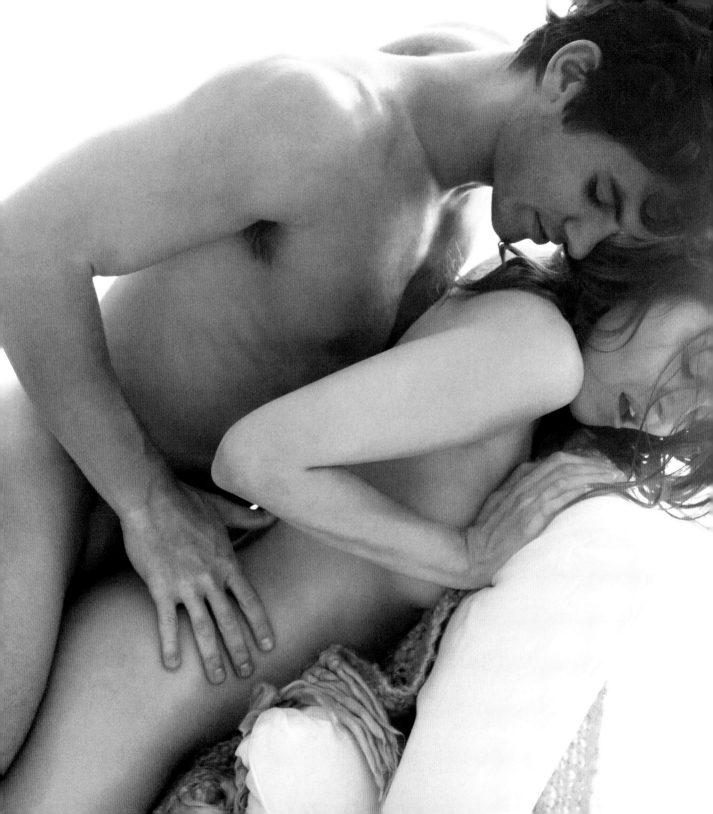

His Body/Your Map

INNER THIGHS

The back of the knee and inner thighs are highly sensitive to men. Start licking and kissing behind the knee, slowly advancing north. Switch to the other leg for variety. Again, slowly, slowly. Glance up at him as you lick and get closer to his sack without touching for as long as he can stand it. It's the sweetest torture he'll ever endure.

PERINEUM

The third most surprising erogenous zone described by men in our survey is the perineum, a patch of skin filled with nerve endings located between the anus and the testicles. Try running one of your silk scarves delicately between his legs and over his perineum, which will send shivers throughout his body.

BUTT

One large survey showed that women enjoy holding his butt in the palms of her hands. A survey of Men's Health readers suggests to go right ahead. They love it. When having sex, wrapping your hands around his cheeks and pulling him in forcefully with a squeeze will make him feel wanted.

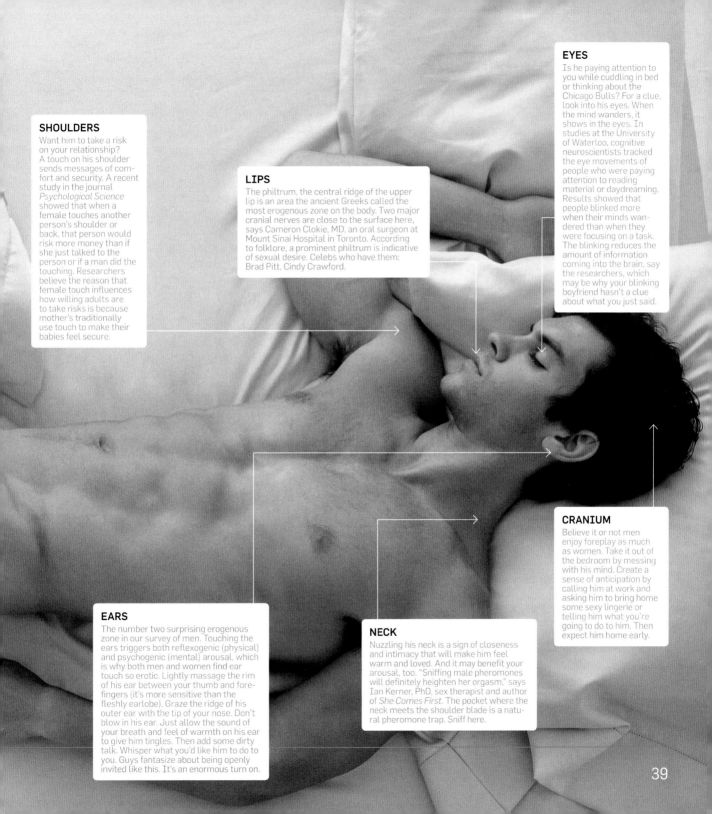

SHOULDERS

Want him to take a risk on your relationship? A touch on his shoulder sends messages of comfort and security. A recent study in the journal *Psychological Science* showed that when a female touches another person's shoulder or back, that person would risk more money than if she just talked to the person or if a man did the touching. Researchers believe the reason that female touch influences how willing adults are to take risks is because mother's traditionally use touch to make their babies feel secure.

LIPS

The philtrum, the central ridge of the upper lip is an area the ancient Greeks called the most erogenous zone on the body. Two major cranial nerves are close to the surface here, says Cameron Clokie, MD, an oral surgeon at Mount Sinai Hospital in Toronto. According to folklore, a prominent philtrum is indicative of sexual desire. Celebs who have them: Brad Pitt, Cindy Crawford.

EYES

Is he paying attention to you while cuddling in bed or thinking about the Chicago Bulls? For a clue, look into his eyes. When the mind wanders, it shows in the eyes. In studies at the University of Waterloo, cognitive neuroscientists tracked the eye movements of people who were paying attention to reading material or daydreaming. Results showed that people blinked more when their minds wandered than when they were focusing on a task. The blinking reduces the amount of information coming into the brain, say the researchers, which may be why your blinking boyfriend hasn't a clue about what you just said.

EARS

The number two surprising erogenous zone in our survey of men. Touching the ears triggers both reflexogenic (physical) and psychogenic (mental) arousal, which is why both men and women find ear touch so erotic. Lightly massage the rim of his ear between your thumb and forefingers (it's more sensitive than the fleshly earlobe). Graze the ridge of his outer ear with the tip of your nose. Don't blow in his ear. Just allow the sound of your breath and feel of warmth on his ear to give him tingles. Then add some dirty talk. Whisper what you'd like him to do to you. Guys fantasize about being openly invited like this. It's an enormous turn on.

NECK

Nuzzling his neck is a sign of closeness and intimacy that will make him feel warm and loved. And it may benefit your arousal, too. "Sniffing male pheromones will definitely heighten her orgasm," says Ian Kerner, PhD, sex therapist and author of *She Comes First*. The pocket where the neck meets the shoulder blade is a natural pheromone trap. Sniff here.

CRANIUM

Believe it or not men enjoy foreplay as much as women. Take it out of the bedroom by messing with his mind. Create a sense of anticipation by calling him at work and asking him to bring home some sexy lingerie or telling him what you're going to do to him. Then expect him home early.

39

20 Things Men Wish Women Knew About Them

1. He loves when you laugh at his jokes. **2.** He'd like you to enjoy watching the Stooges with him, even if you're faking it. **3.** You can have sex with him pretty much anytime, anywhere. **4.** He will welcome taking his hand and showing him just the right spot and rhythm. **5.** He likes when you initiate the handhold. **6.** He notices when guys check you out … and likes it. **7.** Tell him what you'll do to him tonight and you will make his day. **8.** He craves hugs and other signs of affection, even if they don't lead to sex. Honest. **9.** He loves when you wear his T-shirt and boxers. **10.** You can cook for him anytime. **11.** He loves to cook for you. **12.** He's skittish about initiating dirty talk and would like your enthusiastic help. **13.** He can't help but look at other women and it has nothing to do with his lack of love or desire for you. **14.** He's thinking about you when he's masturbating. **15.** Kissing him in a crowded bar is an amazing turn on, cupping his butt while you do it, even better. **16.** He is not evaluating your body. **17.** Your confidence in bed is really hot. **18.** Oral sex is great. Intercourse, better. **19.** There is no better sound in the world than you having an orgasm. **20.** He will do just about anything to have sex with you twice as often as you are having it now.

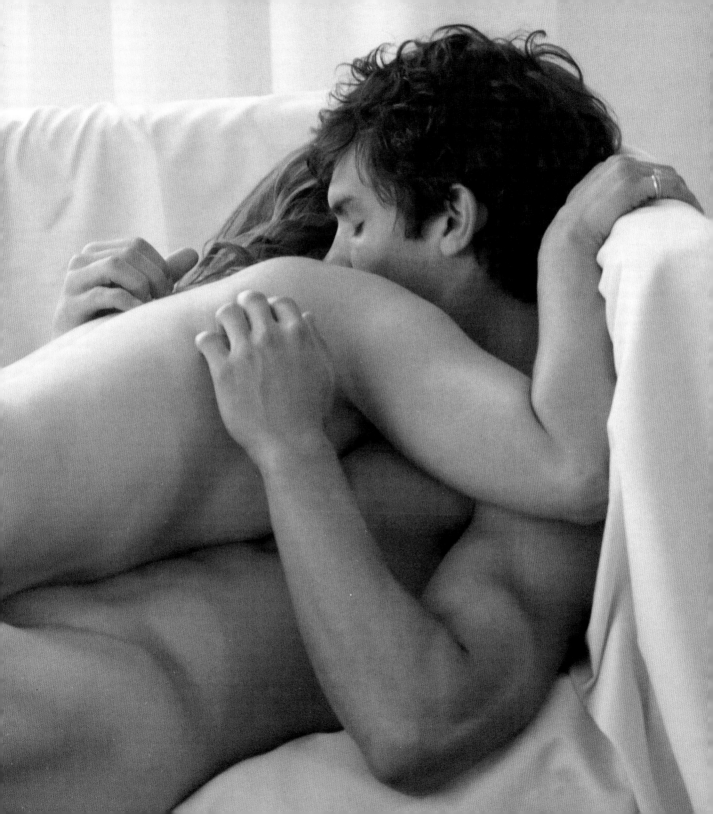

Ask The Guy Next Door

ANSWERS TO FREQUENT QUESTIONS ABOUT MEN
BY *WOMEN'S HEALTH* RELATIONSHIPS COLUMNIST MATT BEAN

Q. What exactly makes a woman good in bed?

A. Enthusiasm trumps experience and tricky moves, and the best sex can't be measured by one person's performance. It's about give-and-take, understanding your partner, and unpredictability—so pounce on him when he least expects it.

Q. My guy swears he has no sexual fantasies. He's lying, right?

A. Through his teeth. You can't blame him though: Transparency isn't always easy when it comes to the kinky stuff. He's probably worried you'll react badly, get jealous over a daydream about his Pilates instructor at the gym, or judge him for being into something that you're not. So if you're going to push this conversation, you have to keep an open mind. The best way to get him to spill the beans? Cop to a fantasy of your own first—something tame to start. If that goes well, you can take turns, ratcheting up the raunch factor and maybe even trying a thing or two along the way.

Q. Date nights for married couples: totally cheesy or are they actually a good idea?

A. Calling it date night is cheesier than a bad chick flick. But the occasional night out is a great idea—a necessity even. Just don't let it become part of your rut. Hit the newest cocktail joints in your area and keep the babysitter up late. Or make out in the car for a while before you head into the house. You'll inject your relationship with some new life and give yourselves enough fresh memories to carry you through until the next escape.

Q. How do I ask my guy to trim the 'fro down below?

A. Most guys would rock a pink pubic Mohawk if they thought it would get them more sex. We're pretty easy that way. Bring it up in a casual non-bedroom setting: "I'm due for a trim down there. How about you do the same and we'll compare later?"

Q. Our down-there hair: totally bare, fancy landing strip, or au natural?

A. Less is definitely more, but rather than stick with a signature 'do, switch it up. Change keeps us guessing—and guessing keeps us interested. So maybe you start with a trimmed-down triangle. After a few weeks, whack it down to a landing strip. Then wait for a special occasion and take it all off. Wait a while, then let the grass grow back the same way it came off—start with a strip, then allow it to gradually fluff up and widen out.

Q. My boyfriend has slept with tons of girls. How do I get over it?

A. Like a bad haircut, you're going to have to wait this one out. Sucks, I know, but once his number is out of the bag, this pointless—but potent—piece of sexual intel will stop warping your brain only after you've established a track record together. And that takes time. Think about it this way: Why would he be so honest about his past if he wanted to repeat it? And if you're worried about not measuring up, don't. Those girls—all of them—are sexual history for a reason.

Q. The only time my husband wants to have sex is at night, when I'm too tired. Why can't he be more flexible?

A. You both ought to be more flexible. If you're into wake-up sex, ask him what it will take for him to rise to the occasion. He may be more willing if you accommodate him once in a while too. Sure, it's tough to summon the energy for a drawn-out sex session after a long day, but you can take the pressure off with an after-work quickie before exhaustion settles in. Or ask him for a 5-minute massage to help you shed the tension of the day—and you both get in the mood.

Q. Do guys like it when a woman is loud in bed?
A. Guys slobber over surround sound and subwoofers for a reason: We like aural. Loud sex doesn't just add something to the physical and visual sensations we receive, it's also proof you're enjoying yourself—and when you're turned on, we're turned on.

Q. I caught my husband masturbating. Why does a guy who can have sex whenever he wants need to do this?
A. Caught? Well, it's not as if you found him stashing a dead body. I know this is hard to believe, but even sex with a gorgeous woman like you won't make a guy forget about the fun factory between his legs. (There's no pressure to perform on solo excursions, which is why guys like them.) But if it bothers you, lay down some rules. One: He should choose his moments wisely (when you aren't likely to interrupt). Two: Like a backpacker, he should leave no trace—in the garbage, the computer's cache, etc. And three: He's augmenting his sex life, not replacing it. If there's something he wants in bed, he needs to ask.

Q. My guy is never romantic. How can I get him to step it up?
A. Lame hints or jabs about your coworker's massive orchid delivery will only add to the pressure he probably already feels. Take the stress off by telling him you're okay with whatever he comes up with, whether it's watching the sunset together or mowing a heart into the lawn. That said, it's fair to tell him your favorite kind of flower or the name of a restaurant you want to try.

Q. What outfit do guys find hottest?
A. I'm partial to a well-worn Chicago Cubs T-shirt and a come-hither look. But you can't go wrong if you follow these three rules. One: Less isn't necessarily more. A snug fit can conjure up more daydreams than an eyeful of thigh. Two: Ditch the six-inch heels and contortionist bras. If you're not comfortable in your clothes, we won't be comfortable watching you in them. And finally, when in doubt, go with jeans that hug your ass and a soft cotton shirt—one just tight enough for us to imagine how you'd feel in our hands.

Q. My guy and I used to have steamy make-out sessions, but now he skips the kissing and goes straight for the main event. How can I get him to slow down?
A. He's jumping the gun because he knows he can. Slow his roll the next time he tries skipping steps, then remind him just how hot it was before he'd seen the promised land. Your best bet: taking things outside, like to a park. There's no better time than late summer to sprawl out on a picnic blanket, pop a bottle of white, and start whispering dirty ideas in his ear and kissing a little. The public setting will cuff his wandering hands. Wait until he's frothing at the mouth, then tell him it's time to go home. You'll break 14 traffic laws en route, rock the bed off the box springs, and make your point: Good things come to those who wait.

Q. I have a role-playing fantasy, but I'm not sure he'll be into it. How should I bring it up?
A. If you're shy about revealing your raunchier daydreams or if sex between you has been vanilla so far, start small. Maybe you slip on a pair of four-inch pumps and suddenly you're his sexy secretary, or a pair of cowboy boots turns him into a rough rider. "Finding" something in the room to spark the role-play makes it seem less premeditated, and will ease the transition for both of you.

Q. Does expensive lingerie really turn guys on, or is it just a big waste of money?
A. Ever see a 10-year-old tear into a Christmas present? That's pretty much what lingerie does to a guy. The better the packaging, the sooner it's stripped off, so think twice before dropping half your paycheck on velvet hems, tulle trim, or mother-of-pearl clasps. Though guys do appreciate the effort, most are satisfied with the simple stuff: silky favorites and skimpy cuts that hug your curves like a roadster on the California coast.

Chapter 4
The Better Sex Workout

A 4-WEEK PLAN TO FIRM UP, FIRE UP,
AND LOOK AND FEEL GREAT

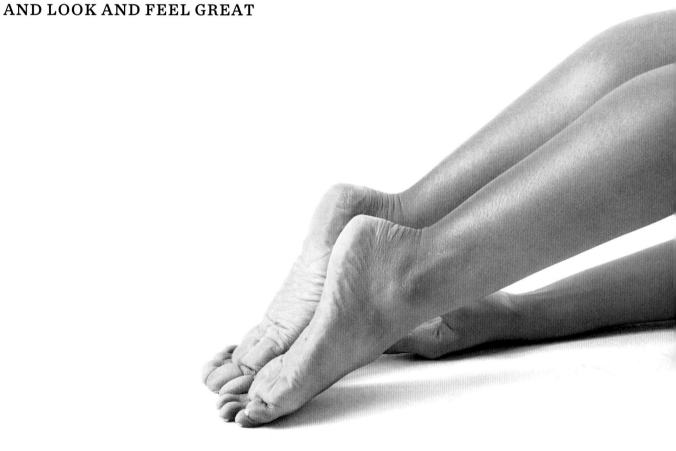

Women'sHealth

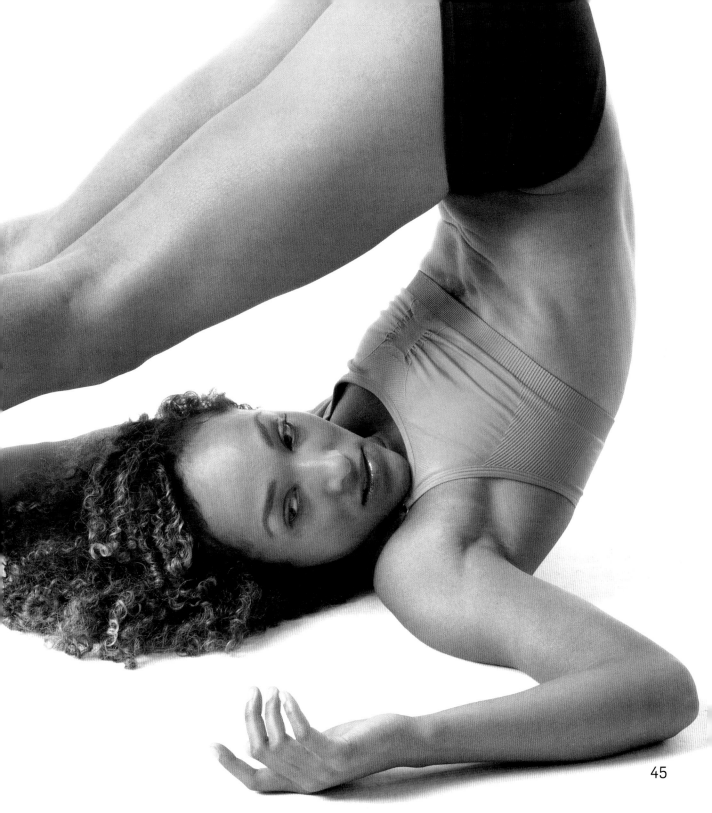

A quick

show of hands, ladies: Who has felt more than a teensy weensy bit of anxiety the first time they slipped into a new swimsuit and stepped onto the beach? Exactly. Now, who among you has wondered—even for an instant—what he might be thinking about your body as you shimmy out of your tight jeans? Thought so.

The point is that when you're thinking about cellulite, your mind is hard pressed to focus on his tongue action. For many women, body self image has a huge bearing on their sexual lives. Numerous studies have shown that women who are unhappy with their weight and shape are less likely to have sexual partners, have sex less frequently, and are less inclined to experiment sexually than are women who feel comfortable with their appearance. It can be a significant problem, especially considering how common it is for women to feel uncomfortable in their own skin.

One national survey of 30,000 married and single women found that a stunning 55 percent felt dissatisfied with their bodies.

One of the top sexual psychology research labs in the country recently explored the connection between body image and sexual function in a study of 85 college women. Researchers from the Meston Sexual Psychophysiology Laboratory at the University of Texas at Austin gave the women a body-image questionnaire designed to gauge their feelings about their sexual attractiveness. Next, the women were sent to private rooms with some erotic literature and instructed to rate how sexually turned on the story made them feel. The analysis of the responses showed that those women with high body self-esteem reported much greater sexual desire after reading the stories than women who felt unhappy with their weight or attractiveness. What's more, the women who were happy with their bodies reported a greater urge to get it on with their partners after reading the sexy lit.

"Being worried about how your body looks or anxious about how he might be evaluating your body can distract you from the pleasurable sensations that can help you become aroused," says researcher Cindy M. Meston, PhD, the lab's director.

Isn't it the truth?

On the flip side, when women experience a boost in self-esteem through weight-loss, a self-improvement achievement, or some other positive therapy, they are more likely to report a boost in sexual function and satisfaction.

And that's what this chapter is about.

Sex can be the best motivation to lose weight and stick with an exercise routine. Think about exercising this way: It holds the keys to feeling great about your body and enjoying the love life you've always dreamed of. Exercise can deliver all those benefits and more—starting, well, immediately. As soon as you elevate your heart rate and rev up your respiratory system by moving your muscles, cobweb-clearing oxygen floods your brain. Your body releases feel-good hormones called endorphins that lift mood, repel stress, and reduce anxiety. The sense of accomplishment that follows a workout helps you swell with feelings of self-worth. Even the healthy flush in your face gives your skin a youthful glow. All of these things provide instant, positive feedback and future motivation to stick to a lifestyle of regular exercise and healthy eating. And weight loss, if that's your goal, will work wonders in helping you feel comfortable and happy in your skin. When you like how you feel naked, your body and brain are fully synchronized to enjoy all the pleasures of sex.

On the following pages, you'll find a 4-week metabolism-boosting workout program that will help you feel terrific about your body. The plan is designed to help you quickly lose weight, especially from the tummy, and tone your muscles, especially the backs of the arms, thighs, and butt (so you'll look fabulous in and

TOP

3

THINGS THAT GIVE THE AVERAGE WOMAN A CONFIDENCE BOOST

1. **A workout**

2. **Compliments**

3. **Seeing a flattering photo of herself**

The Better Sex Workout | HERS

SAMPLE WEEK SCHEDULE

MONDAY
Superset/brisk walk or run

TUESDAY
Cardio circuit

WEDNESDAY
Yoga/brisk walk or run

THURSDAY
Superset/brisk walk or run

FRIDAY
Cardio circuit

SATURDAY
Interval training

Warm-Up 1
- Low Side-to-Side Lunge
- Inchworm
- Standing Hip Thrust
- Gluteal Bridge

Warm-Up 2
- Hinge
- Lower-Back Lie-Down
- Plié
- Gluteal Bridge

Kegels
Pelvic floor strengtheners, described on page 61, should be done at the end of every workout.

out of your jeans). The workout is organized as a superset (more on that later); for now all you need to know is that it's quick and effective.

There's also a cardio workout to boost your aerobic capacity for sexual endurance and a special warm-up sequence that will return a youthful flexibility to muscles and tendons stiffened by sedentary desk jobs. Finally, we've built your Kegel exercises right into the program to ensure that you strengthen the muscles of the pelvic floor that increase arousal, enjoyment, and the likelihood of orgasm.

How to do the workout

- Do the superset resistance workout twice a week on nonconsecutive days.

- Complete the first superset, 8 to 10 repetitions of exercises 1A and 1B with no rest in between. Then rest for 1 minute and proceed to the next superset, exercises 2A and 2B, and so on.

- Do the cardio circuit twice a week—just not on the days you do the superset workout.

- Begin each training session with a good warm-up to ready your muscles for the rigors of resistance training and to avoid injury. The warm-up, designed by Jeff Bell, owner of Bell Fitness Company in New York, includes moves designed to lengthen and strengthen muscles that typically get a workout during sex. We've altered the mix of warm-up exercises for each workout to keep things fresh so you'll never get bored.

Warm-Up Exercises

This quick routine will warm your muscles and loosen your joints while stretching and strengthening the stabilizing muscles of the lower body, pelvis, and core—all used when you get busy. You might be tempted to jump right into the main workout. Don't. Take it slow. Think of this as foreplay for your workout. Warm-ups will prepare your muscles so they can work harder and get more from the main workout. And they'll help you avoid injuries. We've broken the warm-up into two groups so you can alternate. The boxed letters match the instructions to the photos.

Low Side-to-Side Lunge

Improves strength and flexibility of lower body, especially hips, glutes, and groin.

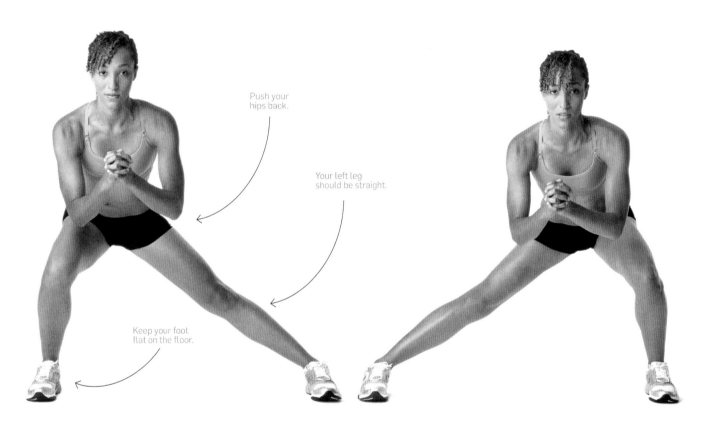

Push your hips back.

Your left leg should be straight.

Keep your foot flat on the floor.

 A

- Stand with your feet spread wide, about twice shoulder-width apart, your feet facing straight ahead. Bend slightly at the waist and clasp your hands in front of your chest. Shift your weight over to your right leg as you push your hips backward and lower your body by dropping your hips and bending your right knee.

 B

- Your lower right leg should remain nearly perpendicular to the floor. Your left foot should remain flat on the floor. Without pausing, reverse the movement and raise yourself back to a standing position. Next, repeat to the left side. Alternate back and forth. Do 10 to 20 reps on each side.

Inchworm

Loosens thighs, hips, obliques, back, and shoulders.

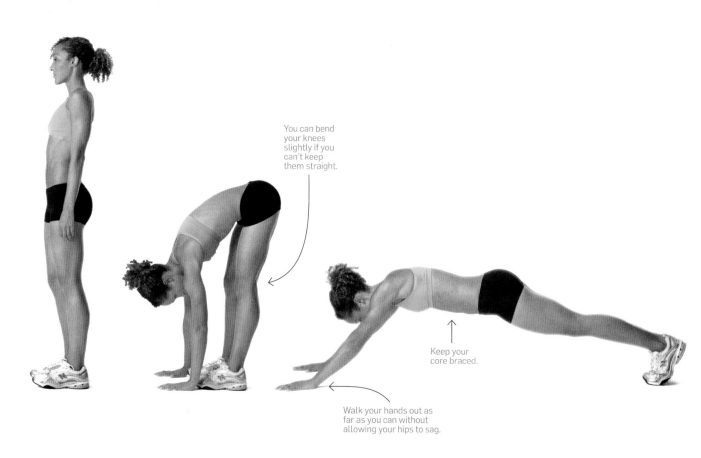

You can bend your knees slightly if you can't keep them straight.

Keep your core braced.

Walk your hands out as far as you can without allowing your hips to sag.

A
- Stand with your legs straight, feet hip-width apart.

B
- Bend at the waist and place your hands on the floor.

C
- Keeping your legs straight, walk your hands forward while keeping your abs and lower back braced. Then take tiny steps to walk your feet back to your hands. That's 1 repetition. Do 6.

Standing Hip Thrust

Stretches the hip flexors.

A

- Stand with your feet together, hands on your hips. Step forward with one foot so that your feet are a couple of feet apart. Keep your toes facing forward and your knees slightly bent.

B

- Gently push your pelvis forward until you feel a very mild stretch in your hips. Although this move seems too subtle, don't overdo it: The hip flexors are attached inside the legs in such a way that it takes very little effort to stretch them. Hold the stretch for 30 seconds then reverse leg positions and repeat.

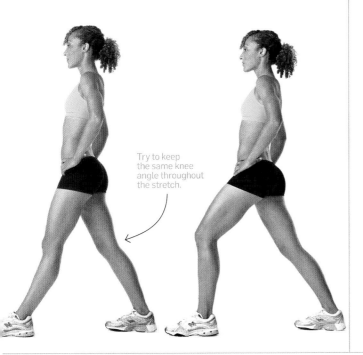

Try to keep the same knee angle throughout the stretch.

Gluteal Bridge

Enhances orgasm by strengthening, and boosting endurance of, the pelvic muscles.

A

- This exercise is also known as a hip raise. Lie on the floor, arms at your sides, knees bent, and heels on the floor.

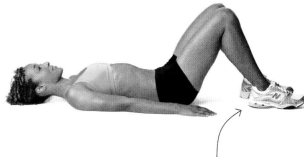

Press with your heels, not toes, when you begin to lift up.

B

- Lift your hips off the floor until your knees, hips, and shoulders form a straight line. That's 1 repetition. Do 20.

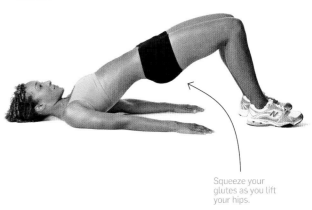

Squeeze your glutes as you lift your hips.

51

The Better Sex Workout HERS

Hinge

Stretches and strengthens the core, quadriceps, and hip flexors.

A

- Kneel on the floor with your hands at your sides. Resist the urge to sit back and rest your weight on your heels. Your back should be straight and your knees bent at a 90-degree angle.

B

- Keeping your head and spine in line with your thighs, slowly lean back a few inches. Hold for 3 seconds then return to the starting position. Do 5 to 10.

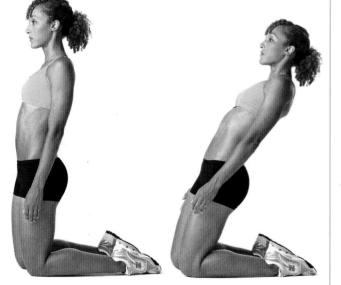

Lower-Back Lie-Down

Stretches the lower back muscles.

A

- Lie flat on your back with your legs bent, feet flat on the floor, and arms at your sides.

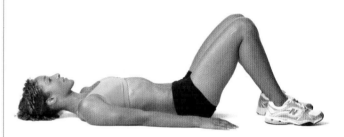

B

- Draw your knees up to your chest and gently grab your legs just below the knees. Slowly pull both knees toward your chest as far as you can comfortably go, keeping your back flat on the floor at all times. Hold the stretch for 2 to 3 seconds, and then slowly lower your legs. Repeat the stretch for 10 reps.

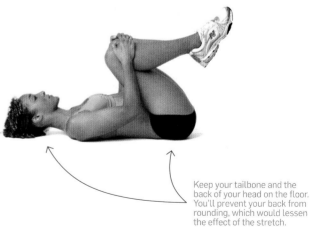

Keep your tailbone and the back of your head on the floor. You'll prevent your back from rounding, which would lessen the effect of the stretch.

Plié

Strengthens the hamstrings, calves, and quads and improves flexibility.

FIRE DRILL

Just 10 minutes of moderate exercise dials up your metabolism for an hour or longer.

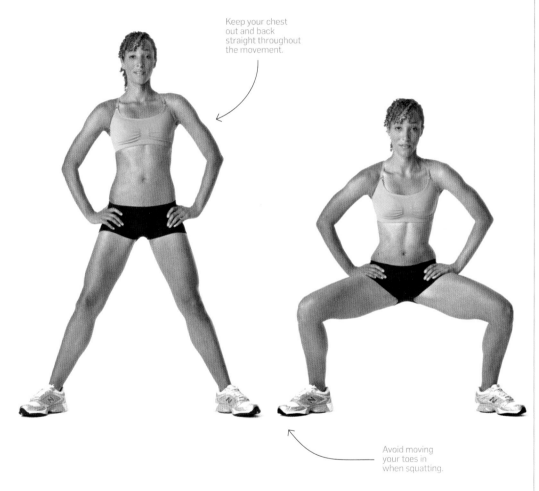

Keep your chest out and back straight throughout the movement.

Avoid moving your toes in when squatting.

A

- Stand with your feet wider than shoulder width apart, toes pointed out and hands on your hips.

B

- Slowly bend your knees until your thighs are parallel to the floor. Press up through your heels to stand. That's 1 repetition. Do 12 to 15.

The Better Sex Supersets

The beauty of this workout is its simplicity and effectiveness. You can do it in the privacy of your home, so it's extremely convenient. All you need are a pair of 5- to 10-pound dumbbells, a stability ball, and a bench or step. The resistance workout was designed by regular *Men's Health* and *Women's Health* contributing trainer Craig Ballantyne, author of *Turbulence Training*.

The secret to its speed is doing sets of two exercises back to back with no rest. (You rest only after completing a superset.) Trainers call this technique a "superset," and it can increase your calorie burn by 13 percent. The pairs of exercises are chosen specifically to work different muscle groups. This way, the muscles you just exhausted while doing exercise one get a break when you're doing exercise two. This allows you to trim workout time while adding an aerobic-fitness aspect to the workout.

The Program

EXERCISES	REPETITIONS	REST
SUPERSET 1		
A Dumbbell Step-Up	8-10	0
B Stability Ball Ab Pike	8-10	1 min
SUPERSET 2		
A Dumbbell Chest Press	8-10	0
B Stability Ball Leg Curl	10-15	1 min
SUPERSET 3		
A Dumbbell Row	12 with each arm	0
B Cross-Body Mountain Climber	24 total leg lifts	1 min
SUPERSET 4		
A Dumbbell Lunge	12 with each leg	0
B Stability Ball Plank	Hold for 30 seconds	1 min

SUPERSET 1A
Dumbbell Step-Up
Targets the glutes and hamstrings.

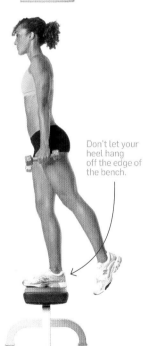

The step should be high enough that your knee is bent at least 90 degrees.

A

- Hold a pair of dumbbells at arm's length, palms facing in, and stand facing a bench or step. Put your right foot on the bench.

Don't let your heel hang off the edge of the bench.

B

- Push down through your right heel and lift your left leg up, keeping the left foot off the bench. Return to start. That's 1 repetition. Do 8 reps leading with your right leg, then 8 reps leading with your left leg.

SUPERSET 1B
Stability Ball Ab Pike
Strengthens the hip flexors.

Keep your head in line with your spine throughout the movement.

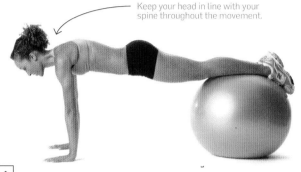

A

- Start in a pushup position with your shins resting on a stability ball. Brace your abs and keep your back straight from head to heels.

Push your hips toward the ceiling.

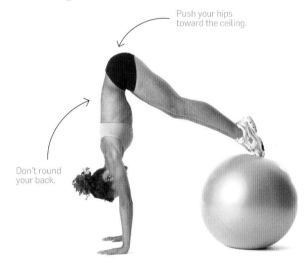

Don't round your back.

B

- Keep your legs straight as you raise your hips toward the ceiling, drawing the ball toward your arms. Hold for 1 second and roll back to start. That's 1 rep.

The Better Sex Workout

SUPERSET 2A
Dumbbell Chest Press
Strengthens the chest and arms.

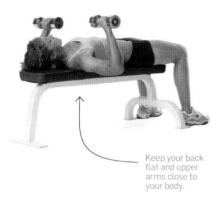

Keep your back flat and upper arms close to your body.

A

- Lie on a workout bench with your feet flat on the floor. Hold a dumbbell in each hand on either side of your chest, upper arms parallel to the floor, and palms facing your feet.

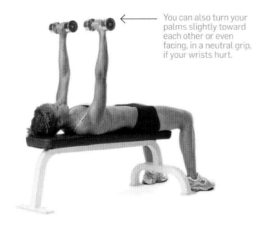

You can also turn your palms slightly toward each other or even facing, in a neutral grip, if your wrists hurt.

B

- Press the weights straight up. Pause, then slowly lower back to start. That's 1 rep.

SUPERSET 2B
Stability Ball Leg Curl
Tones the glutes and hamstrings.

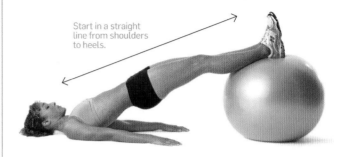

Start in a straight line from shoulders to heels.

A

- Lie on the floor, calves on top of a stability ball, arms flat on the floor at your sides. Squeeze your glutes and raise your hips so your body forms a straight line from shoulder to heels.

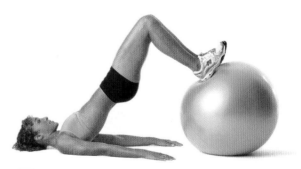

B

- Bend your knees to roll the ball toward you. Straighten your legs to roll the ball back, then lower your body to the floor. That's 1 rep.

SUPERSET 3A
Dumbbell Row
Works the upper back.

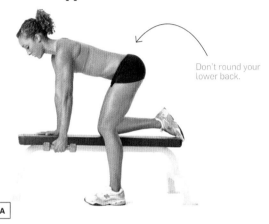

Don't round your lower back.

A

- Place your right knee and right hand on an exercise bench. Hold a dumbbell in your left hand, palm facing the bench.

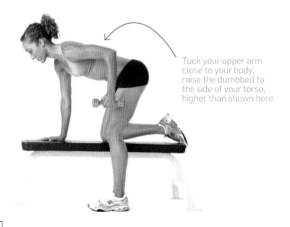

Tuck your upper arm close to your body; raise the dumbbell to the side of your torso, higher than shown here.

B

- Slowly bend your elbow and pull the dumbbell up as far toward your shoulder as possible. Pause then lower the dumbbell back to start. That's 1 rep. After completing all reps, repeat the exercise using your right arm.

SUPERSET 3B
Cross-Body Mountain Climber
Exercises the muscles that stabilize the spine.

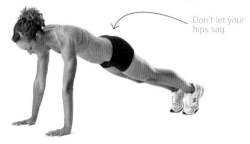

Don't let your hips sag.

A

- Assume a pushup position with your arms straight and hands on the floor directly under your shoulders.

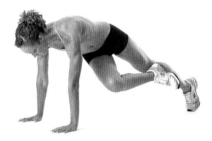

B

- Keeping your abs braced, pick up your right foot and slowly bring your right knee toward your left shoulder. Return that foot to the starting position.

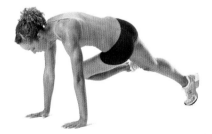

C

- Repeat the move with your left leg. Continue to alternate legs this way quickly but using good form. Complete 12 reps per leg.

The Better Sex Workout | HERS

SUPERSET 4A
Dumbbell Lunge
Builds the quadriceps and calves.

- Stand with your feet hip-width apart and hold a dumbbell in each hand at your sides, palms facing in.

Stand as tall as you can, chest up, shoulders back.

Brace your core and hold it that way for the entire exercise.

- Step forward with your right leg, bending your right knee until both legs form 90-degree angles—your left knee should nearly touch the floor. Push back to the starting position. Repeat, this time stepping forward with your left leg. Alternate legs for a total of 12 lunges on each side.

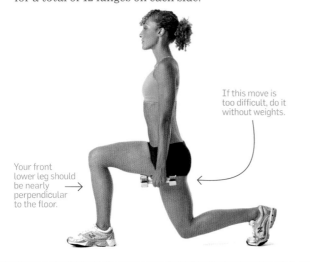

If this move is too difficult, do it without weights.

Your front lower leg should be nearly perpendicular to the floor.

SUPERSET 4B
Stability Ball Plank
Works the lower back muscles and abs.

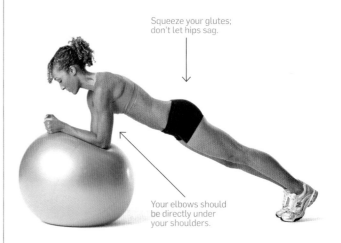

Squeeze your glutes; don't let hips sag.

Your elbows should be directly under your shoulders.

A

- Get into an elevated plank position on a stability ball by resting your forearms and elbows on the top of the ball. Your elbows should be directly under your shoulders. Keep your shoulder blades back and down and your body in a straight line. Brace your abs and hold the position for 30 seconds.

  Make it easier: Do the plank without a stability ball; place your elbows and forearms on the floor.

  Make it harder: From a plank on the ball, bring one knee toward your chest and return it to the floor, then do the same with the other knee. Alternate knees for 10 repetitions per leg.

The Cardio Circuit

You don't have to cover large expanses of territory to get a decent cardio workout. Heck, you don't need a treadmill or a stationary cycle either. Calisthenics are terrific for boosting your heart rate, blasting calories, and building muscle, especially if you do them in circuit fashion—going rapidly from one move to the next without resting between exercises. Do the following four moves for the prescribed number of repetitions. When you finish the fourth exercise, catch your breath for 3 minutes. Then start another circuit. At week three of this 4-week plan, add another circuit for a total of three, resting between each. If you go beyond 4 weeks, you can add additional circuits or increase the number of repetitions or hold times per exercise.

Jumps

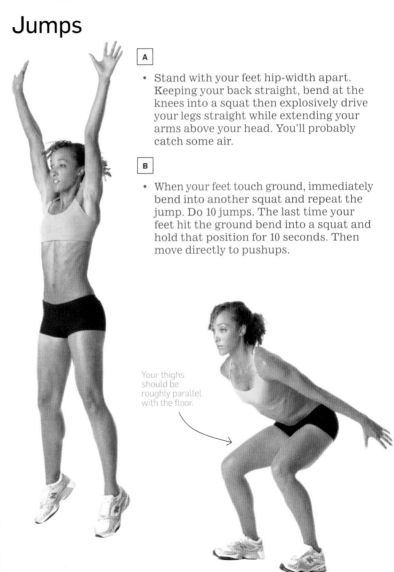

Your thighs should be roughly parallel with the floor.

A
- Stand with your feet hip-width apart. Keeping your back straight, bend at the knees into a squat then explosively drive your legs straight while extending your arms above your head. You'll probably catch some air.

B
- When your feet touch ground, immediately bend into another squat and repeat the jump. Do 10 jumps. The last time your feet hit the ground bend into a squat and hold that position for 10 seconds. Then move directly to pushups.

The Better Sex Workout |

Pushups

A

- Place your hands on the floor, shoulder-width apart, and directly under your shoulders.

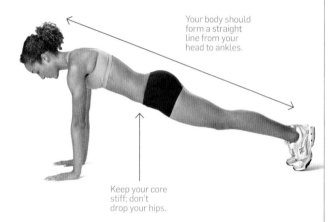

Your body should form a straight line from your head to ankles.

Keep your core stiff; don't drop your hips.

B

- Keeping your back straight and abs drawn in tight, lower yourself to touch your chest to the floor. Press up into the starting position and repeat. Do 10 pushups. Hold at the top of the last pushup for 20 seconds.

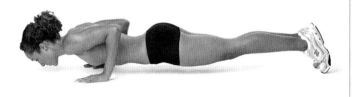

Plank-Side-Plank

Perform the following as one movement without rest.

A

- From your pushup position, assume a plank. Bend your arms and support your body with your elbows and forearms. Your upper arms should be perpendicular to the floor, elbows directly under your shoulders. Hold this position for 20 seconds.

If you were to place a broomstick on your back, it should make contact with your head, upper back, and butt.

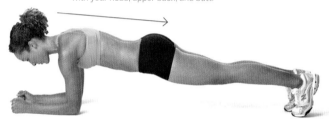

B

- Move into a right-side plank: shift your weight onto your right forearm and the outer part of your right foot. Rest your left leg on top of your right leg, keeping both straight. Move your left hand on your hip. Hold for 10 seconds. Return to the standard plank and hold for 20 seconds, then shift to a left-side plank and hold for 10 seconds.

Keep your hips raised and pushed forward.

Stack your feet.

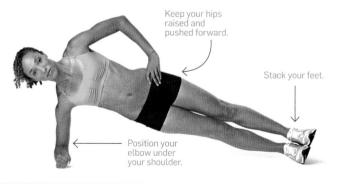

Position your elbow under your shoulder.

Mountain Climber

KEGEL EXERCISES
(to be done at the end of every workout)

Lie on your back on the floor with knees bent 90 degrees and feet flat on the floor. Find the PC muscles, the pubococcygeus muscle that you use to stop the flow of urine when peeing. Without tightening your glutes, squeeze your PC muscles and hold for 15 seconds. Then release. Do up to 20 at the end of every workout.

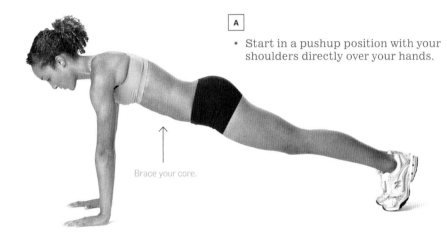

A

- Start in a pushup position with your shoulders directly over your hands.

Brace your core.

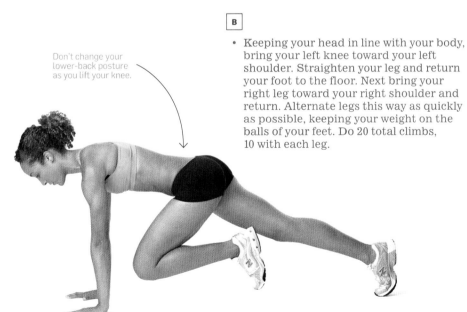

B

- Keeping your head in line with your body, bring your left knee toward your left shoulder. Straighten your leg and return your foot to the floor. Next bring your right leg toward your right shoulder and return. Alternate legs this way as quickly as possible, keeping your weight on the balls of your feet. Do 20 total climbs, 10 with each leg.

Don't change your lower-back posture as you lift your knee.

The Flat-Tummy Interval Workout

Fire up your metabolism and burn tummy fat by fitting one high-intensity interval-training (HIIT) workout into your weekly fitness plan. Recent studies show that short bouts of high intensity physical effort interspersed with periods of easy-pace recovery effort burn more fat calories than long aerobic sessions do. One Australian study found that women who did HIIT training 3 days a week for 15 weeks dropped significantly more weight than those who exercised for the same period of time at a lower intensity. Because you're already doing 2 cardio workouts per week, we recommend only 1 day devoted to intervals. Here's what a typical interval looks like. You can run, bike, or use the cardio machine of your choice.

- Warm up by running or biking for 3 minutes at an easy pace.
- Run or bike for 30 seconds at 90 percent of your best effort.
- Slow down to a little less than half speed for 2 minutes to recover.
- Repeat this sprint/recovery sequence five times.
- Cool down for 3 minutes.

Using that plan as a guide, increase the length of your sprints and decrease the length of your easy-pace intervals each subsequent week, while adding reps. Begin and end each interval session with a warm-up and a cool-down.

	SPRINT PACE	EASY PACE	REPS
WEEK 1	30 seconds	2 minutes	5
WEEK 2	30 seconds	90 seconds	6
WEEK 3	1 minute	90 seconds	8
WEEK 4	1 minute	1 minute	10

BONUS EXERCISE

Tone Your Arms

STAY STRONG ON TOP

A lot of women dislike their arms. What they really hate is their triceps, the flabby backs of their arms. If yours continue to wave long after you've said goodbye, grab a dumbbell and do this triceps-building exercise every other day. It's called the dumbbell overhead triceps extension and it's the best way to firm up these muscles.

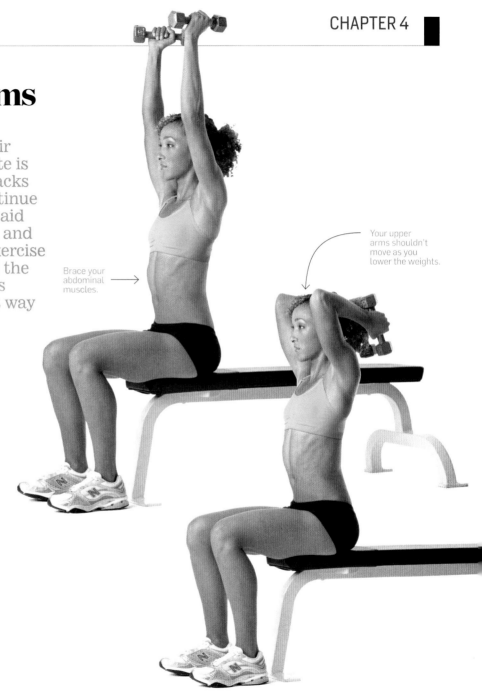

Brace your abdominal muscles. →

Your upper arms shouldn't move as you lower the weights.

- Sit on the edge of a bench and hold two lightweight dumbbells in your hands above your head, palms facing.

- Without moving your upper arms, lower the weights slowly behind your head. Pause, then straighten your arms to the starting position. Do 10 reps.

Women's Health®

Chapter 5
The Sexual Diagnostic

FROM BODY-IMAGE WOES TO LOW LIBIDOS,
A TROUBLESHOOTER'S GUIDE TO HEALTHIER SEX

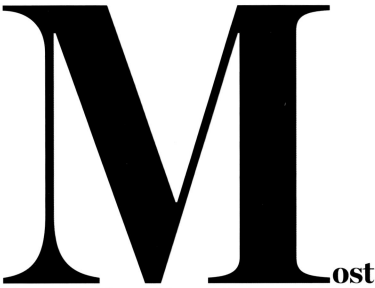

Most of you probably would agree that women tend to be more knowledgeable, mature, and less childish about their private parts than men. Do an internet search of penis jokes. It turns up more than double the number of vagina jokes. That tells you something.

Still, no one loves to strip naked in front of someone wearing a cold stethoscope. Not surprisingly, one in five women admits to feeling uncomfortable discussing their vaginas with their doctors, according to a national survey by the Association of Reproductive Health Professionals. Well, we hope to change that with this chapter by creating a private forum for sexual-health information to help you troubleshoot sex-related physical and psychological issues, and make them easier to discuss with your partner and your doctor. Plus, we'll share the most frequently asked questions from the readers of *Women's Health* and answers from our experts.

A Trip to the Clinic

ONE COUPLE'S DIARY

Sexual dissatisfaction affects nearly every woman at some point in her sexual life. And it can present itself in many ways. Sexual health clinics specialize in investigating the roots of sexual dissatisfaction and suggesting solutions. You can go solo or as a couple. *Women's Health* sent writer Leslie Goldman and her husband Dan to The Clinic at The Berman Center to see what they could learn and improve upon. For the record, their sex life is anything but broken. But it could be better—and hotter. And that's what they were after.

Gripe No. 1: I believe I should orgasm faster than a 14-year-old boy with a copy of *Penthouse*. When I can't, I give up.
Gripe No. 2: Dan and I have different schedules, which means I'll return from a late workout, endorphins blazing, just as he's polishing off a chihuahua-size burrito.
Gripe No. 3: Despite being a professional body image speaker and author, I'm as self-conscious about my butt as Nora Ephron is about her neck. When naked, I insist on walking backward away from the bed in a sort of modified grapevine, terrified that my husband will catch a glimpse of cellulite.

Sex therapy may be an obvious fix, but I'd always pegged it as one of those things normal people don't do. I'd never even considered it until the magazine asked me to investigate the Chicago Clinic run by Laura Berman, PhD, the Dr. Phil of getting your freak on. Apparently my misgivings gel with popular opinion: "I've found that 50 percent of people are not satisfied with their sex lives," Berman says. "But only 10 percent of men and 20 percent of women seek help." Well, change begins with me, so I e-mail my concerns to Berman, and she recommends I sign up for an intensive 3-day retreat that will address everything from sexual inhibitions to stress management. Which brings me to my Q&A with The Sex Swami.

I meet Berman in her brightly lit downtown office, which looks more like a spa than a medical institution. Sitting in a red chair, her blonde hair held back with a black headband, Berman makes eye contact, shoots me an easy smile, and hands me a binder filled with my personalized schedule, journal, and a slew of questionnaires, including a "depression inventory" and a "genital image scale." Holy crap, what have I gotten myself into?

I sink into the couch and set my water glass down. Before I know it, we're discussing my sexual background (four male partners plus a short-lived stint of drunken heteroflexibility that culminated in my waking up with a raging hangover and a naked 21-year-old named Valerie); the cues I received about sex and love from my family (tons of laughter and affection, no divorces, and "Put an aspirin between your knees and never let it fall" from my father before every high school date); and how Dan and I ultimately came to be (8 years of best-friendship followed by his dogged pursuit). It's a lot to cough up so soon, and just as we really start to dig in, she tells me we have to stop so that I can get to my Tantra lesson.

11 a.m. to 1 p.m.
Booty Breathing

To help me rethink my orgasm-centric mentality, Berman has sent me to the TantraNova Institute, a Chicago clinic that teaches "the ancient art of sacred Tantric sexuality." I'm greeted by "beloveds" and business partners Elsbeth Meuth, EdD, 58, petite with ultra-short blonde hair and a thick German accent, and Freddy Zental Weaver, 51, a towering,

handsome man with rich, chocolate-brown skin. They lead me into a studio filled with candles, silk pillows, and a floor-to-ceiling painting of a figure with seven chakras ablaze. (For those of you who don't have the token yoga-obsessed friend, chakras are "energy centers" that run roughly from the base of the spine to just above the head. They're associated with a wide range of physical and mental states—the throat chakra with communication, the heart chakra with love, and so on.)

I sit cross-legged on the floor; the Tantric duo faces me. Freddy guides us through a meditation exercise. His voice is so smooth I can't believe it's not butter. As we inhale, Elsbeth explains the importance of breath: By circulating it through our bodies, we create energy, enhancing sex and, for the truly practiced and fortunate, paving the way to whole-body orgasms.

My homework, Freddy tells me, is to "self-love," perhaps the most PC term ever for masturbation. But orgasm is not the goal. I should encounter myself as my own lover, setting the scene with flowers, music, oils. The purpose of this exercise, Elsbeth explains, is to enjoy the sensations rather than rushing to completion. After caressing my hands, arms, and stomach, I may wish to move on to my "yoni" (Sanskrit for "cooch"). "Start by massaging her," Freddy encourages as I scribble down notes. "Dance on the edge of orgasm." I want to blurt out, "Didn't I see that in a Hallmark card?" but keep mum, engrossed in thoughts of

CHAKRA CAN

Sit cross-legged on the floor. Close your eyes and visualize your breath as a stream of light entering your body. Imagine this light flowing through your sexual chakra, near the lower abdomen and vagina. Having trouble feeling your breath anywhere but your nose? Touch your hand to the chakra to focus on the sensation of breath there.

tonight's assignment. Before my yoni gets any self-loving, though, I need to cab it back to Berman's to meet my husband for our first and only couples session.

"So, Dan, how would you classify your sexual relationship?"

My guy is such a sport. He really didn't want to air our sexual laundry on a national clothesline, but he's so supportive of my career—and our relationship—that he folded. He opens up to Berman immediately, describing it almost exactly as I would. "We're happy, extremely affectionate . . . lots of kissing and cuddling." He concedes that we are intimate less often than we used to be, due to dueling schedules and his back injury, and that he'd like to get it on more often.

We brainstorm ways to become more sexually proactive. Berman suggests scheduling sex, but we deplore the idea of PDAing our PDA. She counters, "Most young couples today have to make a paradigm shift: Instead of saying, 'Ugh, scheduling sex is a chore,' make it something you can look forward to." Or we can encourage nooky to occur more organically by freeing up time at night. I need to set boundaries between my work and personal life, Dr. B. explains, for the sake of my mental and sexual health. Can I put aside 2 hours at night with no work? I balk. "Think about it as productive time for your relationship and it won't feel so gluttonous," she says. We compromise on an hour.

Then she brings up the rear: "What do you think about her butt issue?" she asks, looking at Dan.

SQUEEZE PLAY

Show your partner how buff your love is with this couples Kegel: During sex, tighten your pelvic muscles as if you were starting and stopping the flow of pee. Ask him to do the same. Breathe deeply together for an "arousing and connecting" experience, says Elsbeth Meuth of Chicago's TantraNova Institute.

He laughs, describing it as firm and strong, but I blurt out that he's lying and before I know it, I'm crying. This is ridiculous. I was anorexic in college but have been recovered for over a decade.

Berman posits that my caboose complex is a remnant of self-loathing I experienced with my eating disorder. For tonight I am assigned the charming task of standing before him, naked and ass-backward. Oh, and to have sex too.

8 to 9 p.m.
I Touch Myself

That night, I am surprisingly psyched for self-love. I close the bedroom door and cue up Sade. A citrus tea light twinkles from my dresser, guiding my way toward the bed, which I've covered with an old beach towel to protect the sheets from massage oil.

I take a few deep breaths and am ready to love all my 2,000 parts. "Smooth Operator" plays in the background as I stroke my arms, discovering that my wrists are pleasingly sensitive, especially when lightly tickled. I drizzle more oil over my stomach and breasts and enjoy dreamy rubbing for about 10 minutes. I know orgasm isn't the goal of this assignment, but a vibrator beckons from my bedside drawer, so I succumb, self-loving myself three times in a row. Bad student! I was supposed to massage my entire body but skipped my legs, back, and butt. I should have paid more attention to the directions rather than jump to my fast and furious conclusion. Obviously, this is an area I need to work on. But, hey, it was much easier to climax after all that caressing.

10 to 11 p.m.
Bringing Sexy Back

I steel myself for the butt exercise. I position Dan on the edge of the bed, proudly presenting my front half—I love my perky breasts and toned stomach. I don't know what scares me more: that my man, who loves me unconditionally, might be turned off, or that I might realize he really does love all of me—and then what will I have to obsess over? After a few frustrating minutes I say, "F@&! it," and rotate. Words like "cellulite" and "nutcase" zap through my mind. Dan kisses my back and whispers I am beautiful. We wind up having a nice heart-to-heart in bed, during which he gently confronts my perfectionism, asking me if I would love him less if his butt were, say, not up to Brad Pitt standards. Okay, he's got a point. He kindly calls supermodel Gisele "an airbrushed freak," and because we're already horizontal, we switch off the light and continue the oral conversation.

Day 2: 9:30 to 10:30 a.m.
Q&A, Take Two

I recount the butt experiment to Berman, explaining how caring Dan was and how hypocritical I, as a body image speaker, felt having to admit this eating disorder leftover. She explains that with my perfectionist tendencies, my tush is symbolic of my need for control. "When you have really high expectations—of how you look, what you're supposed to accomplish, how you do at work—you set yourself up for failure and disappointment," she says.

Same goes for orgasms: If they're not happening right now, I think I've failed. Ironically, the more someone worries about climaxing, the more stress it creates, Berman explains. "An orgasm is the epitome of letting go." I need to be easier on myself and relinquish control.

This is starting to resemble conventional therapy, and I suggest we focus more on sex. Berman smiles firmly and shakes her head no. "Who you are is the sum of your life experiences—psychological, emotional, and sexual." While sex therapy, in its purest form, addresses sexual challenges in a relationship by helping you relearn behaviors, Berman likes to intertwine it with general as well as couples therapy, which explores the inner workings of the relationship.

My hour of psychoanalysis flies by in what feels like 10 minutes, and it's time for me to shut up and dance. Enter Miss Exotic World 2005, Michelle "The Ass That Goes Pow!" L'amour.

2 to 3 p.m.
Burlesque Is Best

I warm up in the Berman Center yoga studio, swiveling my hips to drum-thumping music with L'amour, 27, a tiny, hazel-eyed brunette. You might think you'd be too shy to faux-striptease with a total stranger, but that's because you've never met L'amour. She's like the straight-talking love child of Eartha Kitt and Shakira, sexy and unassuming in a

DESPISE YOUR THIGHS?

Got a least-favorite body part? For 1 week, jot down notes about when it bothers you most, then see if you can find patterns. Is it when you're with your girlfriends, at home with your guy, walking by your office crush? Identifying those circumstances is the first step to replacing negative thoughts with positive ones.

pint-size package. She hands me a pink boa and satin gloves and shows me how to shimmy, to "present" my breasts (by cupping and lifting from beneath), and to tug my gloves off with my teeth. We talk about how burlesque appeals to women because it explores different definitions of "sexy": intelligent, humorous, playful. She describes it as "a very encouraging way to showcase curves." I can see why Berman has clients with body image issues try it. L'amour runs me through my routine once more and sends me home to show my husband some T&A.

11 p.m. Meet the Next Pussycat Doll . . . Meow

Back home, Dan is waiting for me in the living room while I check myself out in the bathroom mirror. Black push-up bra, check. Matching thong, check. Gloves,

check. Pink Hello Kitty boa from my 30th birthday party, check.

As "Fever" plays from my computer, I totter over to the couch in my patent-leather heels, a nervous smile plastered across my face. But I channel my inner Dita Von Teese and begin with a slow hip rotation, stroking my boa and sliding my satin gloves down my neck and around my breasts. I even do the move where I turn around, bend over, and slap that ass. I end up straddling Dan's lap. He has enjoyed the show. And even though the elaborate moves were seductive, he says the best part was seeing my near-naked body.

Day 3: 10 a.m. to noon Final Session

Back at the center, the topic of the day is control. Berman suggests that the

HEALTH RESOURCES FOR WOMEN

American Academy of Clinical Sexologists:
3203 Lawton Road
Orlando, FL 32803
407-645-1641
esextherapy.com

American Association for Marriage and Family Therapy:
112 South Alfred Street
Alexandria, VA 22314
703-838-9808
aamft.org

American Association of Sexuality Educators, Counselors and

Therapists (provides referrals for experts in your area):
P.O. Box 1960
Ashland, VA 23005
804-752-0026
aasect.org

American Psychiatric Association (online resource for anyone seeking mental health information):
HealthyMinds.org

American Psychological Association:
750 First Street, NE

Washington, DC 20002
800-374-2721
apa.org

Centers for Disease Control National AIDS Hotline:
800-342-2437

CDC National STD Hotline:
800-227-8922

Federal Government Source for Women's Health Information:
Womenshealth.gov

The National Breast Cancer Foundation:
www.nationalbreast
cancer.org

National Herpes Resource Center Hotline:
919-361-8488

National Kidney and Urologic Diseases Information Clearinghouse:
3 Information Way
Bethesda, MD 20892
800-891-5390

SHARE Breast and Ovarian Cancer Support (supportive network of breast and ovarian cancer survivors):
Breast Cancer Hotline
212-382-2111;
Ovarian Cancer Hotline
212-719-1204;
Sharecancersupport.org

control freak in me might surrender if Dan were extra-aggressive in the bedroom. In fact, she says, the most common fantasy women have is feeling powerless. Because I feel safe with Dan, I can give up the wheel and enjoy the ride. This will be therapeutic, Berman promises, so I deviously plot charging handcuffs and a whip to his Flexible Spending Account.

I dash off an e-mail to Dan—Subject: Your Mission, Should You Choose to Accept It—and stop at Freddy and Elsbeth's for a rousing round of Kegels, designed to enliven my sexual center and enhance orgasm. We do them together, chanting, "Squeeze, release, squeeze, release." It's Genital Jazzercise! They encourage me to do these every day: in the car, while writing. Soon my vagina will drop a size and crave protein bars.

Feeling tingly, I return home. I can't wait for tonight's hard-hitting homework assignment: caveman sex.

10 p.m.
Neander-Thrall
We're snuggling harmlessly in bed, and I get up to pee. When I come back, the room becomes a blur of bathrobe, boxer shorts, and bed sheets. Next, I'm against the wall, arms pinned overhead. Then I'm launched through the air, landing on a pile of pillows. Now I'm on my knees—but despite prior concerns I'm pretty sure my ass looks great. The sex is rough, and after all this talking and reflecting, I can finally let go and say, "Ahhhh."

TUNE-UP CENTERS FOR YOUR SEX LIFE

CHICAGO
The Clinic The Berman Center
The Sex Scholar Laura Berman, PhD
The Specialty Customized 3- or 5-day retreats for couples, singles, or women-only groups
Contact 800-709-4709; bermancenter.com
Cost $500 to $750 per day

MONTREAL
The Clinic Sex and Couple Therapy Service at McGill University Health Center, Royal Victoria Hospital
The Sex Scholar Yitzchak Binik, PhD
The Specialty This hospital-based program covers the spectrum of sexual, couple, and marital problems (from pain during sex to intimacy issues). Also offered: "Making Love Better," for those in good relationships who want to get even closer.
Contact 514-398-6094; sexandcoupletherapy.com
Cost Up to $55 per session (income-based sliding scale)

PASADENA
The Clinic The Center for Relationship, Marriage, and Sex Therapy
The Sex Scholar Lori Buckley, PsyD, CST
The Specialty Group sessions include "Passion & Tantra," a day-long workshop for couples; "Love Strategies," and "The Art of Passion and Intimacy for Couples."
Contact 626-893-4208; drloribuckley.com
Cost $400 per couple per month for the weekly couples groups

PHILADELPHIA
The Clinic The Pelvic and Sexual Health Institute
The Sex Scholars Susan Kellogg-Spadt, PhD, and Kristene Whitmore, MD
The Specialty 100 percent medical—pelvic pain and all types of sexual dysfunction
Contact 215-893-2643; pelvicandsexualhealthinstitute.org
Cost $90 to $2,000 per session

SEATTLE
The Clinic The Gottman Relationship Institute
The Sex Scholars John M. Gottman, PhD, and Julie Schwartz Gottman, PhD
The Specialty The Gottman's present "The Art & Science of Love" couples workshop five times a year in Seattle. Certified Gottman Therapists offer the same workshop in other locations.
Contact 888-523-9042, ext. 1; gottman.com
Cost $725 per couple

Troubleshooting Your Va-Jay-Jay

SOME COMMON, SOME STRANGE THINGS THAT CAN GO AWRY & WHAT TO DO ABOUT THEM

NOT GETTING ANY?

You're not alone. Women today have less time for sex than their 1950s counterparts. And it's estimated that 40 million Americans have what experts call a sexless marriage (having sex fewer than 10 times a year).

You seem to be getting more yeast infections now that you've been wearing thongs regularly.

The cause: That thin strip of fabric may save you from the dreaded visible panty lines, but it also serves as a superhighway for microbes. When the underwear hits your perineum (the patch of skin between the vagina and the anus), bacteria hitch a ride straight to your vagina. "A thong is actually a connector," says Adelaide Nardone, MD, an OB-GYN in Providence, Rhode Island. As you move, the fabric shifts and before you can say "Monistat," you've got a yeast infection. To make matters worse, thongs tend to rub, causing tiny tears in the delicate skin around your vulva and clitoris, creating access for microbes.

The cure: You don't have to toss your thongs as long as they're cotton or have a cotton crotch. The breathable fabric keeps you drier, so bacteria can't grow as easily. You might also consider growing out that Brazilian bikini line: Hair serves as a barrier between you and your panties, so leaving more carpet on the floor provides cushioning for your vulva, says Nardone. And don't wear thongs when you exercise. Invest in some workout bottoms with cotton crotches and go commando at night.

You haven't had a period since you went off the Pill (and you're not pregnant).

The cause: The hormones that are used in birth control pills can interfere with those your body naturally produces to cause ovulation and menstruation. They can do this for some time after stopping the pill. The absence of a menstrual period, called post-pill amenorrhea, is not uncommon, especially if your cycle was irregular to begin with, explains Christos Coutifaris, MD, PhD, chief of reproductive endocrinology and infertility at the University of Pennsylvania School of Medicine.

The cure: If you still haven't gotten your period within 3 months of tossing your last pill pack, schedule an appointment with your gynecologist. Amenorrhea can be a symptom of other health issues.

It feels like a tiny water balloon is growing in your vagina.

The cause: A clogged Bartholin duct. These

two tiny tubes on either side of your vagina secrete lubrication in conjunction with the Bartholin's glands (two pea-sized organs under the skin) when you become sexually aroused. Sometimes secreted lubrication gets trapped in the duct, causing a soft, squishy cyst that swells near the vaginal opening.

The cure: Clogged Bartholin ducts are usually benign and don't require treatment. You may be able to unplug the duct simply by sitting in a warm bath for 20 minutes two or three times a day. "If it looks like a pea and goes away on its own, then it was probably temporarily clogged, and I wouldn't worry about it," says Colleen Kennedy, MD, assistant professor of obstetrics and gynecology at the University of Iowa. If the cyst becomes painful or increases in size, see a doctor, who will most likely recommend a procedure called marsupialization. This in-office treatment involves draining the cyst, then sewing the cyst wall to the outer skin to create a new duct. It will heal in about a month.

Lately, even when you're turned on you're not very lubricated.
The cause: Vaginal dryness can result from lots of different things, including but not limited to dehydration, taking certain medications (even over-the-counter antihistamines), nursing, or a thinning of mucosal tissue and changing hormone levels during menopause.
The cure: Personal lubricants. Always have them on hand for getting wet and wild. Choose water-based lubricants;

they are safer if using condoms. Oil-based lubes can damage the integrity of condoms. And avoid colored, scented, and flavored lubricants, which can trigger yeast infections and may ultimately exacerbate dryness.

You think you gave your guy a yeast infection.
The cause: It's uncommon, but it does happen, according to David Weiner, MD, a urologist at St. Luke's-Roosevelt Hospital in New York. A man can develop similar symptoms—redness, itching, or unusual discharge—after having unprotected sex with an infected partner. He's especially at risk if he is taking antibiotics, has diabetes, or has an impaired immune system (all of which can allow yeast to flourish) or if he's uncircumcised. "The foreskin creates a moist environment that is conducive to yeast growth," Weiner says.
The cure: Over-the-counter antifungal medicine can be used to treat the condition, but it's best to hold off on having sex until your symptoms—and his—are completely gone. That way, you won't risk re-infecting each other.

Sex in the missionary position is painful.
The cause: Certain sex positions could be more painful than others if you have a tilted uterus. Some 20 percent of American women have a retroverted uterus, which is when the top of the uterus naturally slants toward the spine or tailbone instead of up toward the belly button.

ARE YOUR MEDS STEALING YOUR SEX DRIVE?

Oh, the irony. You start taking oral contraceptives (OCs) so you can have worry-free sex. Then the magic little pills start sapping your sex drive. Why? OCs contain estrogen, which increases the production of a protein called sex-hormone binding globulin (SHBG), says Michael Krychman, MD, medical director of sexual medicine at Hoag Hospital in Newport Beach, California. SHBG can trap testosterone, affecting your sex drive. Other potential sex-drive-stalling meds: those that reduce blood pressure, anxiety, and acid reflux, and antidepressants. **SEX RX:** Ask your doc about the sexual side effects of all of your drugs. You may also want to try a contraceptive method that doesn't use hormones, such as condoms, a diaphragm, or an IUD.

The Sexual Diagnostic

The cure: Visit your gynecologist for an exam to determine if yours is tilted. A sharply retroverted uterus can make using tampons or a diaphragm difficult because they can dig into the body of the uterus. Sex can be painful for the same reason. "Different positions, such as woman on top, can alleviate the discomfort," says Mary Jane Minkin, MD, an OB-GYN at Yale University School of Medicine. If you're trying to conceive and have a tilted uterus, lying on your tummy after sex may help sperm swim into your cervix.

Your libido has hit the road.
Possible cause: You've hit perimenopause. Prior to menopause, hormonal shifts—specifically decreasing estrogen—lead to physiological changes that can make sex seem about as appealing as running a marathon with a pebble in your sock. Sensitive vaginal tissues become less lubricated, the ensuing dryness leads to pain, and painful sex quickly turns into no sex. Hot flashes don't help either.
The cure: Talk to your physician about the pros and cons of hormone replacement therapy (HRT), which may lessen menopausal symptoms. New research shows an estrogen cream or suppository may ease dryness without the risks of HRT. Lubricants can also help, especially if pain during intercourse is a problem.

There's a burning sensation when I pee after having sex.
Possible cause 1: The friction of thrusting could have irritated the urethra, which is a common thing. Vaginal dryness and prolonged intercourse could contribute.
The cure: Soaking in a warm bath after sex can provide some relief. Using lubricants during sex may prevent this from happening again.
Possible cause 2: An infection in the urinary tract or vagina. If you notice pain only after the urine touches your vulva, it's likely the latter. Pain that persists or gets worse as you continue to empty your bladder is more likely to be a bladder infection.
The cure: Visit your doctor. Typically, antibiotics are prescribed. You can reduce your chances of getting a urinary tract infection by urinating before and after sex.

Often after intercourse, you detect a strong fishy odor and some itching but have no other symptoms.
The cause: It could be bacterial vaginosis, a very common vaginal infection in which the normal balance of bacteria in the vagina is disrupted by an increase in harmful bacteria. Bacterial vaginosis can be triggered by douching or by new or multiple sex partners. Other symptoms include vaginal discharge, itching and a burning sensation. Untreated, BV can lead to significant health problems, including premature delivery, postpartum infections, pelvic inflammatory disease, and increased vulnerability to HIV infection. It's estimated that up to one-third of pregnant women in the United States have BV.

PREVENT STIs

For a chart describing sexually transmitted infections (STIs), prevention, and treatment, see "Better Safe Than STI" on page 95 in Chapter 5/HIS: The Sexual Diagnostic.

The cure: While BV can clear up on its own, treatment with the antibiotics metronidazole or clindamycin is recommended. Women who've had a premature birth or low birth weight baby should be checked for bacterial vaginosis regardless of symptoms.

You lack energy and have trouble getting and staying asleep. And you have little interest in sex.
The cause: You could be suffering from depression. When you're feeling down in the dumps, desire can take a big hit. Women tend to isolate themselves and that can strain even the strongest of romantic relationships.
The cure: Antidepressants may lift the dark cloud, but some affect your ability to have an orgasm. If you notice your sex drive takes a nosedive after you start a new medication, tell your doctor; she may be able to prescribe an alternative. And consider seeing a psychologist for talk therapy. Exercise also helps; it enhances mood and energy, and it boosts blood flow to the genitals.

You're a mom, an employee, a wife and you're too stressed for sex.
The cause: You're a mom, an employee, and a wife. Besides totally tuckering you out, the chronic stresses of modern life can also trigger a cascade of hormonal changes that mess with your body's sexual-response cycle. And here's another modern sex buster that adds to all the craziness: today's always-connected technology.

The cure: With spontaneous sex almost out of the question, you need some serious "life management," experts say. Put a lock on the master bedroom door and set a technology time limit. Shift gears with a soothing bath, suggests Los Angeles–based sex therapist Linda De Villers, PhD. Plunging into warm water takes you away from the laptops and cell phones that clog up your day.

You've just had a baby and you're not interested in sex.
The cause: See "You're a mom, employee, wife," above. Give yourself a break; you're tired. Also, you may not feel happy with the new shape of your body due to pregnancy. Many women find themselves withdrawing or not willing to experiment sexually if they're overweight or shaped differently postpartum. Emotionally, you may have bought into the media's idealization of what is really sexy: that you have to look a certain way in order to have really good sex.
The cure: Bask in the feel-good glow of compliments. Feel free to ask the new dad what he likes about your body; his praises can help you feel more positive. "Women have a talent for disliking the very things about themselves that other people find very attractive," says sex therapist Linda De Villers, PhD. But, also, don't underestimate the mental boost of shedding some pounds. Surveys and studies show that losing weight helps women feel sexy. In fact, even a 5-pound weight loss has been shown to jump-start sex drive.

BUZZ WORTHY

Do you find that you are reaching for your Rabbit more often than your honey bunny? It's fairly common for some women to prefer using their vibrators to having intercourse. A vibrator is simpler and more accessible than a cooperating penis. While there's nothing wrong with incorporating sex toys into your love life, becoming reliant on a vibrator—or even preferring it over your partner—can be a serious problem. If you really are addicted to your vibrator at the expense of your relationship with your partner, talk to a therapist to gain some insight about your relationship. If the vibrator gives you more satisfaction than sex with your partner, talk about trying some new moves or even using the vibrator together.

The Big Book of Sex Birth Control Guide

	THE PILL	EMERGENCY PILL	IUD	RING	
Popular Brand(s)	Ortho Tri-Cyclen; Yaz; Lo/Ovral; Loestrin; TriNessa; Ocella	Plan B One Step; Next Choice; Ella	Mirena; ParaGard	NuvaRing	
Approximate Cost*	$10 to $50 per month	$30 to $60	$200 to $600 (device and insertion)	Up to $50 per month	
How to Use	Oral pills; must be taken daily	Oral pill; taken with in 72 hours after failed contraception; Ella works up to five days after intercourse	Small T-shaped device that is inserted into uterus by professional; monthly self-check for placement; lasts 5 to 10 years	Plastic ring inserted into vagina monthly, remains in place for 3 weeks, then removed for 1 week (during period)	
Effectiveness**	98 percent	87 percent	99 percent	98 percent	
Best For	Temporary, but long-term birth control	Women who need a backup to failed contraception	Women who wish to delay pregnancy by 5 or more years	Women who dislike daily pills	
Not Recommended For	Smokers, women with a history of cardiovascular problems or breast cancer	Women who think they may have been pregnant before the failed contraception, women looking for a routine birth control method; Ella is not recommended for nursing mothers	Women who want short-term protection or who have a history of fibroids	Smokers, women with a history of cardiovascular problems or breast cancer	
Risks	Increased risk of blood clots and stroke, risk of heart attack if you have a history	May increase blood sugar levels in women with diabetes	Infection, expulsion; ParaGard: increase in menstrual flow; Mirena: blood clots and stroke	Increased risk of blood clots and stroke, risk of heart attack if you have a history	
Potential Side Effects***	Weight gain, bloating, breast tenderness, spotting	Changes in your period, nausea, lower abdominal pain, fatigue, headache, dizziness, breast tenderness	Cramping after insertion, weight gain, bloating, breast tenderness, spotting	Vaginal infections, irritation, and secretions, headache, weight gain, bloating, breast tenderness, spotting	
Prescription Needed?	Yes	No for Plan B One Step or Next Choice; Yes for Ella	Yes	Yes	
When Are You Protected	Immediately if started on the first day of your period, otherwise backup is needed for one week	After taking, within allotted 72-hour window for Plan B One Step and Next Choice; after taking and within allotted five-day window for Ella	ParaGard: immediately; Mirena: immediately if injected during first 7 days after start of period, otherwise backup needed for 1 week	Immediately if inserted on first day of period, otherwise backup needed for 1 week	
Active Ingredients	Estrogen and different progestins—some pills contain only progestin	Progestin (levonorgestrel) for Plan B One Step and Next Choice; Ulipristal acetate (a progesterone agonist/antagonist) for Ella	Mirena: progestin (levonorgestrel); ParaGard: copper coil	Estrogen and progestin (etonogestrel)	

SHOT	PATCH	IMPLANT	SPONGE	DIAPHRAGM
Depo-Provera	Ortho Evra	Implanon	Today Sponge	Ortho All-Flex; Milex Wide Seal
$35 to $75, plus exam fees	$15 to $50 per month	$400 to $800 (device and insertion)	$9 to $15 for three	$15 to $50 plus cost for office visit (fitting required by professional); $7 to $18 for spermicide
Injection administered by a professional into upper arm or butt; lasts up to 4 months	Bandage-like patch applied to skin every 7 days, then removed; each month has 3 weeks of patches, then a week without (for period)	Matchstick-sized rod implanted under inner-arm skin by professional; lasts up to 3 years	Foam disk inserted up to 24 hours before sex; can be left in up to 30 hours total; no doctor fitting required	Reusable latex or silicone disk inserted into vagina with spermicide before sex; lasts up to 2 years
99 percent	98 percent	99 percent	84 to 91 percent for those who have not previously given birth; 68 to 80 percent for those who have	92 to 96 percent
Women who cannot take estrogen or are breastfeeding	Women who prefer topical medications or dislike daily pills	Women who cannot take estrogen or are breast-feeding	Women who dislike daily pills or can't take hormones	Women who dislike daily pills or can't take hormones
Women who want short-term protection	Smokers, women with a history of cardiovascular problems or breast cancer	Women who want short-term protection	Women who have had a recent childbirth, abortion or miscarriage, or have a history of toxic shock syndrome; those allergic to spermicides	Women allergic to spermicides, women on their periods
Delay in pregnancy after discontinuing, calcium loss from bones, increased risk of blood clots and stroke, risk of heart attack if you have a history	Increased risk of blood clots and stroke, risk of heart attack if you have a history	Increased risk of blood clots and stroke, risk of heart attack if you have a history, shift of implant in arm	Toxic shock syndrome	More frequent urinary tract infections, increased risk for toxic shock syndrome, may be dislodged by the male partner in certain sexual positions
Weight gain, irregular periods, breast tenderness, bloating, nervousness, depression, slowed hair growth	Irritation at the application site, weight gain, bloating, breast tenderness, spotting	Irregular bleeding (may stop completely), irritation at the application site, weight gain, bloating, breast tenderness, spotting	Allergy to spermicide; vaginal irritation, may cause sex to be messy or too dry	Allergy to diaphragm material or spermicide
Yes	Yes	Yes	No	No (however, fitting required by doctor)
Immediately if injected within first 7 days of period, otherwise backup needed for 1 week	Immediately if applied during the first 24 hours after start of period, otherwise use backup for 1 week	Immediately if inserted during the first 5 days of period, otherwise use backup for 1 week	Immediately and for the next 30 hours—must stay in place at least 6 hours after sex	Immediately after insertion; more spermicide may need to be reapplied—must stay in place at least 6 hours after sex
Progestin (medroxyproges-terone acetate)	Estrogen and progestin (norelgestromin)	Progestin (etonogestrel)	Spermicide and protective plastic foam barrier	Spermicide and protective latex or silicone barrier

The Big Book of Sex Birth Control Guide (continued)

	CONDOM	FEMALE STERILIZATION	FEMALE STERILIZATION	VASECTOMY
Popular Brand(s)	Durex; Trojan; Lifestyles; etc.	Adiana	Essure	N/A
Approximate Cost*	$2 to $6 for three	Check with your healthcare provider	Check with your healthcare provider	$350 to $1,000
How to Use	Latex or lambskin sheath applied to penis every time before sex; one time use only	Professional inserts silicone device into fallopian tubes causing scar tissue to form and block sperm from reaching egg	Professional threads small metal and fiber coils into fallopian tubes; system blocks tubes and causes scar tissue to form around coils, blocking sperm	In an out-patient procedure, doctor cuts and seals tubes that carry sperm into semen
Effectiveness**	98 percent	98 percent	99 percent	99 percent
Best For	Men; women who have multiple partners or cannot take hormones	Women who want permanent sterilization but prefer minimally invasive treatment when compared to the invasive surgery of tubal ligation; procedure cannot be reversed	Women who do not want to become pregnant and cannot or do not wish to use other forms of birth control; procedure is permanent	Men who don't want to father a child
Not Recommended For	N/A	For those women who may want to become pregnant someday, have already had a tubal ligation, are taking immunosuppressive drugs, have certain conditions involving the uterus or fallopian tubes, have had pelvic infections	Women who might want to become pregnant, have recently given birth or had an abortion, previously had a tubal ligation, are sensitive to nickel, or have had pelvic infections	Men who may want to someday become a father; should be considered permanent, although it can be reversed
Risks	None	Small risk of pregnancy; incorrect placement, infection	Perforation of uterus or fallopian tubes, pelvic pain, infection	Those associated with major abdominal surgery such as damage to bowel, bladder, or blood vessels; wound infection; reaction to anesthesia; abdominal pain
Potential Side Effects***	Irritation if allergic to latex (use lambskin instead)	Cramping, pelvic or back pain, nausea, headache, bleeding, spotting	Cramping, abdominal pain, nausea, dizziness, bleeding, spotting	Swelling, bruising of the scrotum, bleeding or blood clot in scrotum, blood in semen, infection of surgery site
Prescription Needed?	No	Yes	Yes	Yes; procedure typically done in doctor's office
When Are You Protected	Immediately	Backup contraception must be used for 3 months and then x-ray or ultrasound is used to verify that fallopian tubes are blocked	Must use backup contraception for 3 months following procedure, and then x-ray or ultrasound is taken to confirm successful blockage	Doesn't provide immediate protection; Backup contraception must be used for at least three months and until doctor confirms there are no sperm in the semen through two samples examined weeks apart
Active Ingredients	Protective latex or lambskin barrier and sometimes spermicide	Silicon implant	Metal and fiber coils that cause scar tissue blockage	N/A

TUBAL LIGATION	RHYTHM METHOD	WITHDRAWAL	ABSTINENCE
N/A	N/A	N/A	N/A
$1,000 to $2,500	None	None	None
Professional cuts or blocks fallopian tubes to permanently prevent pregnancy	After several months of charting to establish reliable patterns, sex is permitted only on "safe" days, when woman is not ovulating	Man attempts to withdraw from intercourse before ejaculation	Man and woman abstain from sexual intercourse but may decide to engage in non-insertive sexual play (petting, dry-humping, masturbation, oral sex)
98 percent	14 to 47 percent	Risky; 4 to 19 percent	100 percent when observed completely
Women who want permanent, surgical sterility	Women who cannot use hormonal methods and couples who do not wish to use any unnatural form of birth control	When safer methods are not available or possible	Those who want to avoid risk of pregnancy
Women who might want to become pregnant, are obese, have cardiac or pulmonary disease, blood clots, internal abdominal scarring, preexisting gynecologic conditions	Those not willing to invest the time to learn and do the required record keeping or uninterested in accepting periodic abstinence	Anyone seeking to avoid pregnancy	N/A
Those associated with major abdominal surgery such as damage to bowel, bladder or blood vessels; wound infection; reaction to anesthesia; pain	Can have a high failure rate if not accurate and consistent	High risk of failure and unwanted pregnancy; requires great self-control and may result in reduced pleasure; pre-ejaculate fluid may contain sperm	Sexually-transmitted diseases are still possible
Abdominal pain or cramping, fatigue, dizziness, bloating, shoulder pain, sore throat	N/A	N/A	N/A
Yes; general anesthesia surgery	No, but professional help is useful in estimating "safe" times	No	No
Immediately, but must avoid sex for one week to allow healing	N/A	N/A	Immediately; conception is not possible during complete abstinence
N/A	N/A	N/A	Willpower; mutual conviction

*   depending on insurance coverage

** when used correctly

*** doesn't include all side effects, just the most common ones

(Consult your doctor for additional information that can help you make the safest birth control choice.)

Chapter 6
Lovin' Spoonfuls: The Better Sex Diet

HOW TO EAT TO LOOK YOUR BEST
AND FEEL INCREDIBLE

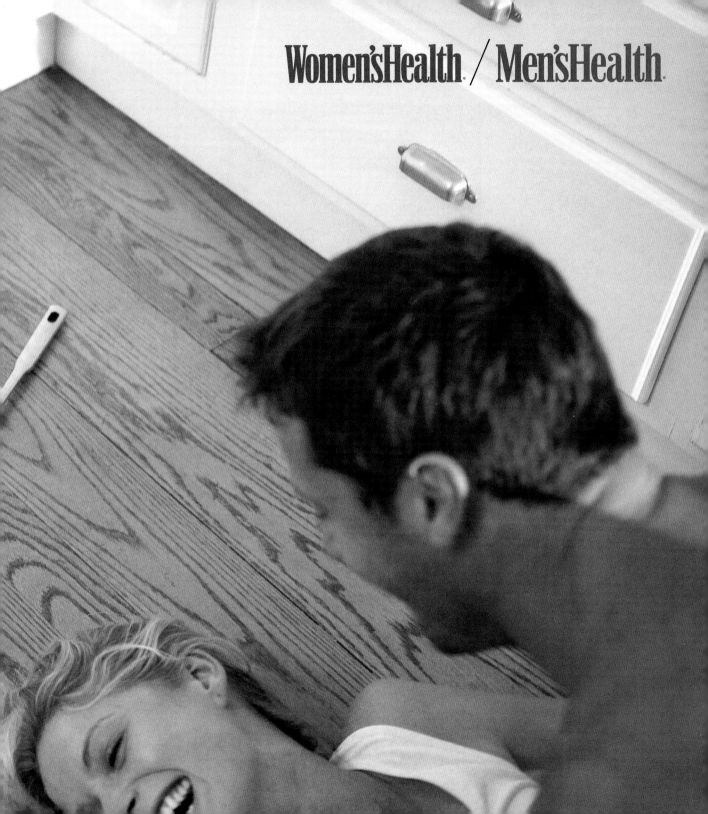

Women'sHealth / Men'sHealth

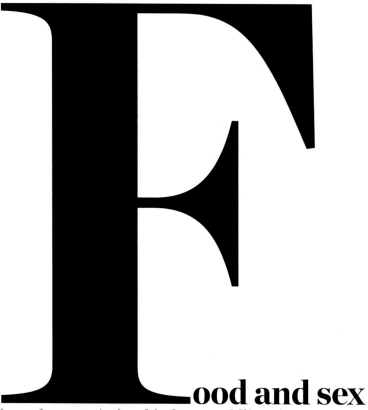

Food and sex

have been entwined in lore and literature ever since Eve ate the apple. Or was the Forbidden Fruit a pomegranate, grape, or fig, as some Renaissance masters have depicted in their artwork?

From the ancient Greeks to the Chinese and the Aztecs to, well, you, the two appetites have been closely connected. Hippocrates prescribed honey to fuel the libido. Montezuma supposedly drank 50 cups of cacahuati, a bitter chocolate drink, before making love to women. In 1749 Henry Fielding fed lobster, oysters, and beef to his lovers in a highly sensual (for the time) chapter in *Tom Jones*. Casanova ate oysters daily to keep

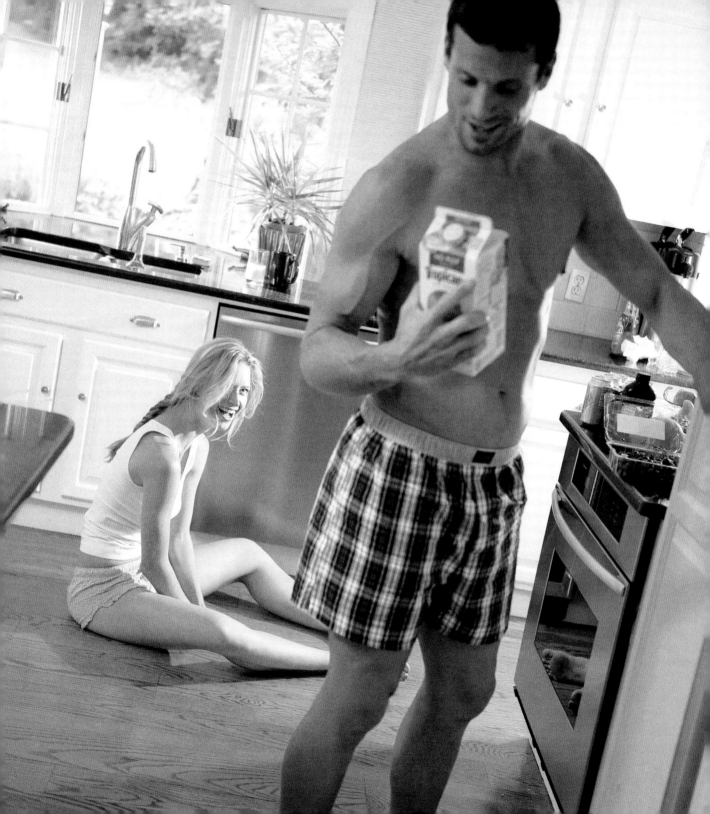

the ladies satisfied. Mickey Rourke fed maraschino cherries to Kim Bassinger in that famous scene from the film *9½ Weeks*. And how can you forget the orgasmic dinner scene in *Like Water for Chocolate*? Tita prepares roast quail in rose petal sauce to seduce Pedro, but the whole dinner table becomes turned on by the sensual meal, especially sister Gertrudis. That isn't a napkin on her lap she's reaching for! She escapes to the privacy of a shower stall, which bursts into flame, and then runs naked through the agave until she's picked up by a Mexican revolutionary on horseback. And they live happily ever after.

If food could only do that perhaps there would be no more wars, no more loneliness, and we'd be having sex instead of watching *What Would Brian Boitano Make?* on the Food Network.

Alas, the notion of food as aphrodisiac is short on science. Triggering an instant hunger for sex by eating, say, a banana or an oyster just isn't going to happen.

But ... go ahead and eat those sexy foods. It is well documented that delicious food and sex activate the exact same pleasure and reward receptors in the brain. Functional MRI studies (analyzing brains scans taken when people do stuff) show that when humans eat a decadent meal, their neocortex lights up with fireworks just as it does when they are having an orgasm.

While food as aphrodisiac may be speculative, it is clear that some foods are very good for your genitals, encouraging blood flow to the region and triggering feel-good hormones that fan the flames of passion. And some foods—fried Twinkies, for example—are just very bad for your genitals, especially if you want to keep them in excellent working order for sex.

Too much of a good-tasting-but-artery-clogging thing can be a bummer in bed. All the side effects of being overweight or obese—high blood pressure, elevated LDL (bad) cholesterol, and atherosclerosis, the accumulation of plaque that restricts blood flow through arteries—are linked to sexual health problems.

Atherosclerosis, in particular, damages the endothelium layer that lines the arteries. When that happens, the arteries' ability to produce nitric oxide production declines, and nitric oxide is crucial to erections. "The penis is the thermometer for a man's overall health," says Ridwan Shabsigh, MD, director of the division of urology at Maimonides Medical Center. "The penile artery is half the size of coronary arteries, so plaque build up there will show up symptomatically before it does in other major arteries.

Impaired blood flow is not just a man's problem. "Many of the same health issues that cause erectile dysfunction in men, such as diabetes, high blood pressure, and high cholesterol, as well as many medications used to treat these conditions can cause sexual dysfunction in women," says sexual health expert Jennifer R. Berman, MD, director of The Berman Women's Wellness Center in Los Angeles.

How to Eat for Better Sex

Sexologists, cardiologists, and psychologists agree: how much you consume has a huge impact on your sexual health. Exactly what you eat is critically important, too.

"Essentially, what's good for your heart is good for better sex," declares Steven Lamm, MD, a faculty member at New York School of Medicine, and author of *The Hardness Factor: How to Achieve Your Best Health and Sexual Fitness at Any Age.*

And what exactly are those sexy eats? We're glad you asked. On the following pages, you'll find your menu of SUPER SEX FOODS to prepare your body and brain for the bedroom. Building more of these SUPER SEX FOODS into your daily diet is one of the easiest (and tastiest) ways to improve your health for optimal sex. If trimming down is one of your goals, then we suggest you also adopt the six principles of losing weight found in the Slim and Sexy Weight-Loss Plan on page 106. This combo meal of nutritional advice will help you achieve a fitter body quickly and easily so get down to doing something much more fun, like . . . cooking.

S.U.P.E.R. S.E.X. F.O.O.D.S.

S pinach and other green vegetables
U nsweeted tea
P eaches and other fruit
E ggs
R ed wine and meat

S eeds and nuts
EX tra protein

F atty fish
O atmeal and other whole grains
O ysters and other shellfish
D ark chocolate
S trawberries and other berries

Spinach
and Other Green Vegetables

Spinach is a potent source of magnesium, which helps dilate blood vessels, according to Japanese researchers. Better blood flow to the genitals, as you've learned, creates greater arousal for men and women. Spinach and other green vegetables like broccoli, Brussels

WITH THIS ONION RING, I THEE WED

An unhappy marriage may be as bad for your health as a fast-food diet. Investigators found that women in rocky relationships were up to 40 percent more likely than happily married women to have metabolic syndrome, a cluster of health issues that can lead to diabetes and heart disease. Chronic stress stimulates the release of the hormone cortisol, which causes the body to store fat in the belly.

SUPER SEX

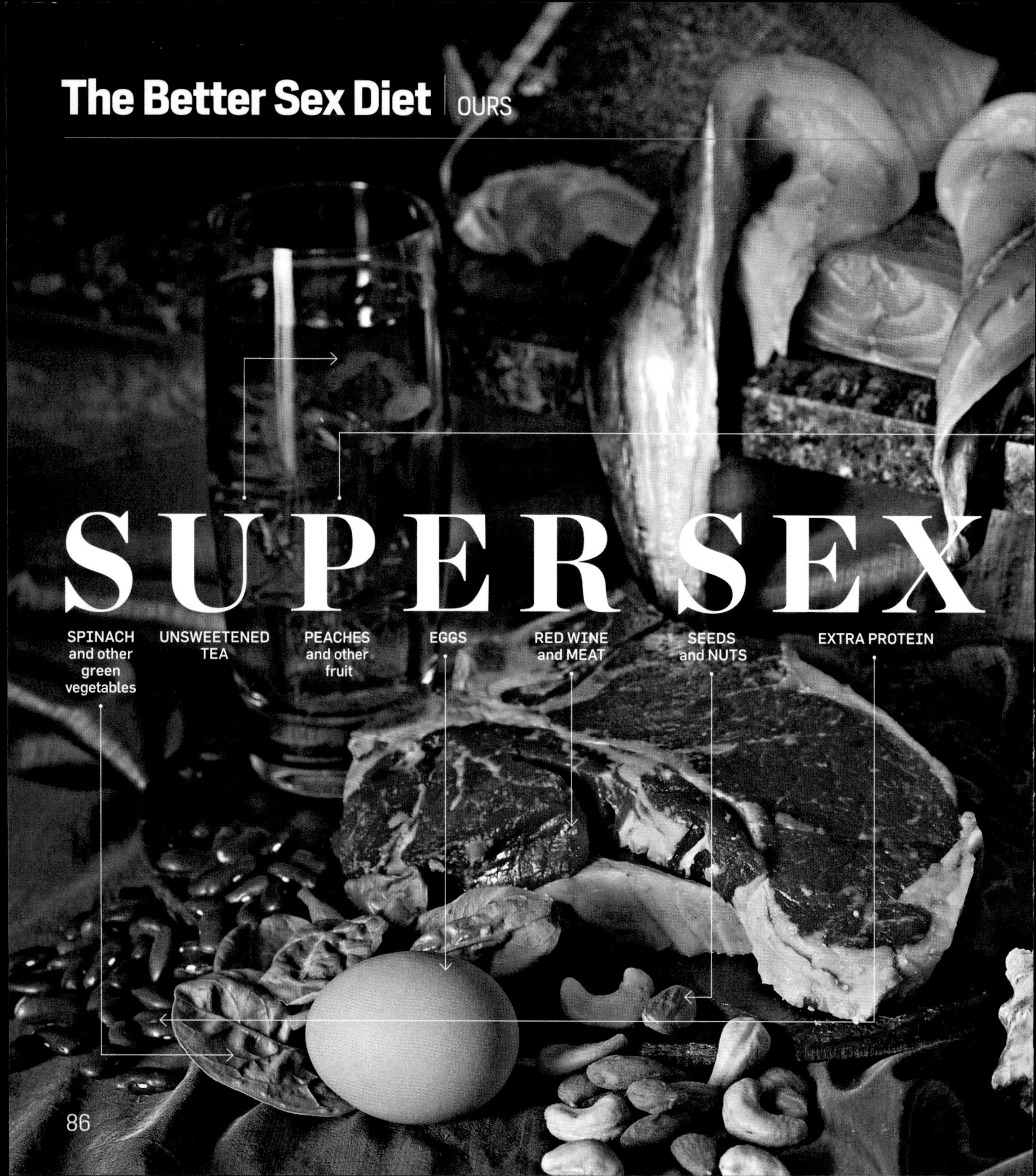

SPINACH
and other
green
vegetables

UNSWEETENED
TEA

PEACHES
and other
fruit

EGGS

RED WINE
and MEAT

SEEDS
and NUTS

EXTRA PROTEIN

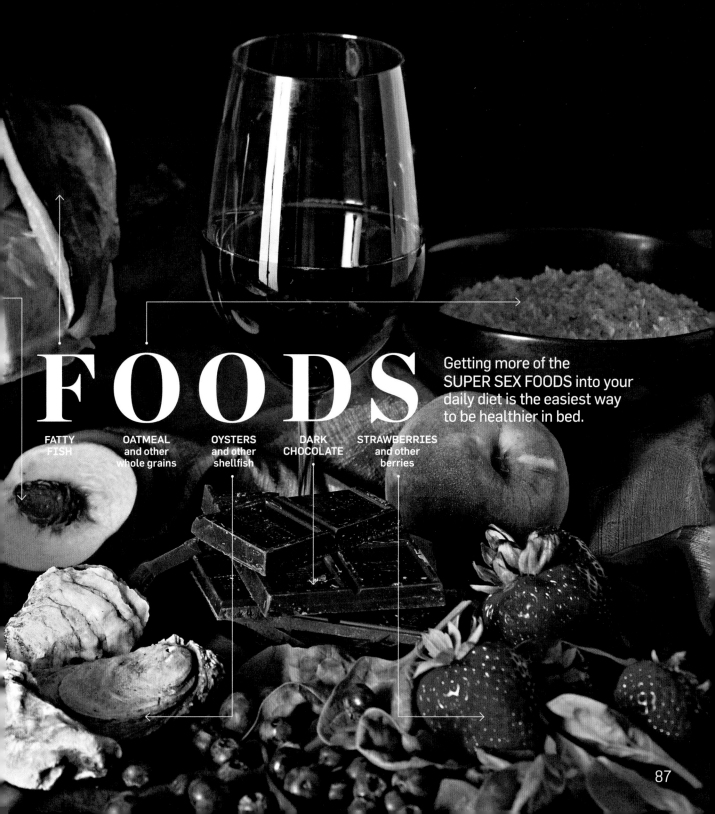

FOODS

Getting more of the SUPER SEX FOODS into your daily diet is the easiest way to be healthier in bed.

FATTY FISH

OATMEAL and other whole grains

OYSTERS and other shellfish

DARK CHOCOLATE

STRAWBERRIES and other berries

87

sprouts, kale, cabbage, Swiss chard, and bok choy are also good sources of our favorite sex nutrient—folate. Extra insurance for good reproductive health, folate may lower blood levels of a harmful substance called homocysteine. This abrasive amino acid irritates the lining of arteries and encourages plaque to adhere to it. A high level of homocysteine is a significant risk factor for peripheral arterial disease (PAD). But it appears that dietary folate is protective. In a study of 46,000 men, Harvard University researchers found that those who consumed the most folate daily were 30 percent less likely to develop PAD than men who ate the fewest folate-rich foods.

Unsweetened Tea

The antioxidant catechin found in tea promotes blood flow all over the body for sex power and brainpower; it enhances memory, mood, and focus. One particularly potent catechin, a compound called ECGC prevalent in green tea, is thought to increase fat burn. A study in the *Journal of Nutrition* found that people who consumed the equivalent of three to five cups of green tea a day for 12 weeks experienced nearly a 5 percent reduction in bodyweight. Drink freshly brewed green or black tea every day— hot or iced. Bottled teas don't offer the same benefits. And keep the sugar out of it. Unsweetened tea is an excellent alternative to high-calorie, sugar-laden soft drinks and juices. One 12-ounce

can of soda has about 10 teaspoons of sugar in it. America is drinking itself into obesity! The high-fructose corn syrup in many soft drinks raises insulin levels, which can over time develop into diabetes. Studies also show that getting too much sugar lowers the body's ability to produce endorphins. Low endorphins can lead to depression, and know that depression sucks the life out of our sex drive.

Peaches
and Other Fruits

One study shows that vitamin C may increase libido in women. Another finds that people who eat foods high in vitamin C report better moods and have more sex. We'll take that as another good reason to eat more vitamin C-rich fruits and vegetables. But there are many other sex and heart-healthy reasons to get enough of this antioxidant. It helps boost blood flow, meaning that both sexes can get friskier, faster.

And, gentlemen, if you are looking to add some deductions to your 1040 form, eat more grapefruit, oranges, and peaches. Men who consume at least 200 milligrams of vitamin C a day improve their sperm counts and motility, according to research at the University of Texas Medical Branch. In the study, 75 men ages 20 to 35 (all heavy smokers with poor sperm quality) were divided into three groups: two that took 200 and 1,000 mg of vitamin C, respectively, and a group that took a

1

Percentage your risk of stroke increases for each fast-food restaurant that's in your neighborhood.

dummy pill. The daily vitamin C takers significantly improved the quality of their sperm, with the 1,000 mg group showing the greatest boost in sperm counts. In a later study, 30 infertile men were able to impregnate their partners after just 60 days of vitamin C supplementation. In some men, fertility was restored in just 4 days.

Vitamin C also keeps sperm from clumping, so they have a better chance of reaching their destination, says Marc Goldstein, MD, director of the Cornell Center for Male Reproductive Medicine and Microsurgery. Grapefruit contains 120 percent of the recommended daily allowance of 90 milligrams of vitamin C for men. Other excellent sources are watermelon, kiwi, mango, oranges, cantaloupe, strawberries, broccoli, tomatoes, leafy greens, and ascorbic acid supplements.

When in the produce aisle, also pick up some watermelon too. They are filled with high concentrations of the good-for-your-heart, good-for-sex phytonutrients lycopene, beta carotene, and, the big one, citrulline. Citrulline is particularly exciting for its ability to relax blood vessels, according to studies at Texas A&M University. When you eat watermelon, the citrulline is converted to the helpful amino acid arginine. "Arginine boosts nitric oxide, which relaxes blood vessels, the same basic effect that Viagra has, to treat erectile dysfunction and maybe even prevent it," explains Bhimu Patil, PhD, director the Texas A&M's Vegetable

and Fruit Improvement Center. Patil says the citrulline-arginine relationship may be especially beneficial to people who suffer from obesity and type 2 diabetes because it may boost their circulatory and immune systems. You've known how to eat a watermelon since you were three, but there are other ways to enjoy summer's sweet treat besides slurping and spitting seeds. Make a watermelon shake: Dump 1 cup of seedless watermelon chunks in a blender, add 6 ounces of plain Greek yogurt, 1 teaspoon of either honey or agave sweetener, and 6 ice cubes. Blend well. Makes one serving.

Eggs

Over easy, hard-boiled, or scrambled, eggs aren't the most sensual food on the menu, but it's hard to beat them for a fit and healthy body inside and out. Their nutrients, including folate, iron, phosphorus, and selenium, are heart healthy and also known to maintain the health of epithelial tissues, which line the vagina and uterus in women. Eggs are rich in vitamins B_6 and B_5, which help balance hormone levels and ease stress, and are important for a healthy libido. Calorie for calorie, eggs deliver more biologically usable protein (if you eat the yolks) than any other food, including beef. Eggs are an excellent part of a weight-loss strategy thanks to their protein and B_{12}, a vitamin that studies have shown is necessary for breaking down fat. One study in the *International Journal of Obesity* found

LOVE STINKS

The more garlic you eat, the less likely you are to have heart disease and compromised blood flow to your genitals. (Tip: eating parsley will help neutralize the garlic odor.)

that when overweight people ate two eggs or a bagel for breakfast 5 days a week for 8 weeks, those who ate the eggs lost 65 percent more weight (and lost it faster) than the bagel eaters.

Red Wine
and Meat

Sounds like the makings of a good time to us! Italian researchers recently found that women who drink red wine in moderation enjoy higher levels of sexual interest and respond with more lubrication than women who don't drink or drink less. The researchers believe that the antioxidants and alcohol in the wine may trigger the production of nitric oxide in the blood, which helps artery walls to relax, increasing blood flow to the genitals. Just limit yourselves to a glass or two. More alcohol than that can put a damper on sexual performance and lead to bed spins of a not-very-sexy nature. Worth noting: even teetotalers can benefit from the red grape. Dark grape juice contains antioxidant polyphenols that protect the cardiovascular system and help keep skin flexible and elastic.

That brings us to the meat of this entry. Red meat. Lean cuts are great sources of zinc, a mineral that curbs production of a hormone called prolactin, which at high levels can cause sexual dysfunction, according to Berman. Zinc is also a key muscle-building nutrient, and the high concentrations of conjugated linoleic acids (CLA) in beef, studies show,

may spur weight loss. Choose filet mignon or other deep red cuts with round or loin in the name, because they are the leanest.

Seeds and Nuts

Pumpkin and sunflower seeds, almonds, peanuts, walnuts, and other nuts all contain the necessary monounsaturated fats with which your body creates cholesterol—and your sex hormones need that cholesterol to work properly. That's something the ancient Romans didn't know when they tossed walnuts at newlyweds for good breeding luck. Long linked to fertility—the shell, of course, resembles a man's cojones; the inside meat is vulvalike in form—nuts make a perfectly sexy snack. Packed with muscle-building protein and filling fiber, they are a heart-healthy, albeit calorie-dense, treat.

Pistachios contain plant cholesterol that can produce a 10-point drop in your triglycerides and a 16-point decline in your LDL (bad) cholesterol, reports the *Journal of the American College of Nutrition*. Brazil nuts are the richest source of selenium—a mineral that has been linked to preventing cancers of the prostate and colon—you can eat. Pecans deliver the most antioxidants of any nut. Adding them to your diet may reduce your risk of cancer, heart disease, and Alzheimer's disease. Walnuts, almonds, and other nuts also reduce levels of LDL cholesterol, and a compound called lipoprotein(a) that increases clotting

THE SUGAR SOLUTION

Black tea reduces the glycemic index of a meal, according to a study in the *Journal of the American College of Nutrition*. How? An active compound in tea triggers a greater secretion of insulin, a hormone that lowers blood sugar.

and can lead to a stroke, according to a study published in *Annals of Internal Medicine*. (Are you getting the point yet why we're nuts for nuts?) Sunflower seeds pack the highest natural vitamin E content of any food. "No antioxidant is more effective at fighting the aging effects of free radicals," says Barry Swanson, PhD, a professor of food science at Washington State University.

Extra Protein

There just aren't many sexy foods that begin with the letter X. But the benefits of adding more protein to your diet outweigh this small editorial reach. Protein is so important to weight maintenance that you should eat it with every meal and snack. Proteins boost metabolism a little more during digestion than any other type of food. Plus protein increases metabolism by helping to build muscle and stall the muscle loss that naturally happens as we age. Muscle is more metabolically active than fat is, so the more lean muscle on your body the better at burning calories it will be. Plus, well-toned abs and thighs are nice to look at when unadorned by clothing. So, how do you eat more protein without going overboard on eggs and meat? Beans— they're good for the heart and your glutes. Kidneys, garbanzos, black beans, and navy beans are full of muscle-building protein. While they may not be the best choice for a side dish if you plan on sex for dessert,

building your meal plan around a foundation of beans and legumes will ultimately pay off for you sexually. Many studies show that bean eaters are leaner and healthier than people who don't eat beans. According to one study in the *Journal of the American College of Nutrition,* people who eat ¾ cup beans or legumes a day have lower blood pressure and smaller waists than people who get their protein from meat. Beans are also full of cholesterol-lowering soluble fiber. A quarter cup of red kidney beans delivers 3 grams of fiber, plus more than 6,000 disease-fighting antioxidants. Navy beans are particularly rich in potassium, which regulates blood pressure and heart contractions, something you'll need as your heart starts racing when he does that special move that makes you melt.

Fatty Fish

If, as doctors like to say, what's good for your heart is good for your love life, oily coldwater fish like salmon, mackerel, sardines, and tuna should figure heavily into your weekly meal rotation. The omega-3 fatty acids DHA and EPA found in fish help to raise dopamine levels in the brain that trigger arousal, according to Yvonne K. Fulbright, PhD, a sexologist and *Women's Health* columnist. Other health benefits: anti-inflammatory properties that fight blood clots and heart arrhythmias, better brain function, and protection against dementia. Studies

20

Percentage of women who eat right before they go to bed.

show that omega-3s can also reduce symptoms of depression. Research from the University of Pittsburgh showed that people with high omega-3 blood levels were happier and more agreeable. Tell us that can't help you get more sex! Fish is one of the many healthy foods that contain the amino acid L-arginine, which stimulates the release of growth hormone among other substances and is converted into nitric oxide in the body. It's worth repeating: nitric oxide is critical for erections and it can help women's sexual function as well by causing blood vessels to open wider for improved blood flow.

Oatmeal
and Other Whole Grains

Eating oatmeal is one of the few natural ways to boost testosterone in the bloodstream. The male hormone plays a significant role in sex drive and orgasm strength in both men and women. Oats (as well as seeds, ginseng, nuts, dairy, and green vegetables) contain L-arginine, an amino acid that enhances the effect nitric oxide has on reducing blood vessel stiffness. L-arginine has been used to treat erectile dysfunction. Like Viagra, it helps relax muscles around blood vessels in the penis. When they dilate, blood flow increases so a man can maintain an erection. Studies show that L-arginine also improves blood flow to the clitoris and tissue surrounding the vulva. Oatmeal and other whole grains like whole-grain bread, brown rice, and barley also qualify as good-for-the-heart, better-for-the-gut foods. They are slow-burning, complex carbohydrates that won't drive your blood sugar through the roof. They keep you feeling fuller longer and provide excellent energy. Try a bowl of steel-cut oatmeal with fresh berries and bananas with a drizzle of honey before your next marathon sex session. These kinds of carbs are also ideal for fueling your brain. And as we all know, sex begins in your gray matter. If your prefrontal cortex (central station for decision making and personality expression) is running on empty, you're not going to get very far in your excursion to the bedroom. The brain needs a constant supply of glucose for you to be sharp enough to woo her or him. Whole grains will provide an even flow of that brain energy, and their B vitamins also nourish the nervous system. University of Toronto researchers recently determined that eating carbohydrate-rich foods like whole-grain bread is equivalent to a shot of glucose injected into your brain. According to the study, the higher the concentration of glucose in your blood, the better your memory and concentration—so you can remember and rock that Kama Sutra position you read about.

One of the best whole grains you can eat is quinoa (pronounced *keen-wah*), and it's becoming hugely popular so you're starting to see it front and center in grocery stores. This nutty-tasting grain is a good substitute for rice or pasta. It has fewer carbohydrates than regular cereal grains and, even better, it contains all the essential amino acids of a "complete" protein like eggs.

Oysters
and Other Shellfish

In addition to their reputation as the ultimate aphrodisiac (thanks to their resemblance to female genitalia), raw oysters actually do have a connection to sexual function. Oysters hold more zinc than most any other food, and it is believed that this mineral may enhance libido by helping with testosterone production—higher levels of the hormone are linked to an increase in desire. Zinc is also crucial to healthy sperm production and blood circulation. While Casanova reportedly ate 50 raw oysters a day, about six will provide double the recommended daily allowance of 15 mg of zinc. To spice things up a bit, try a few dashes of hot sauce on your raw oysters. Other good sources of zinc are shrimp, red meat, pumpkin seeds, poultry and pork, eggs, and dairy products.

Dark Chocolate

Devouring something gooey and decadent is incredibly sensual. Dark chocolate, in particular, contains a compound called phenylethylamine that releases the same endorphins triggered by sex, and increases the feelings of attraction between two

people, according to research published in the *Journal of the American Dietetic Association*. In fact, brain scans in a British study showed that eating chocolate causes a more intense and longer brainbuzz than kissing does. In this study researchers monitored the brains and heart rates of couples while they kissed passionately or ate chocolate. The brains of both men and women showed greater stimulation while the chocolate melted on their tongues than when their tongues were tied in a passionate kiss.

Chocolate does appear to boost heart health. Scientists at the Harvard University School of Public Health examined 136 studies on cocoa and found heart-health benefits from increased blood flow, less platelet stickiness, and reduced bad cholesterol.

What's the "healthiest" chocolate? The disease-fighting flavonols that make dark chocolate good for the body also cause the bitterness. To balance flavor and health benefits, try dark chocolate with 70 percent cacao, recommends Jeffrey Blumberg, PhD, who directs the Antioxidants Research Laboratory at Tufts University. A 2-inch square chunk, at about 100 calories, will deliver a healthy treat without messing with your weight-management efforts.

Strawberries
and Other Berries

Red is sexy. Red roses, sports cars, slinky red dresses. Strawberries.

9
Percentage of Americans who eat the daily recommended five to seven servings of fruits and vegetables.

The Better Sex Diet | OURS

OURS

BEST BEDTIME SNACK (IF YOU WANT TO SLEEP)

A small bowl of bran cereal with fat-free milk or a fiber-filled piece of fruit, like a pear. Both snacks contain enough carbohydrates to soothe you into slumber but not enough to make you toss and turn.

Researchers at the University of Rochester conducted experiments on undergraduate students to see if there was any real connection between the color and sex. In one, male and female students viewed images of women on red or white backgrounds. The men found a woman's image on red more attractive than on white, while the female students did not. In another test, men were asked to rate attractiveness of pictures of women on red, white, gray, green, or blue backgrounds. As expected, the men scored the women on red as more sexually attractive. They also said they would spend more money on the women in red than on those in the other colors. Strawberries can be considered sexy for another reason besides their sensual color: they are high in the B vitamin folate that helps prevent birth defects, and vitamin C, a potential libido booster. Strawberries dipped in melted dark chocolate anyone? Or how about the classic strawberries and whipped cream? Blueberries (and blackberries) are just as sexy. Ideal for a great morning-after breakfast in bed, so you have energy for round 2, both berries contain compounds that are thought to relax blood vessels and improve circulation for a natural Viagra-like effect. Plus, they are tremendous workhorses for pushing excess cholesterol through your digestive system before it can be broken down, absorbed, and deposited along the walls of your arteries.

More Lovin' Spoonfuls

Man and woman cannot fornicate on spinach and strawberries alone. Fortunately, they don't have to. There are dozens of delicious foods that will help you burn fat, protect your heart, and achieve rock-hard abs—and other hard things, too.

Avocado

The ancient Aztecs called them testicles. Hanging in pairs from trees, the fruit is so suggestive that Catholic priests in Spain once forbade parishioners from eating them. But beyond their shape, avocados have a strong connection to the testes, the production center of sperm, due to their high folate content. Men planning to have children should consider loading up on avocado (as well as leafy greens) because folate may protect sperm from mutations. A study at the Lawrence Berkeley National Laboratory in a 2008 issue of the journal *Human Reproduction* analyzed the sperm of 89 men for chromosome abnormalities, and then compared the results to a food frequency questionnaire the men completed. The researchers found that men with the highest folate intake had the lowest frequency of sperm with

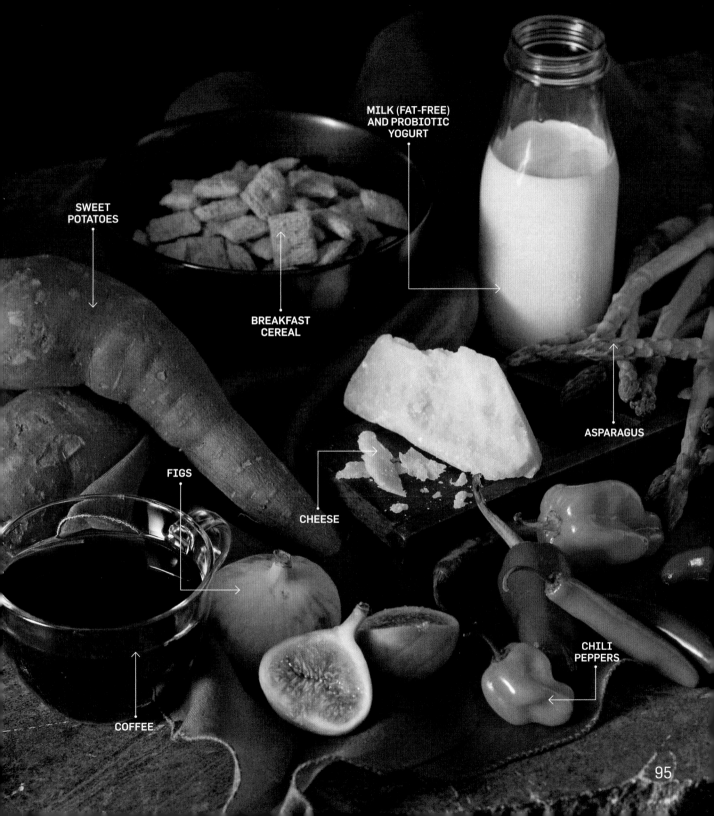

SWEET POTATOES

MILK (FAT-FREE) AND PROBIOTIC YOGURT

BREAKFAST CEREAL

ASPARAGUS

FIGS

CHEESE

COFFEE

CHILI PEPPERS

95

extra chromosomes compared with men who had lower consumption.

Asparagus

This phallic vegetable has been associated with sex since the first hunter-gatherer spotted shoots popping out of the forest floor and cried, "Hey, you know what those remind me of?" It's hard to argue. The springtime shoots are loaded with B vitamins that increase levels of histamine, a neurotransmitter that facilitates orgasm. Green asparagus spears are rich in rutin, a potent scavenger of free radicals. The crowns also have high levels of the chemical protodioscin that may improve sexual function. "Protodioscin has been shown to boost arousal and even help combat erectile dysfunction in some men," says Lynn Edlen-Nezin, PhD, coauthor of *Great Food, Great Sex*.

Bananas

If you suffer from a bit of sexual anxiety, eat a banana before you hook up. Bananas deliver the feel-good neurochemical serotonin into the blood stream, which elevates mood and calms the nervous system. "Bananas contain potassium, a mineral that increases muscle strength, an element crucial to orgasm," says Lou Paget, author of *The Great Lover Playbook*.

Breakfast Cereal

Fortified breakfast cereals and breads contain niacin, a vitamin that's essential for the secretion of histamine, a chemical our bodies need in order to trigger explosive sneezes—and orgasms. They are high in thiamin and riboflavin, too, vitamins that help you use energy efficiently and that are important to proper nerve function, which translates into more stimulation and pleasure during sex.

Celery

Every stalk of this Bloody Mary swizzle stick is packed with androstenone and androstenol, two pheromones that can help men attract women. "When you chew a stalk of celery, you release androstenone and androstenol odor molecules into your mouth. They then travel up the back of your throat to your nose," says Alan Hirsch, MD, author of *Scentsational Sex: The Secret to Using Aroma for Arousal*. "Once there, the pheromones boost your arousal, turning you on and causing your body to send off scents and signals that make you more desirable to women." This crunchy natural breath freshener can benefit anyone. Packed with the right combination of water, sodium, and potassium, celery has been shown to reduce blood pressure and calm anxiety. And since it's 90 percent water, you can eat as much of this low-calorie, high-fiber food as you want without regret.

Cheese

One of the first body parts the opposite sex looks at when scoping out a potential date: the teeth. Keep them bright and healthy by eating cheese. Cheese is a good source of calcium, to keep your teeth strong, plus it can lower the levels of bacteria in your mouth and keep teeth clean and cavity-free. The American Dental Association recommends eating at least two servings of block cheese every week to maintain tooth health.

Chili Peppers

Curry, Mexican salsas, and chili peppers contain the chemical capsaicin, which triggers the release of endorphins. It also stimulates nerve endings, increasing metabolism, raising the heart rate, causing flushed cheeks, sweating, and other physical affects that mimic arousal.

Coffee

A few years back, women flooded local Starbucks and Dunkin' Donuts shops after a study titled "Coffee, Tea and Me" from a researcher at Southwestern University in Texas found that caffeine may boost female desire for sex. However, her study was conducted on 108 female . . . rats. Caffeine seemed to shorten the amount of time it took for the females to be motivated to seek out the male rats. While it may be temping to speculate that it would have the same effect on humans, the researcher cautioned that, unlike most women, the rats had never been exposed to caffeine before. The researcher said that, therefore, the sexual enhancement might work only for women who aren't habitual users. And it may take a lot more caffeine. However, caffeine has been shown to have health benefits. After a sip of a caffeinated beverage, the brain releases dopamine, a neurochemical that stimulates areas of the brain responsible for alertness, problem solving, and pleasure. A cup before a workout has been shown to help athletes exercise longer and harder. And although researchers don't know exactly why, they speculate that the large amounts of antioxidants in coffee and other compounds in caffeine may be responsible for improved insulin resistance and reduced diabetes risk.

Figs

Considering their resemblance to female genitalia (when sliced in half), it's no surprise the fig has been historically lauded as a sexual symbol. It's been written that Adam and Eve used its leaves to cover their privates, the ancient Greeks are said to have celebrated the arrival of the fig crop with wild sex rituals, and the great seductress Cleopatra loved to eat them from the fingers of buff young male attendants. Nutritionally, figs make sense as a sex snack. Like blueberries, they contain more soluble and insoluble fiber than most fruits and vegetables and they are rich in many nutrients important to good sexual health, including potassium, magnesium, iron, manganese, calcium, and antioxidants. High in simple sugars, a quarter-cup serving will boost your serotonin levels and provide a quick energy lift.

Flax Seeds

Sprinkle flax seeds on your cereal, yogurt, or ice cream for a shot of omega-3 and omega-6 fatty acids, which are the major building blocks of all sex hormones. One tablespoon of the nutty-tasting seeds helps increase testosterone, the chemical with the most direct libido-boosting effect, according to Rutgers' sexuality researcher Helen Fisher, PhD, an advisor to *Women's Health*. Another good plant-based source of these essential fatty acids is walnuts.

Garlic

Garlic may be the last thing you want on your breath when you're ready to have sex. But garlic may be something you want to get more of on other occasions due to its high concentration of the compound allicin. Numerous small clinical studies suggest that regular garlic consumption may reduce cholesterol, blood pressure and risk of certain cancers, and work against peripheral artery disease, improving blood flow particularly to the lower extremities.

Honey

Honey's B vitamins aid the production of testosterone, and its boron content helps the body use estrogen, which is a key factor in proper blood flow and arousal. In the kitchen, drizzle it on your oatmeal. In the bedroom, drizzle it on any warm, lickable surface.

Milk (Fat-Free) and Probiotic Yogurt

The calcium in milk is essential for bone building. The vitamin D in fortified milk helps calcium keep your muscles, heart, and nervous system humming. Recent studies show that calcium also influences fat metabolism. In a 12-week study at the University of Tennessee, two groups of people were put on a diet plan that cut 500 calories from their daily intake. One group consumed 1,100 mg of calcium every day by eating yogurt. The other group got 500 mg of calcium a day, which is typical for the average American diet. It turned out that the yogurt eaters lost 61 percent more bodyweight than the low-calcium group, with 81 percent coming from the belly area. The research team determined that human fat cells carry a gene that causes the body to produce fat when calcium levels are low, but that high calcium levels turn off this fat-causing gene. Yogurt is another great source of calcium. But when choosing your yogurt, reach for the probiotic kind. Hint: the label will read "live and active cultures." This yogurt contains beneficial organisms that work with the bacteria in your gut to boost your immune system. What's more, yogurt is one of the few foods with conjugated linoleic acid, a special type of fat that some studies show can reduce body fat.

Pomegranate Juice

Throughout the ages the pomegranate has been revered for its medicinal qualities. Many world religions consider the fruit sacred. In Judaism, its many seeds symbolize fertility and prosperity, relating to the first commandment of the Torah: "be fruitful and multiply." In the

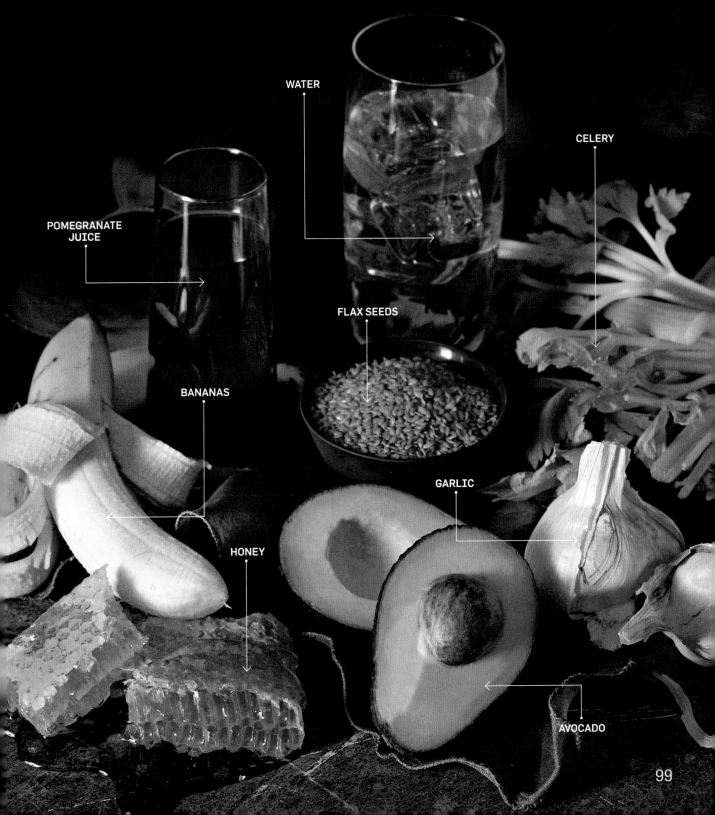

WATER

CELERY

POMEGRANATE JUICE

FLAX SEEDS

BANANAS

GARLIC

HONEY

AVOCADO

99

Old Testament, The Song of Solomon compares the cheeks of a bride behind her veil to the two halves of a pomegranate. In China, a picture of an open pomegranate is a popular wedding gift. With such a fertile cultural history, you might expect the many-seeded fruit to have powerful sexual properties. Indeed, a study in the *Journal of Urology* found that pomegranate juice was good for healthier erections—in rabbits. So far, human studies haven't been very promising. Still, there are a lot of good reasons to eat and drink of this fruit. When scientists at the University of California, Los Angeles studied this ruby-red fruit, they found that pomegranates are rich in polyphenols, antioxidants that allow blood to flow through your veins—a key component of good sex. And Israeli researchers discovered that men who drank 2 ounces of pomegranate juice a day for a year lowered their systolic blood pressure by 21 percent and dramatically improved blood flow to their hearts.

Sweet Potatoes

Your skin is your largest sex organ. Keep it soft, supple, and wrinkle-free by limiting exposure to the sun, one of the primary reasons men and women age prematurely. In addition to applying the sunscreen cream, ingest some SPF by eating sweet potatoes. European researchers recently found that pigments from beta-carotene-rich foods—like sweet potatoes and carrots—can build up in your skin, helping to prevent damage from ultraviolet rays.

FEEL YOUR FIGS

When shopping for fresh figs, make sure they have a slight bit of give when you squeeze them and they will ripen nicely. If they are too hard, they may remain hard.

Really Happy (Ending) Meals

HOW TO MAKE LOVE IN THE KITCHEN

Everyone knows the way to a man's heart is through his stomach, but a romantic meal homemade by him for her, well, that may be the ultimate strategy for seduction. A recent survey we conducted showed that 70 percent of *Women's Health* readers are more turned on by a romantic dinner prepared by a man than by a meal at a fancy restaurant.

That doesn't surprise Amy Reiley, a master of gastronomy and author of the books *The Love Diet* and *Fork Me, Spoon Me*. "Cooking for someone is the ultimate gift of love," she says. "And sharing a meal together at home can be a powerfully sensual experience that calls upon all of our senses at once."

That experience can be the perfect prelude to a passionate night of lovemaking, says Beverly Whipple, PhD, professor emeritus at Rutgers University and coauthor of *The Science*

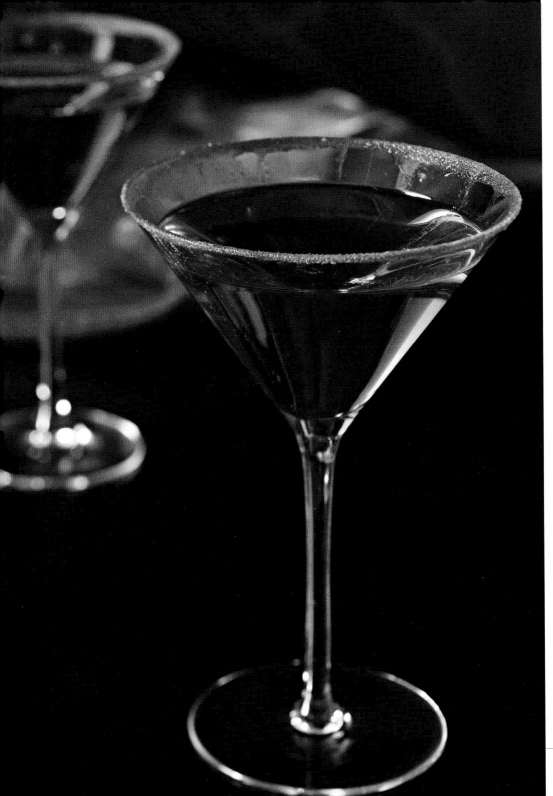

LOVE POTION #9

You don't need a PhD in biochemistry to know that a little booze can loosen the bikini strings. The cayenne pepper in this sexy cocktail contains capsaicin, which raises your heart rate and makes you sweat—simulating the physiological effects of sexual arousal.

GET NAKED MARTINI

1½ ounces chilled
   Absolut Peppar
   Vodka
   Splash of grenadine
   Cinnamon sugar

Combine vodka and grenadine in a shaker with ice. Run an ice cube around the rim of a martini glass, then place the glass rim-down on a plate sprinkled with cinnamon sugar. Set glass upright and strain in liquid.

"Cooking is like sex; it's about giving pleasure. You can't climax too early."

—Chef Gordon Ramsay

of *Orgasm*, because "we literally taste, smell, and consume our lovers." Before you head off into the kitchen, keep these tips in mind so that heat in the kitchen equals heat in the bedroom.

Leave room for dessert.

Avoid heavy foods like a big bowl of pasta or a steak and baked potato, and desserts with tons of sugar. "You can't eat like that and expect to have sex later on; you'll fall asleep first," says Reiley. Keep dessert very light and simple. Reiley recommends already-made strawberries dipped in dark chocolate or her personal favorite: fresh figs at room temperature dipped in ice cold sour cream and then rolled in brown sugar.

Keep it simple and quick.

Put your energy into romancing your partner, not slaving over a stove. If you want to impress with an elaborate meal, make it in advance.

Mix various textures and temperatures.

Cool and hot, creamy and crunchy, "the more contrasts in a dish, the greater the aphrodisiac quality of the meal to stimulate the senses," says Reiley.

Ready to put theory into practice? Try the following romantic meal selection on your partner. Loaded with sexually beneficial ingredients, it was developed by Reiley and her *Love Diet* coauthor Juan-Carolos Cruz, host of The Food Network's *Calorie Commando* and *Weighing In*.

SAVORY WATERMELON SALAD

Makes 2 servings as an appetizer or side dish.

- 2 cups watermelon (about 1 pound), cut into bite-sized pieces
- 1 tablespoon rice wine vinegar
- 2 tablespoons fat-free feta cheese
- ½ cup finely chopped Vidalia or other sweet onion
- ¼ teaspoon salt
- 1 tablespoon fresh chopped mint

Toss the ingredients together.

RED CURRY SHRIMP WITH RIPE MANGO

Makes 2 to 3 servings.

- ½ ripe mango
- 12 large shrimp
- Pinch of salt
- 1 teaspoon paprika
- ½ teaspoon coriander powder
- ¼ teaspoon cumin
- ¼ teaspoon freshly ground black pepper
- ¼ teaspoon cinnamon
- ½ teaspoon powdered ginger
- 1 tablespoon grape seed or other neutral oil
- 1 small diced red onion
- 1 large diced tomato

1. Peel and dice mango then chill in the refrigerator.

2. Peel the shrimp and sprinkle with a pinch of salt.

3. In a small mixing bowl, combine paprika, coriander, cumin, black pepper, cinnamon, and ginger. Add shrimp and toss until coated.

4. Heat the oil in a nonstick sauté pan over high heat.

5. Add shrimp to the pan and sauté until they begin to curl and change color.

6. Add the onion and tomato and continue to cook for an additional 2 minutes, tossing occasionally. (Onions should still have some crunch.)

7. Remove from heat and transfer to a serving platter. Top with cold mango and serve immediately for a hot/cold/spicy/sweet sensation.

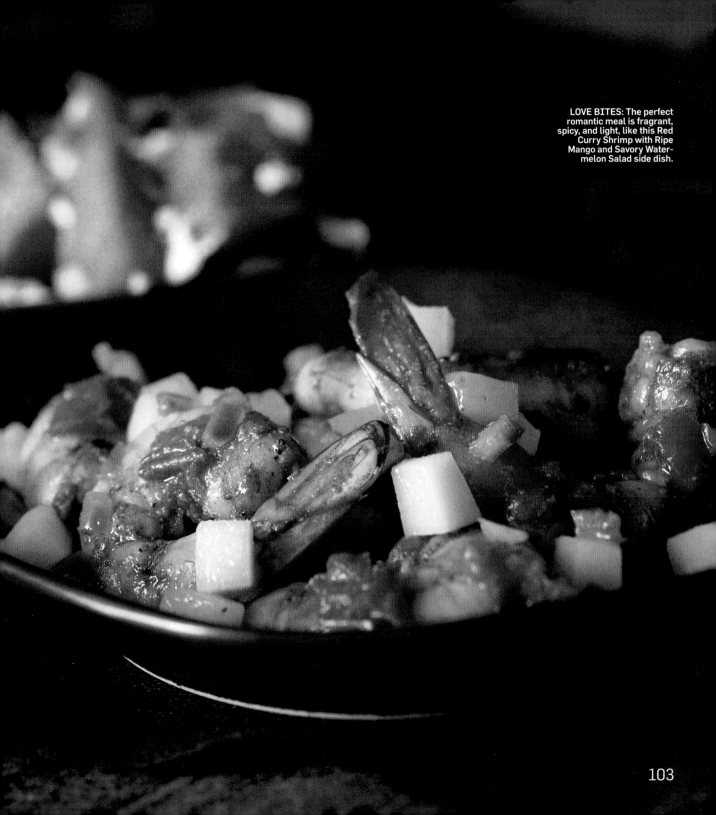

LOVE BITES: The perfect romantic meal is fragrant, spicy, and light, like this Red Curry Shrimp with Ripe Mango and Savory Watermelon Salad side dish.

103

WHAT'S RED AND BLACK AND SEXY ALL OVER?

CHOCOLATE-COVERED STRAWBERRIES

Makes 2 servings (with plenty extra to snack on in the a.m.).

1 carton fresh straw-berries, washed and fully dried

8 ounces high-quality dark chocolate

A few sheets of parchment paper

Make a double boiler by filling a pot with an inch or two of water, covering it with a metal or glass mixing bowl, and bringing the water to a boil. Break the chocolate into chunks and add it to the mixing bowl. Using a rubber spatula or a wooden spoon, stir the choco-late until completely melted and smooth. Dip the strawberries in the melted chocolate, swirling them around to ensure they are evenly covered. Lay the fruit on a baking sheet (or even just a few plates) covered with the parchment paper and refrigerate for at least an hour.

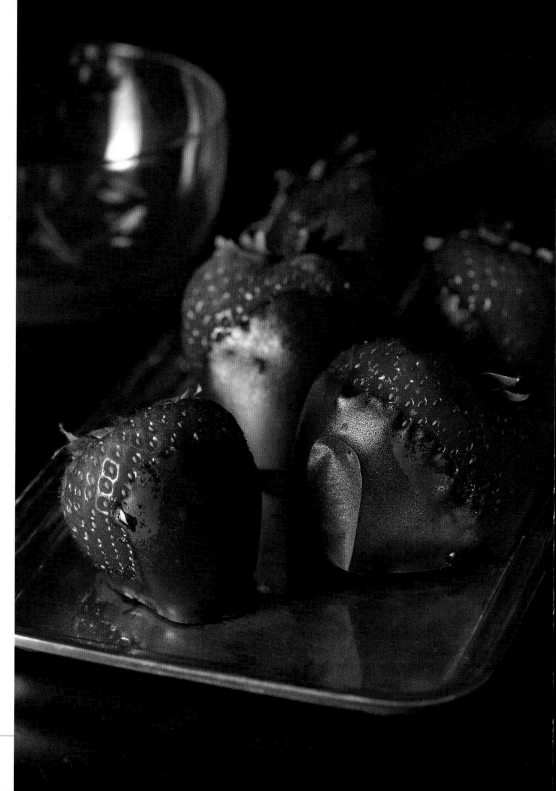

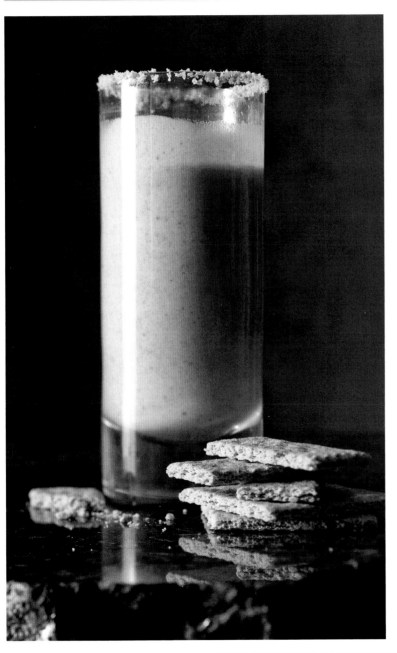

MORNING AFTER DATE SHAKE

Dates are a source of magnesium—essential for sexual hormone production—and a great source of fiber. Be sure to prep the dates at night for a long, slow morning in bed. Makes 2 servings.

- 5 dried dates soaked in milk overnight
- 1 graham cracker crushed into crumbs
- 2 pinches cardamom
- ½ cup plain Greek-style yogurt
- 1 teaspoon honey
- 8 ice cubes

1. Pit and chop dates and soak overnight in milk in the refrigerator.

2. Combine graham cracker crumbs and 1 pinch of cardamom in a shallow dish or plate. Moisten the tops of two glasses with milk, then dip the rims of both glasses in the crumb mixture.

3. Put dates and soaking milk in a blender. Add yogurt, honey, 1 pinch cardamom, ice and blend.

4. Carefully pour liquid into two rimmed glasses. Tastes best drunk in bed.

The Slim and Sexy Weight-Loss Plan

THE FASTEST WAY TO DROP POUNDS AND LIFT YOUR LIBIDO

Losing weight can do more to improve your love life than finding George Clooney or Angelina in your bed wearing nothing but chocolate mousse.

Even if you've struggled with weight all of your life, even if you have yo-yoed on and off diets before, we at *Women's Health* and *Men's Health* magazines know that you can get into better shape quickly and more easily than you think is possible. See, we've been in your shoes and those of many, many others who do battle with their bellies and backsides and thighs. We've interviewed the top weight-loss experts in the United States, and we know that dropping pounds is not about eating rice cakes and tofu, or about starving yourself and beating yourself up when you eat a brownie in a "moment of weakness." You're not weak. You're human. And, like the rest of us humans, you like to eat good food. That pleasure—like the pleasure of sex—is too strong to deny. It goes against nature. So, don't sacrifice. Instead, learn how to enjoy food the right way. Indulge intelligently, so that you can live your life to the fullest while staying fit, trim and healthy.

Sound too good to be true? It's not.

We've seen it happen time and time again in our readers who follow the eating strategies in our pages. Need inspiration? Check out the You Lose, You Win! column in *Women's Health* or The Belly Off! Club in *Men's Health*. These are stories about people like you who have overcome a reliance on unhealthy foods and a lifestyle of reclining. These people lost weight and found new life, and you can, too, using the same smart tricks and techniques. Our brands' best-selling books, *The Abs Diet, The Belly Off! Diet, Look Better Naked, The Big Book of Exercises*, and *Your Best Body at 40+*, are based on core principals of healthy nutrition that fight fat, build muscle, and turn formerly flabby bodies into lean, healthy bodies.

Step 1. Load up your daily menu with the SUPER SEX FOODS that began this chapter. Not only are they great for libido and sexual function, but they are among the healthiest foods for weight loss.

Step 2. Move your body more. Start today by getting outside and walking briskly for 30 minutes. It's the best thing you can do for your heart and for your love life. Then schedule regular weekly workout times.

Step 3. Follow these six core principles of nutrition that will help you lose weight quickly and safely:

- Eat more, eat often.
- Never skip breakfast.
- Choose slow-burning carbohydrates.
- Burn calories with protein.
- Learn portion control.
- Avoid sugary soft drinks and limit alcohol.

Eat more, eat often.

You know this already from experience, but it's worth repeating: Diets of sacrifice that say "no" to foods almost always backfire because we don't have the willpower to deny ourselves the pleasure of eating certain foods forever. That's why *Women's Health* and *Men's Health* magazines say, "Eat! Eat! Fill up on foods that fill you up and satisfy your hunger longer." These foods are almost always rich in nutrients, fiber and, often, water. We're talking mostly about fruits and vegetables here, including many of the items listed in SUPER SEX FOODS. Eat more food and space out those calories throughout the day, instead of only during the three traditional mealtimes. Studies show that people who eat more frequent, smaller meals throughout the day are half as likely to become overweight as people who eat three or fewer times a day. Why? Because eating either a meal or a snack every 4 or so hours helps keep your body working to digest and absorb foods, increasing that thermic effect of food to boost your metabolism. What's more, eating regularly throughout the day—and making sure your meals and snacks include satiating protein, fat, and fiber—keeps cravings away so you'll be less likely to raid the vending machine or overeat at lunchtime.

Give it a try for a week and you'll feel the difference in your body that eating this way can make. Your chow schedule might look like this:

7:00 a.m.	Breakfast
10:00 a.m.	Snack
1:00 p.m.	Lunch
4:30 p.m.	Snack
7:00 p.m.	Dinner
9:30 p.m.	Snack (optional)

Never skip breakfast.

If you eat dinner at 7, don't have a snack before you go to bed and skip breakfast. You may go as many as 15 hours without food (until your grumbling belly forces you to grab a doughnut at 10 a.m.). When you fast for extended periods like that your body can tap into muscle for fuel instead of fat. Just what you don't want to happen. Your body is hungry. It needs to refuel.

> *"Great food is like great sex. The more you have, the more you want."*
>
> —Food writer Gael Greene

Another thing can happen when you don't break your fast with a good breakfast: your metabolic rate can be diminished by up to 10 percent, according to nutritionist Leslie Bonci, RD, of the University of Pittsburgh Medical Center and a sports nutritionist for the Pittsburgh Pirates. That's why breakfast skippers also tend to have trouble maintaining a healthy weight. In a study at the University of Massachusetts Medical School, researchers found that people who don't eat breakfast are 450 times more likely to be obese than those who do eat breakfast. Here again, your food choices play an important role in how useful your breakfast can be for weight loss and maintenance.

What to eat? How does a cheese and vegetable omelet with whole-wheat toast sound? Make sure you load up on high-quality protein, slow-burning carbohydrates (fruit and whole-grain cereal) and a little healthy fat (like olive oil). Several scientific studies have shown the weight-loss benefits of eating more protein at the morning meal. In one, researchers at Virginia Commonwealth University found that dieters who ate 600-calorie breakfasts rich in high-quality protein lost significantly more weight and kept it off longer than other dieters who consumed a low-calorie breakfast (300 calories) and just a quarter of the protein.

A quick note for people who exercise in the morning before breakfast: Eat a little something before your workout. It doesn't have to be much. Try a half an apple with a peanut butter; a low-carbohydrate meal replacement bar; orange juice cut with water and a scoop of whey protein powder; a hardboiled egg and some green tea; or a smoothie made with whey protein. You need a bit of carbohydrate for energy and the protein accelerates recovery. Smoothies and shakes are terrific choices because the liquid carbs digest quickly to fuel your body and the whey gets into your system as soon as it's needed. Here's a pre-workout morning smoothie to try from *The New Abs Diet Cookbook*.

THE ORANGEMAN
Makes 2 servings.

- 1 cup 1% milk
- ½ cup frozen orange juice concentrate
- 2 tablespoons low-fat plain yogurt
- 1 banana
- 2 teaspoons whey protein powder
- 6 ice cubes

Add milk, OJ, yogurt, banana, protein powder, and ice cubes to a blender, and puree until smooth.

Choose slow-burning carbohydrates.

Carbs aren't the dietary devils they've been made out to be. They're essential fuel for your body and especially your brain. But it's the American way to go overboard, especially in the category of fast-burning carbohydrates like white bread, pasta, rice, potatoes, and—here's the killer—snack foods like chips, candy, and baked goods like cookies, bagels, and cakes. These "white foods" can raise blood sugar quickly, triggering cravings

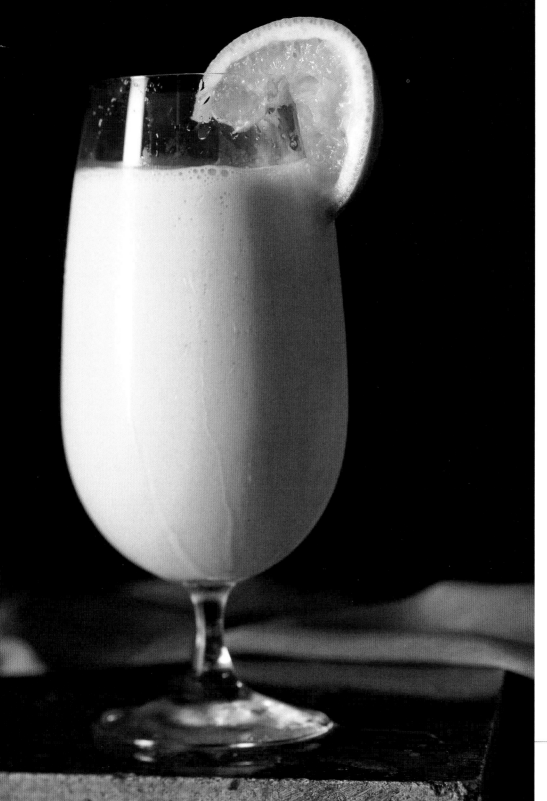

40

Percentage of
couples who report
sex is better on
weekends.

that encourage overeating. What's more, an influx of fast-absorbing carbs switches your body over from burning fat mode to excess-sugar-burning mode and you end up storing more fat. But if you eat slow-digesting carbohydrates, like whole grain breads, oatmeal, and fruits and vegetables, blood-sugar levels remain normal, which allows your body to continue burning fat. That's why even though a big hunk of chocolate cake with sugary frosting and a bowl of oatmeal with strawberries may have the same number of calories, they have very different effects on your body's fat-burning mechanism.

Burn calories with protein.

Protein is so important to weight maintenance that you should eat it with every meal and snack. Proteins boost metabolism a little more during digestion than any other type of food. Plus protein increases metabolism by helping to build muscle and stall the muscle loss that naturally happens as we age. Muscle is more metabolically active than fat is, so the more lean muscle on your body the better at burning calories it will be. You'll find terrific sources for high-quality, muscle-building, hunger-satisfying protein among the SUPER SEX FOODS such as fish, lean meats, chicken and turkey, eggs, dairy products, beans and legumes, and nuts. When you can, try to choose organic meats, poultry, and dairy foods to avoid hormones and gain nutrition. Grass-fed beef, for example, contains upwards of

60 percent more omega-3 fatty acids than regular beef, plus more vitamin E and fat-burning conjugated linoleic acid (CLA). Organic milk, chicken, and eggs also contain more of these essential fatty acids.

Master portion control.

There's a big difference between "dieting" and putting down your fork before you feel full. Dieting is a blockade. Portion control is free trade, with checks and balances. Portion control is your biggest weapon in the war on weight because it allows you to eat whatever you want, really, so long as you are diligent about the quantity you put in your mouth. So, for example, Boston cream pie is not off limits. Go ahead, have a couple of bites to satisfy your craving for Beantown's best. You'll be more likely to stop at a few bites if you've filled up on a healthy fish dinner and a fresh garden salad first.

A visit to any all-you-can-eat buffet restaurant will help you to understand the power of portion control. It doesn't exist at these kinds of places, and you can see that in the clientele, mostly overweight and often obese. People here are eating thousands of calories' worth of food at a sitting because of the sheer volume and variety of food. Dozens of studies have shown that the more variety and the larger the quantity of available food, the more we will eat. Portion control starts by avoiding temptation. Stay out of the all-you-can-eat buffets. Eat more meals at home

BRUSH YOUR TEETH WHEN YOU'RE HUNGRY

The minty toothpaste flavor can take the edge off a sugar craving. Worst case: you'll have a dazzling smile and fresh breath.

where you have greater control over food preparation. USDA scientists say that on average, people eat 500 more calories a day on days when they eat at fast food restaurants compared with days when they don't. When you do eat out, ask your waiter to doggy bag half of your big restaurant meal before it even arrives. Start with a soup or salad to fill yourself up so you won't eat all of your entrée. One of the most effective ways to lose weight is to gradually condition yourself to eat 10 to 20 percent less at every meal. After a few days you'll start to notice the difference on the scale. And consciously cutting back will help reinforce your understanding that you have control over food. You'll find it empowering. Here are more ways to help you control portions:

Eat juicy foods. Vegetables containing high volumes of water and good amounts of fiber bulk up food, increasing their satiating affect. Try replacing some of the meat in your dinners with vegetables like cabbage, zucchini, cucumbers, broccoli, and peppers; it can be an easy way to trick yourself into losing weight. In a study at Penn State University, researchers found that when people cut the amount of roast beef and rice on their dinner plates in half and added lightly-buttered broccoli, they consumed 86 fewer calories and felt just as full.

Don't talk with your mouth full. Talking at the dinner table can help you control portions, if it helps you to slow down your eating. A study at the University of Rhode Island measured a 10 percent decrease in calorie intake in people who consciously slowed down between bites. If you're eating alone, consciously take smaller bites and chew your food thoroughly. It may help to put your fork down between bites. Breathing, researchers say, helps you gauge your level of satiety because it allows you to focus on how your body feels.

Snack on nuts. Peanuts, almonds, and walnuts have lots of calories, so portion control is crucial. But if you are disciplined, nuts and seeds can be a terrific snack choice for people shooting for Mr. Peanut's shapely figure. Spanish researchers monitored 8,865 people about their diets for 28 months and found that those who ate nuts at least twice a week were 30 percent less likely to have gained 11 pounds or more than people who rarely ate nuts. Study author Maria Bes-Rastrollo, PhD, believes it's because nuts are high in protein, unsaturated fat, and fiber, all of which boost metabolism, burn fat, and keep you feeling full longer.

Weigh yourself every day. When researchers at the University of Minnesota analyzed the habits of 1,800 people who lost weight in diet programs, they found that about 40 percent weighed themselves daily or weekly. Those who did it daily lost an average of 12 pounds compared with 6 pounds for those who weighed weekly. Regular weigh-ins work if you have the right attitude about them. They can tip you off when your weight is starting to creep up so you can take action and they can motivate you to keep going as you see the numbers declining. Weighing yourself also makes you more conscious of your body and what you put in it, helping you to master portion control. Try to weigh yourself at the same time same time every day for greater accuracy because weight typically fluctuates through a 24-hour period.

Avoid TV dinners. Watching *The Biggest Loser* while eating may make you gain weight. People who eat in front of the tube tend to eat more food, 288 calories worth, according to one study at the University of Massachusetts. Why? People become so engrossed in what they are watching on TV that they miss brain signals telling that they are full. But not only does TV distract you while you're eating, it may make you forget what you've eaten. A study in the journal *Appetite* reports that women who ate lunch while watching TV and were offered cookies several hours later ended up eating 20 percent more cookies than they did after a no-TV lunch. TV watching may cause you to space out about what you've already eaten, leading you to consume more, says study author Suzanne Higgs, PhD, of the University of Birmingham in England.

Practice yoga for stronger portion control muscles. People who do yoga tend to eat mindfully, that is, they eat when hungry and are able to recognize when they are getting full so they can avoid overeating, according to a study in the *Journal of the American Dietetic Association* conducted at the Fred Hutchinson Cancer Research Center in Seattle.

Avoid sugary soft drinks and limit alcohol.

Drinks go down in the blink of an eye. And because you're not chewing when you're swallowing, it's difficult to realize how much you're consuming with every big gulp. It's a lot; trust us. The journal *Obesity* estimates that Americans consume 222 more calories from liquids per day than we did in 1965. Last year, the average American swallowed more than 52 gallons of soda, juice, and other sugary drinks. Nearly one in every 10 calories we consume comes from soft drinks. And it is impacting both our weight and our health. One study found that people who drank just two sodas a day increased their diabetes risk 24 percent compared to those who limited soda to once a month.

You can overdo it with something seemingly as healthy as juice, too, which is loaded with calories and sugar. Cut your OJ with water. Or use a proper-sized glass: 6 ounces, not 8, is a serving of juice.

While dozens of studies have shown health benefits of moderate alcohol consumption—for the heart, for the mind, for the soul—remember that beer, wine, and liquor contains calories. And even though gin, vodka, and whisky don't carry carbs, the sugary mixers we flavor them with do. Sugary margarita, dacquiri, and lemonade mixers only encourage more drinking and, of course, fried cheese-stuffed jalapeño poppers and other bar food. What's more, alcohol, any alcohol, impairs your body f rom burning fat. So, if you want to lose weight, limit alcohol to one or two drinks per week. And if you really want to drop pounds fast, abstaining altogether is the way to go.

What's the best beverage of all? You guessed it. Water. Sex is athletic, which is why drinking lots of water instead of calorie-filled beverages is smart. Muscle is approximately 80 percent water, so when you are dehydrated, even by 1 percent, your exercise performance can be impaired. In addition, well-hydrated muscle cells are important to proper protein synthesis for muscle recovery and growth.

These six principles form the rock-solid backbone of any smart weight-loss strategy, and they are simply good eating habits to adopt for the rest of your life. By following them, and eating the SUPER SEX FOODS, you'll automatically eat healthier and consume fewer calories every day. And that's the key to sustained weight loss: ending the day with fewer calories than your body needs to function. It takes a deficit of 500 calories a day to lose 1 pound of flab in a week, which is a safe and reasonable goal. That's because a pound of weight equals roughly 3,500 calories. But consuming fewer calories is not the only way to get to that 500-calorie deficit. You can also burn off calories with exercise. By teaming your Better Sex Diet plan with the Better Sex Workouts in this book, you'll find that you can drop pounds without any extreme effort on either path so shaping up and slimming down will feel natural and easy to maintain throughout your life.

■

Chapter 7
Make Lust
Last

MONOGAMY IS THE MOST
CHALLENGING COMMITMENT
YOU'LL EVER MAKE.
KEEP THE FAITH WITHOUT
LOSING THE EXCITEMENT.

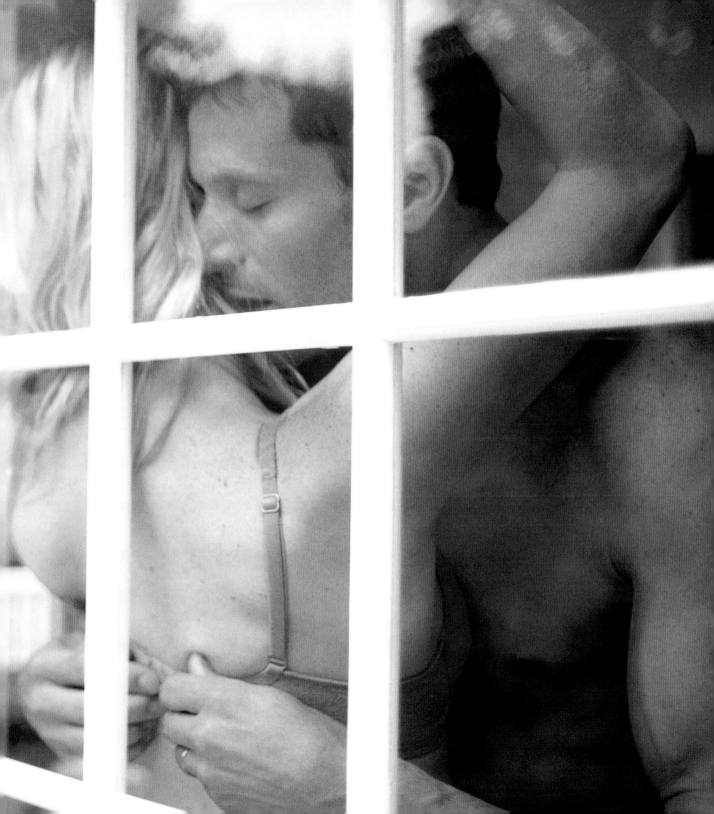

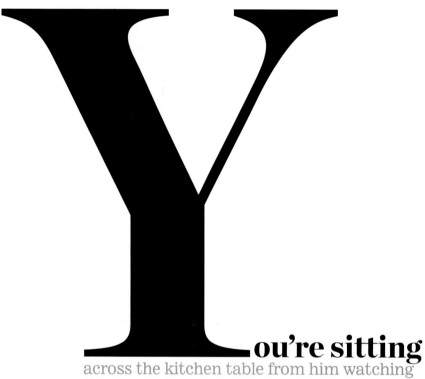

You're sitting

across the kitchen table from him watching the butter melt on your whole-wheat toast and waiting for him to answer your question.

He scratches, turns the sports page. Silence.

You look up at his baggy eyes and bed head and wonder: Is this the gorgeous man who I couldn't wait to get naked? Where did he go? Where did my libido go? Who is this guy, anyway? Did I bring him home by mistake from Walmart?

It's all so intense in the beginning of a relationship. Sex is priority number one—who cares about sleep? Or work? But something happens after the exchange of apartment keys that women and men and sexologists agree on: the obsession starts to wane and the burning lust of new love quickly simmers into real life.

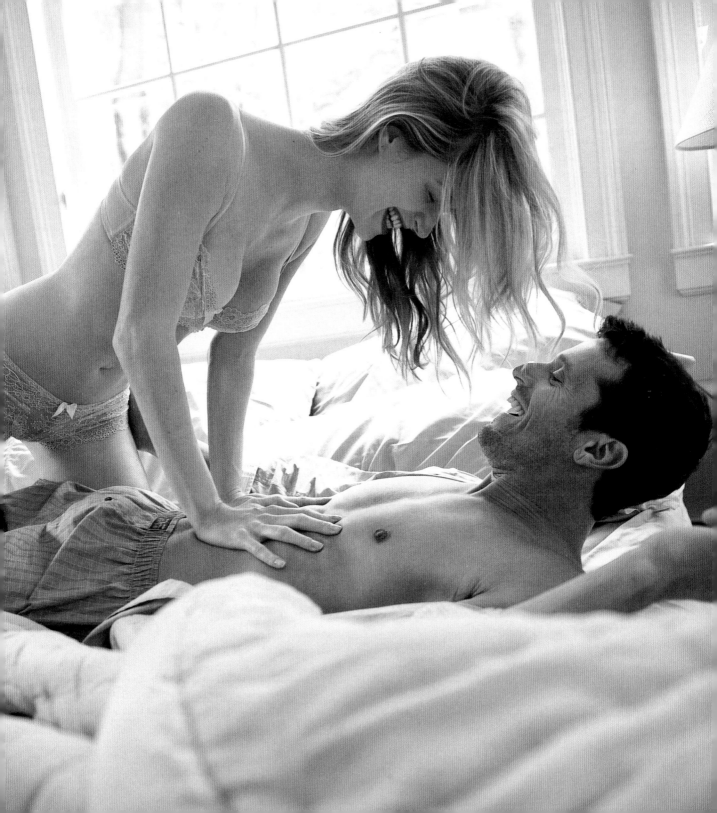

Make Lust Last HERS

Eight months into a relationship or maybe two years into a marriage, the times vary, love's all-consuming sizzle sputters. "As your relationship gets better and more secure, the sexual excitement may fade," says sex therapist Jane Greer, PhD, author of *What About Me?* "Since you know he's not going anywhere, there's little motivation to pull out all the stops in bed to impress him like you did when you first started dating, and vice versa. So sex starts to become routine."

And you begin caring more about who's doing whom on *True Blood* than what's going on in *your* bedroom. To make matters worse, the hormones that are responsible for boosting your bedroom bliss pull a disappearing act right when you need them most. "In the beginning of a relationship, the sex hormones estrogen and testosterone, dopamine (the pleasure neurotransmitter), and oxytocin (the bonding hormone) spike," says Barbara Bartlik, MD, a sex therapist in New York. "But they can decline back to base levels at about 24 months."

Where did that good stuff go and how can you get it back? Before you can figure that out, you need to understand what happened to your brain when you first fell in love.

Scientists aren't exactly sure why things fizzle, but they suspect it has something to do with evolution. Rutgers University anthropologist Helen E. Fisher, PhD, has extensively studied the science of attraction in mammals and birds for more than 30 years and has written five books on sex, love, marriage, and gender differences in the brain. Fisher believes that humans have evolved three distinct brain systems for courtship, mating, and parenting:

- Lust, the sex drive
- Romantic love, the obsessive attraction to a specific partner
- Attachment, deep feelings of union (to channel the energy toward raising offspring)

It's that middle state—passionate romantic love—that can be so fleeting and that we miss so much we want to get it back. The infatuation of early stage romantic love stems from a potent cocktail of brain chemicals whose primarily ingredient is dopamine, a neurotransmitter associated with pleasure, motivation, and reward, says Fisher. (Dopamine also plays a major role in addictions; it's what keeps us hungering for more and more pleasure-inducing stuff like drugs, booze, and Oreo cookies.) Add a shot of norepinephrine, another brain chemical that works like adrenaline, and you get the classic symptoms of being terribly, madly, insatiably in love: the pounding heart, sweaty palms, increased energy, sleeplessness, sexual possessiveness, and a rush of anxious motivation to be with him all the time. But the most important symptom of romantic love is obsessively thinking about your guy.

RED-HOT MONOGAMY TIP

Rent a chick flick. Romantic movies raise levels of oxytocin (the snuggle hormone) in both men and women, and research from Kansas University found that guys like rom-coms, too. (Shh!)

118

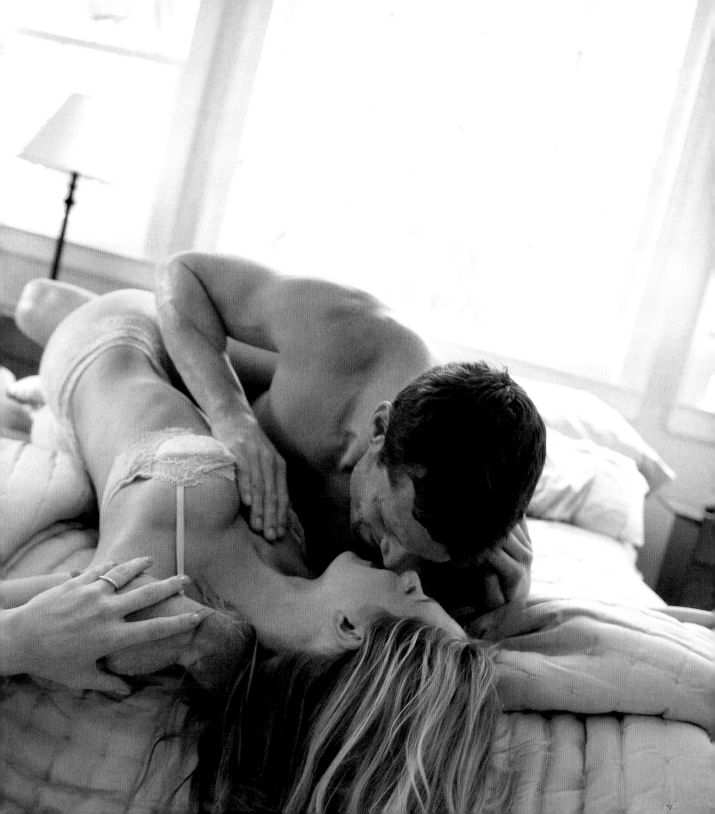

"It's like someone is camping in your head," says Fisher.

In studies, Fisher and colleagues Arthur Aron, PhD, and Lucy Brown, PhD, of SUNY at Stony Brook and Albert Einstein College of Medicine respectively, put people who were wildly infatuated into functional MRI scanners to examine the brain in the throes of early stage romantic love. When they showed the people in the MRI units a photograph of their lover versus a picture of a casual acquaintance, the dopamine-rich area of the brain's reward system lit up like fireworks. What does this suggest? That dopamine is a crucial ingredient in the early part of love. In fact, Fisher believes it's stronger even than sexual desire. "This obsessive, I-can't-get-enough-of-you love has all the characteristics of cocaine addiction," says Fisher.

As amazing as this kind of love feels, it doesn't last forever—a few years, tops, maybe. That's when other brain chemicals, oxytocin (in women) and vasopressin (in men) typically move us from passion into the much less maddening attachment phase of love, a more mature, peaceful connection.

"It's unrealistic to think that you can sustain that kind of idealized passionate sex you experienced in the very beginning," says Peggy Vaughan, author of the *Monogamy Myth* and an expert in affairs and preventing them. That's how affairs can begin; people yearn for that "new love" feeling again, she says, not realizing that new love will change, too. "Couples who come to really know each other can transition into a more accepting love that can actually energize them sexually," she says.

A recent review of 25 studies of short-term and long-term relationships found that, contrary to popular belief, romance could thrive and even grow in monogamous relationships. The findings published in 2009 in the *Review of General Psychology* showed that couples who reported greater attachment-style romantic love versus obsessive love were more satisfied in both short-term and long-term (10 years or more) relationships.

"Romantic love has the intensity, engagement, and sexual chemistry that passionate love has, minus the obsessive component," explains study author Bianca Acevedo, PhD, of the University of California, Santa Barbara. "Obsessive love includes feelings of uncertainty and anxiety; this love drives shorter relationships but not longer ones."

You have a choice to make. You can go back to contemplating the caloric load of the bread and butter combo during breakfast. You can go hunting for that dizzyingly obsessive love high with someone who isn't your partner. Or, you can strive to rekindle the excitement of romantic love without expecting it to feel exactly the same as it did in the beginning—when it was fueled by a dopamine high and caused you to do really crazy, goofy-in-love things.

Life can be good—and monogamy red hot—when you inject some dopamine and norepinephrine and a few other sexy love drugs back into your relationship in strategic doses. No one has the time and energy for the obsessive pursuit anymore, anyway, not when there are careers to nurture, kids to rear, laundry to fold, and tweets to follow. Fortunately, you don't have to. It's never too late to cultivate this more intentional love. "In our latest functional MRI experiment hatched by Arthur Aron we put five people in long-term relationships in the MRI machine," explains Fisher. "We found that areas of the brain associated with intense romantic love still become active 25 years later."

How to tweak those sexy parts of your primal brain once again? A scientific paper published in the *Canadian Journal of Human Sexuality* in 2009 offers some clues. Based on interviews with 20 sex therapists and 44 people who reported having great sex, a team of researchers identified eight key factors of optimal sexuality. They are: being present, psychological connection, deep sexual and erotic intimacy, extraordinary communication, interpersonal risk taking and exploration, authenticity, vulnerability, and transcendence. Optimal sex is fundamentally distinct from the mechanics of sex such as physical sensation and orgasm, according to study author Peggy J. Kleinplatz, PhD. "It takes a lot of effort … The payoff for taking the time to communicate and be intimate with your partner is, as our studies have shown, well worth it."

As for the physical part, experts say that simply switching up the types of sex you have can go a long way to reinvigorating your relationship. "Mixing up erotic styles keeps your sex life in shape, just like mixing up your workouts keeps your body fit and challenged," says Miro Gudelsky, DHS, a sex therapist in New York City.

Not only that, but "continuing to play around with novel types of sex allows you to uncover your sexual preferences—ones you may not have even known you had," says Greer. "And as a couple evolves, adding different dimensions to their sex life will strengthen the relationship overall."

So, try adding these four types of sex to your repertoire: maintenance sex, spontaneous sex, rediscovery sex, and experimental sex. And at the same time, work your way through the 15 smart strategies steamy monogamy you'll find later in this chapter. You'll notice the improvements in your love life almost immediately.

Maintenance Sex

"Think of this as meat-and-potatoes sex—it happens at the end of the day, during the week, when a run-of-the-mill romp is all you have energy for," says Pepper Schwartz, PhD, a professor of sociology at the University of Washington and author of *Prime: Adventures and Advice on Sex, Love, and the Sensual Years*.

Having sex while Jay Leno blares in the background doesn't sound particularly erotic (nothing against you, Jay), but it's a necessary part of every couple's sex life. "This is the kind of sex that connects you

FIGHT RIGHT

Conflict can be good for a relationship. A study at Baylor University suggests that hard negative emotions, such as anger and contempt, help couples instigate conflicts that lead to solutions.

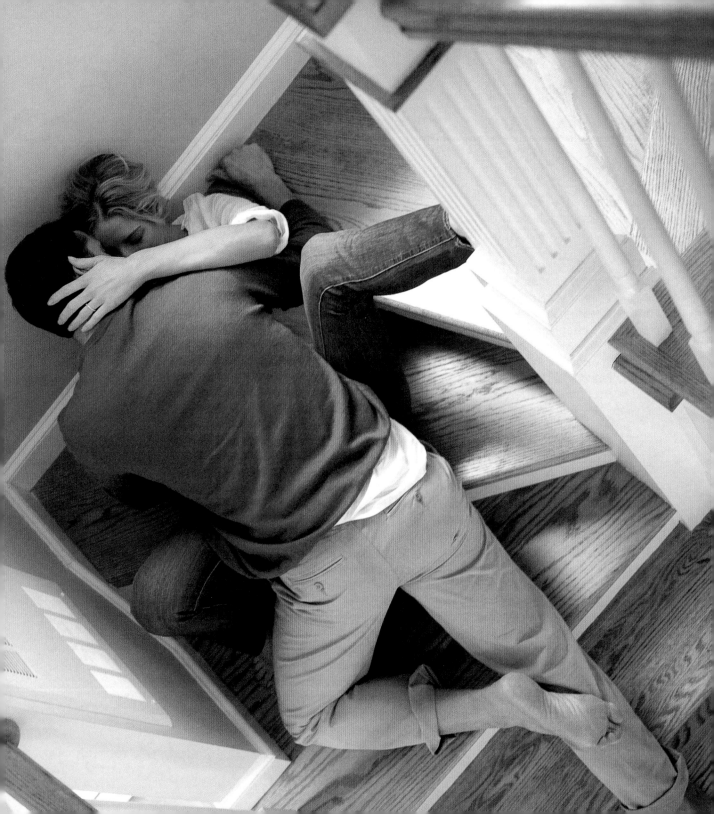

and reaffirms your bond as a couple," says Gina Ogden, PhD, a researcher and sex therapist in Cambridge, Massachusetts, and author of *The Return of Desire.*

On the nights you're too drained for long, drawn-out foreplay, boil it down to a couple of well-placed caresses that you can count on to expedite arousal. When you're both riled up enough for intercourse, the goal is to orgasm—fast. To that end, choose O-friendly positions that lend themselves to clitoral contact. Woman on top is your best bet because it lets you control the pace, but don't count out positions that allow for manual stimulation (side by side, from behind).

You probably won't break the bed or wake the neighbors with this kind of sex, but you'll fall asleep satisfied, which is all that matters. "You don't want this to be the only way you have sex, but you should have it a lot," says Schwartz. "So if you're having sex four times a week, maintenance sex should account for two or three of those times."

Spontaneous Sex

When you're in a new relationship, every surface becomes a potential place to get horizontal. The result? Primal, breathless, passionate sex. Too bad it's the first type to go when hormone levels start to dip. Without those frisky chemicals buzzing around—urging you to jump him anytime, anywhere—sex moves to your brain's back burner. To recapture the animal attraction that leads to spontaneous sex, you need to act like you did when you first got together and were having sex all the time. In other words, keep up with the bikini waxes, wear your pretty underwear (or no underwear at all—your call), get a spray tan, hit the gym. Basically, do whatever it is that makes you feel confident and sexy. "Feeling attractive and desired by your partner promotes arousal," says sex therapist Sandor Gardos, PhD, founder of MyPleasure.com. "It helps prime you for sex."

Seize opportunities when they present themselves and whenever you feel inspired. Join him in the shower before work. Pull over on the side of the road on the way home from a party. Put your hand in his lap while you're sitting on the couch watching TV together. The beauty of sex is that once you put in a little effort, it quickly starts to pay off: An Emory University study found that your body can become aroused physically before you start mentally desiring sex.

Unlike maintenance sex, spontaneous sex doesn't need to happen all the time. "Your sex life isn't a movie," says Schwartz. "Aim for once a week or so."

Rediscovery Sex

Having a big argument (he blew your vacation fund during a friendly game of poker), hitting a major life milestone together (It's a girl!), or weathering a rocky period in your relationship (someone cheated) aren't the kind of events that you'd expect to put you in the mood, but they can inspire sex that's intense, urgent, soulful, and tender.

"Sex that's born from an emotional place has an edge over other types of intimacy," says Gardos. "Because it involves a degree of looking at your partner in a new light, this sex feels like an expression of renewed love." But you don't need to experience a major event to tap into deeper emotions. It just requires a new way of looking at sex—one in which the orgasm isn't the most important thing.

"It's about rediscovering and pleasing each other. Think sensual, not sexual," says Greer. Here foreplay takes center stage. Give each other head-to-toe massages; kiss each other's cheeks, ears, and necks; and pleasure each other orally. "The idea is to make your partner feel important, cherished, and valued," says Greer. Choose positions that allow for eye contact and a slow buildup to orgasm, such as sitting and facing each other or missionary.

"Inspire rediscovery sex every few months by making it a point to think about what made you fall in love and being open to learning something new about him," says Ogden. "Your partner can always surprise you—sometimes you just have to look for it."

Experimental Sex
Daring and boundary pushing, it's the kind of sex that benefits from familiarity and trust. You can break out the sex toys and indulge your fantasies without the fear of being judged. "At the core of experimental sex is novelty, and that's a huge arousal booster," says Gardos. "The more blood that rushes to your genitals, the better your orgasms will be." Also, allowing your partner to see a secret side of you that no one else has access to builds intimacy.

So how do you suddenly start busting out sexual fantasies? You first have to have them. While you're lying in bed, standing in line at the grocery store, or walking to work, let your mind wander to whatever turns you on. It doesn't necessarily have to be stuff you want to act out; studies show that people who simply imagine sexy scenarios are more likely to experiment in bed.

When you want to make your fantasy a reality, broach it by saying something like, "I had a dream you were doing A, B, and C to me," or "I read about this crazy move in a magazine. Want to hear it?" You can also shoot him an e-mail outlining what you want to do to him later. "Writing acts as foreplay for both of you. It forces you to think about what you're saying, which can increase arousal. And he'll be able to read and reread your message, which keeps sex on his mind," says Greer. But there's no better time to introduce something creative than in the heat of the moment; research conducted by M.I.T. and Carnegie Mellon University found that men are more likely to behave boldly when sporting an erection.

"This type of sex is best saved for the weekends, particularly Saturday night," says Gardos. "You've left the stress of the week behind and you have the whole night ahead of you." Break out a spicy move once a month to keep things from getting stale.

Heat the Sheets

15 SMART STRATEGIES FOR SPARKING YOUR DESIRE

Appreciate How Good You've Got It

The grass, as they say, is always greener on the other side of the fence. So is the ass. And you may be tempted, especially when your relationship is in the doldrums, to think how much better sex and everything would be with someone else, someone younger, funnier, smarter, richer, more attentive, and hotter looking.

If you find yourself doing that, realize this: finding someone new, having an affair, and getting a divorce is a lot easier to think about than to do, actually. And just dwell for a moment on the misery of the standard broken marriage: anxiety, animosity, depression, psychological damage to the kids, and the tens of thousands of dollars that go away from you and toward your attorney's new Mercedes. But, hey, look at the bright side; only one in five second marriages fail!

The two leading causes of divorce are lack of communication and lack of patience to work on the marriage; people want a quick fix. But what if you take an affair and divorce completely off the table? Then you are left with only looking for ways to make things better.

The rest of the suggestions in this chapter should help, but start here:

Grab a pad of lined paper and jot down all of the things you love or loved about your partner, the sound of his laugh, how good he is at his job, his ability to pick out just the right gift. Take your time—a few days. Avoid writing down anything negative, only the positives, the things you appreciate about him. Don't leave out the little things. Write it all down.

On a second sheet of paper, write down memorable things you've done together: vacations, parties, trips, dinners, etc. Include situations and brief moments of sadness, tenderness, laughter, love, challenge, and great sex. Think about ways to recreate those times. What can you do to initiate those situations again? Write down your ideas.

Reflect on all the ways you are better off in your relationship than people who are single or divorced. Studies show that committed couples generally are happier, healthier, less overwhelmed by stress, have stronger immune and cardiovascular systems, sleep better, and enjoy more frequent sex.

RED-HOT MONOGAMY TIP

Make out more. Take a trip back to junior high for an evening and restrict yourselves to 10 minutes of kissing and over-the-clothes touching only. Keeping things PG for a set time revs you both up for a more adult encounter.

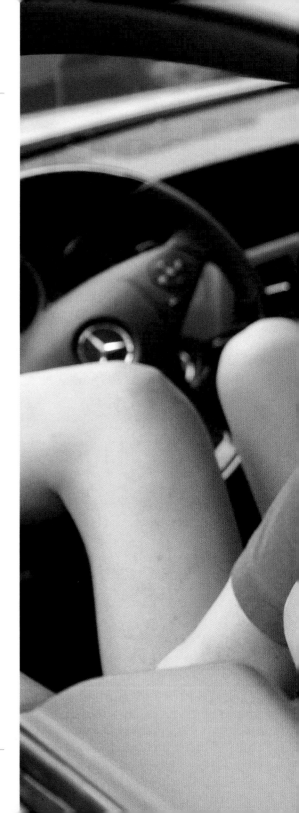

Review your lists every day over the next 2 weeks. In all likelihood, you'll develop a much greater appreciation for your partner and your good fortune. One more tip: Be optimistic about your partnership. Did you know that 70 percent of men and 68 percent of women describe their marriages as "very happy," and 96 percent of men (and 91 percent of women) would marry their current spouse if they had it to do over again? An online survey we recently posted on MensHealth.com and WomensHealthMag.com showed that 77 percent of married women and 78 percent of married men claim to be more in love with their spouses than on the day they were married. Well, what do you know?

Tell Him a Secret

Peggy Vaughan knows a lot about secrets. Many years ago, she discovered one about her husband James: He had been having affairs for years. Since then, they have overcome his infidelities, are happily married and are highly sought-after experts on affairs, having written five books, and the popular and informative website DearPeggy.com. Peggy believes what ultimately saved their marriage—and the critical ingredient to sustaining a loving relationship—is "responsible honesty." What she means by that is having regular, honest communication that goes beyond being truthful in what you say. It means volunteering

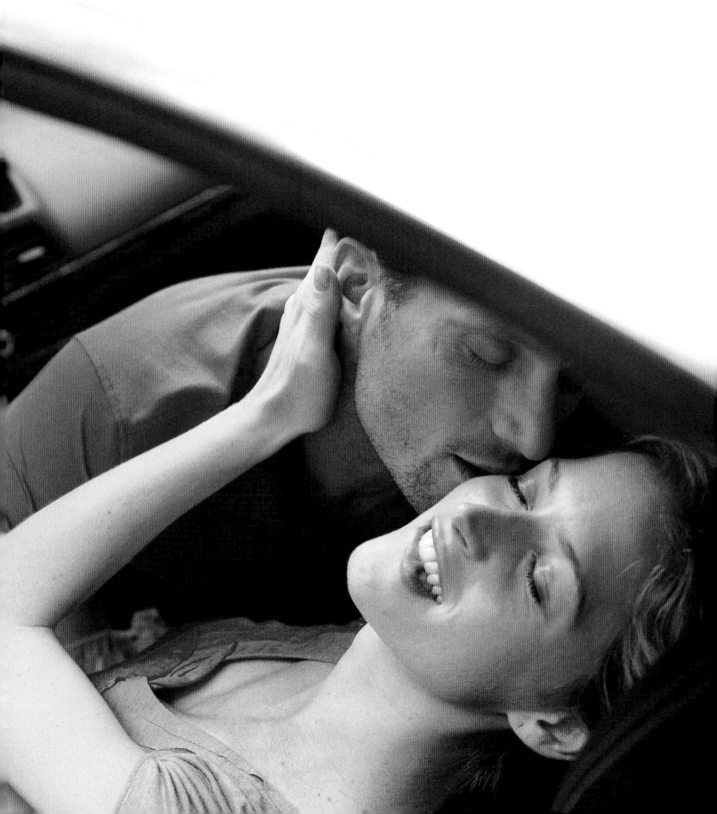

all your thoughts and feelings that are relevant to the relationship.

"A lot of people think being honest is not telling lies; that's not honesty," says Vaughan. "Real honesty is not withholding information relevant to the relationship. Responsible honesty is sharing your deepest hopes, fears, and dreams on an ongoing basis,and it can be sexier than all of the sex manuals combined."

Even little white lies or withholding information out of fear of hurting your partner is poisonous to relationships because it creates emotional distance, says Vaughan. Both men and women do it all the time. It's a way of rationalizing one's unwillingness to devote the time and energy to deal with the complexity of honest communication.

Faking orgasm is one example. "Women do this like crazy out of consideration for their partners and it's one of the huge barriers to really good sex," Vaughan says. "When you are strong enough to expose yourself and make yourself vulnerable, you show your partner the real you." The benefits of such honesty can be life-altering, according to Vaughan:

- It fosters a deeper level of intimacy that leads to a more lasting trust. Vaughan calls trust the most important element for love and good sex.

- It allows your relationship to keep pace with the changes occurring in each of you.

- Honesty also keeps channels of communication open and provides constant challenges that can be used for growth.

- It allows each of you to know yourselves at ever-deeper levels and use all of your resources to build the best relationship possible.

No lie.

Learn His Language

The things that make you feel loved (long walks and talks?) can be very different from what makes your partner feel loved (more oohs and ahhs?). Marriage counselor and best-selling author Gary Chapman says couples often speak different emotional love languages ... as different as Chinese is from English. "No matter how hard you try to express love in English, if your spouse understands only Chinese, you will never understand how to love each other."

Chapman went through 12 years of notes from his counseling sessions and identified five types of emotional languages: Quality Time, Words of Affirmation, Receiving Gifts, Acts of Service, and Physical Touch. They formed the basis for his book *The Five Love Languages,* which has sold more than 6 million copies. "One reason couples argue so much is that they don't feel loved," says Chapman. "And that makes their differences seem so much bigger."

If you feel most loved when he helps you around the house (acts of service), and he feels most loved in bed (physical touch), then you both need to recognize those unique needs in order to achieve a better sex life.

"Love is intentional; it takes work," says Chapman. Start by doing some investigative reporting. Ask your spouse or partner what you do that makes him feel most loved. Or identify your personal love languages by taking Chapman's quiz together. Number the following in order of importance with "1" being what matters most.

— I feel especially loved when a person gives me undivided attention and spends time alone with me.

— I feel especially loved when someone expresses how grateful they are for me, and the simple things I do.

— I feel especially loved by someone who brings me gifts and other tangible expressions of love.

— I feel especially loved when someone pitches in to help me, perhaps by running errands, or taking on my household chores.

— I feel especially loved when a person expresses feelings for me through physical contact.

The statements capture the five types of emotional language; in order: Quality Time, Words of Affirmation, Receiving Gifts, Acts of Service, Physical Touch.

Numbers 1 and 2 are your personal primary and secondary love languages, respectively.

Spend the rest of the week talking and planning with your partner about ways to work toward meeting his and your own top two love needs. The results, Chapman promises, will be dramatic.

Put Sex on the Calendar

Busy couples must be intentional about sex or they will never get around to it. That means scheduling it. Sure, no one wants to schedule sex. After all, it's supposed to be spontaneous, motivated by the heat of the moment, right? Right. In the movies. In college. In your dreams. But not in the reality of today's world with two working partners and a houseful of kids and coaching your daughter's lacrosse team. That's reality. And if you don't have a game plan, you'll end up sitting on the bench. Couples who try carving out time for sex often find that they end up looking forward to it. And even if they are too busy to look forward to it, if they keep that special meeting on the calendar, they are so glad they did afterward. Sex therapists say that if you're in a loving relationship, if you sometimes go ahead with sex even when you don't think you're really in the mood, you'll end up wanting to have sex—and wanting it more often.

That last point dovetails with a new model of female sexual response that suggests for many women the desire to have sex kicks in only after they are in a comfortable place psychologically and are already physically aroused.

Conventional wisdom, based on a model developed by Masters and Johnson in the late '60s, is that desire precedes sexual arousal. That fits men pretty well, but it just doesn't do it for women, according to some sex experts who say that women don't get biologically turned on until much later in the sequence of a sexual encounter. They need to begin with feelings of well-being and emotional closeness, according to Rosemary Basson, MD, a psychiatrist at the Center for Sexual Medicine at the University of British Columbia. The Basson model of female sexual arousal is circuitous with physical drive appearing about two-thirds around the circle.

"The female sexual response is more complex than a man's, requiring motivation and a series of other events including willingness, explains Brooke Seal, PhD, a behavioral therapist in Vancouver. "It helps for women and men to know that it's okay to start sex without desire. It's about putting all those other things in place then the desire will likely come."

Scheduling a time for sex can be an effective strategy because it replaces burning desire as a practical motivator. "If a woman feels comfortable, happy, and loved in a relationship, the Basson model suggests that once you get busy with stimulation, arousal will trigger a hefty dose of "take me right now" desire.

SEX RULES!

Old Rule: Don't Have Sex if You're Not in the Mood
New Rule: Getting Busy Gets You in the Mood

"The whole idea that you have to be in the mood for sex is a fallacy," says Sandra Leiblum, PhD, author of *Getting the Sex You Want: A Woman's Guide to Becoming Proud, Passionate, and Pleased in Bed*. Women often think that to have sex, the stars need to align—it has to be the right moment in just the right place, and they need to be crazy turned on. But fooling around often is the very thing that triggers desire. The act of hooking up pumps out oxytocin—the bonding and attachment chemical—and testosterone, which boosts arousal.

Start Foreplay at 6:30 a.m.

Building on yesterday's concept of planning sex, be intentional about foreplay, too. "To a man foreplay is just the three minutes before insertion," says psychiatrist Louanne Brizendine, MD, author of *The Male Brain: A Breakthrough Understanding of How Men and Boys Think* and *The Female Brain*. "But for a woman foreplay is everything that happens 24 hours before sex."

In other words, getting in the right frame of mind for great sex takes all day long communication, sending frequent signals that say, "I'm thinking about you," "I want to get close to you." Dozens of little things you can do to and for your partner will encourage him to think of you in a positive, romantic way that can trigger desire on a hormonal level. Besides, anticipating sex is sometimes even hotter than the act itself. Try a few of these:
Start the day with a long embrace.
A 20-second hug releases the hormone oxytocin, which produces feelings of trust and attachment, according to researchers at the University of Virgina.

Holding hands triggers it, too.

Send a dirty text message. Slip a note underneath the windshield wiper of your partner's car saying, "I can wait to get my hands all over you tonight." Send a daring text like "Wet4U." A Nielsen survey a few years back found that more than 67 percent of unmarried texters use text messaging to flirt, so why don't you involved people give it a try. Send a daring text like "2Nite0underwear." "Come up with a creative subject line for the e-mail that will make your guy stop in his tracks like … "I'm touching my … " or "You've got me wanting to … " says Yvonne K. Fulbright, author of *Sultry Sexy Talk to Seduce Any Lover: Lust-Inducing Lingo and Titillating Tactics for Maximizing Your Pleasure*. "Use the first line of your text to complete your sexy subject line."

◼ SEX RULES!

Old Rule: Say "I Love You" Every Day

New Rule: Verbalizing Feelings Should be More Than Just a Habit

Mumbling those three little words through mouthfuls of cornflakes every morning or tossing them at the end of every phone call dilutes their importance and impact. To keep them meaningful: Say "I love you" only when you are really feeling it. Better yet, say it in new and interesting ways. For example, try a compliment ("You are seriously

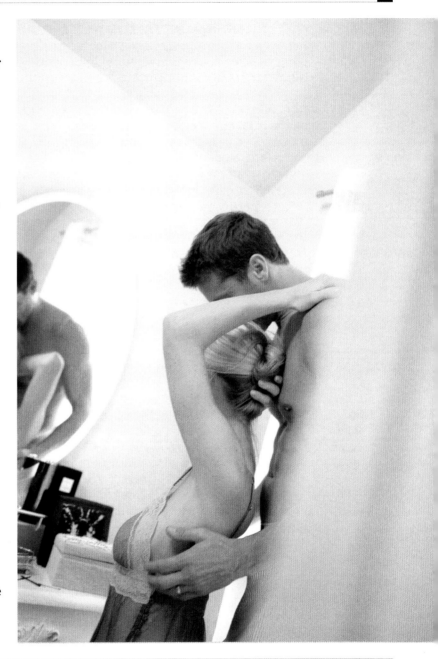

the greatest husband on earth"), a term of endearment ("Honey" or "Babe"), or a statement of appreciation ("It was so thoughtful of you to wash the kitchen floor last night.") They all send the same message of affection without becoming rote.

Schedule a Change of Venue

Your home probably has five or more rooms—a dining room, kitchen, bathroom, living room, heck some even have a home theater room, a rec room, a mudroom. But no dedicated sex room. Not even a sex nook. So why do we feel compelled to have sex in just one place—the bedroom? Why not utilize all 3,000 square feet of that two-story suburban colonial, and the cabana by the pool?

Living room: Have sex on the living room coffee table the night before a party at your house and see if that doesn't bring a naughty smile to his face during hors d'oeuvres.

Laundry: Suggest some oral sex while you're sitting on the edge of the Maytag.

Bathroom: Make use of the mirror and steam things up. Allow him to enter you from behind while holding onto the sink in front of the mirror. The unusual eye-contact during the G-spot-targeting doggy-style creates instant intimacy.

The stairs: He sits on the stairs facing the railing with one leg braced two steps down and the other leg slightly bent. You lower yourself onto him facing the rail and holding it for support.

On the sofa: Straddle the arm of the couch facedown and grind your vagina on the arm as he enters you from behind.

Outdoors: Eighty percent of surveyed *Men's Health* and *Women's Health* readers said they would love to try outdoor sex. "There's something incredibly raw and primal about having sex outside. It awakens the senses," says Gardos. You'll feel the cool breeze on your naked skin, smell the sweet peonies and Aphrodite hostas, hear the crickets, the screech owls, and the neighbors stopping by for a visit. "The fear of getting caught can add to the thrill," says Gardos.

Be Assertive, Not Insertive

Men feel intimate as a result of being sexual; women feel sexual as a result of being intimate. Man or woman, if you can understand the profound truth in that statement, you will be well on your way to building a more romantic and engaging intimacy.

"A lot of women come into the clinic complaining of low libido," says sexual health expert Laura Berman, PhD, founder of the Berman Center in Chicago and a *Women's Health* advisor. "They say they've lost the intimacy in their relationship. They want to cuddle with their guy but the second they do, he thinks it's an invitation for sex. Then the woman has to reject him because she's not in the mood and the whole process begins again. To break this cycle, explore VENIS: "very erotic non-insertive sex." This is sexual contact without penetration, where you focus on romantic, playful eroticism through verbal and physical communication. "It removes the pressure of goal-oriented sex, and as a result sex becomes less predictable and more pleasurable," says Berman.

What kind of activity qualifies as VENIS? It could be as tame as brushing each other's hair or as erotic as covering yourselves in oil and wrestling playfully. Try bathing together by candlelight, massage, licking whipped cream off of each other, cuddling in bed, or masturbating together. "The point is to have one night when intercourse isn't the focus," says Berman.

Have Morning Sex

There's no sweeter wakeup call. "Having sex in the morning releases the feel-good chemical oxytocin, which makes couples feel loving and bonded all day long," says Debby Herbenick, PhD, author of *Because It Feels Good*. Put a smile on both of your sleepy faces by starting the day off very right.

Take advantage of prime "T" time. Your guy's body is hardwired to want sex first thing in the morning. "While he sleeps, the testosterone he'll use for the upcoming day accumulates," says Gabrielle Lichterman, author of *28 Days: What Your Cycle Reveals About Your Love Life, Moods, And Potential*. "From the time he wakes up, he has a three-hour window when he's brimming with peak levels." Don't let them go to waste.

Rise and shag. Set your alarm to play soft music, and as soon as you're roused,

quietly slip out of your pj's. Then try this trick: If he's laying on his back, place your hands on his thighs with your thumbs pointing toward his genitals, suggests acupuncturist Alexis Arvidson. Move your thumbs in a slow, firm circular motion, 2 inches in diameter. According to the ancient teachings of acupuncture, rubbing this thin-skinned area will get the blood flowing straight to his nether regions.

Get fresh. Sneaking off to the bathroom to brush your teeth will do more than ward off dragon breath. The menthol in your toothpaste can give him a tingly thrill during oral sex.

Control Anger

Despite what they say about makeup sex, screaming matches are a poor foreplay choice. Learning how to control major outbursts of anger can go a long way to improving the health of your relationship—and making it hotter.

What gets us so angry? It almost always has to do with feeling disrespected by your partner. Disrespect is just a type of attack, and when we feel threatened and defensive our bodies react as if we are being mugged by a knife-wielding hoodlum, not the person whose bed we share. Your body releases the fight or flight hormones adrenaline and cortisol into your bloodstream and you become so pumped up with righteous indignation that you may explode and say or do foolish things that can be very hurtful to relationships and may take days, weeks, even years to mend.

RED-HOT MONOGAMY TIP

Women who fantasize during sex become more aroused, and they get there more quickly.

"A perceived injustice is a tasty looking bait on the fish hook of anger," says Robert Allan, PhD, a clinical psychologist and author of *Getting Control of Your Anger*. "It can be helpful to recognize reasons for anger as baited fishhooks and realize that when we bite, we lose our freedom."

What to do when you feel anger welling up inside you? Don't take the bait and let loose. "The emotionally intelligent fish swims on by the hooks," says Allan, an expert in cardiac psychology and stress management at Weill Cornell New York Presbyterian Hospital. "As the sixteenth century philosopher Montaigne said, 'there is no passion that so shakes the clarity of our judgment as anger.' Things truly seem different once we have quieted and cooled down."

Thomas Jefferson advised pausing 10 seconds before responding if you are angry, 100 if you are very angry. Not only can that strategy improve your love life; it may save your life. A large clinical trial for treating type-A behavior called the Recurrent Coronary Prevention Project, which reduced second heart attack rates by 44 percent, rated recognizing the hook of anger as the single most effective tool for controlling damaging outbursts.

"Anger management is like toilet training," says Allan, "something we should begin early in life before we get involved with someone."

While controlling outbursts of anger is a useful relationship skill, learning how to argue right is even more constructive.

"It's not the arguing that kills marriages; it's the arguing style," says John Gottman, PhD, the author of *Why Marriages Succeed or Fail: And How You Can Make Yours Last*. Make sure you have five positive interactions for every fight. Smart arguing can even make the heart grow fonder.

Studies have shown that partners can draw closer together during significant arguments when the volley is constructive and demonstrates how much each partner values the other's opinion. That result comes from choosing words carefully and understanding the art of negotiation. Consider a long-term investigation of 154 married couples reported in the journal *Psychology and Aging* that examined their conversation styles by monitoring physiological responses with heart rate monitors and video cameras. During arguments, the research found, couples who more often used the pronouns "we," "our," and "us" tended to be calmer and more emotionally positive than couples who used more individual pronouns such as "I," "me," and "you."

"This is our problem," is one of the most effective things you can say to your spouse in a conflict, according to Kenneth Silvestri, PhD, a psychotherapist in New Jersey. "It puts you on common ground."

Silvestri is all about achieving harmony, having practiced aikido for 20 years. He believes the martial art's principal of redirecting the energy of an attack through graceful blending

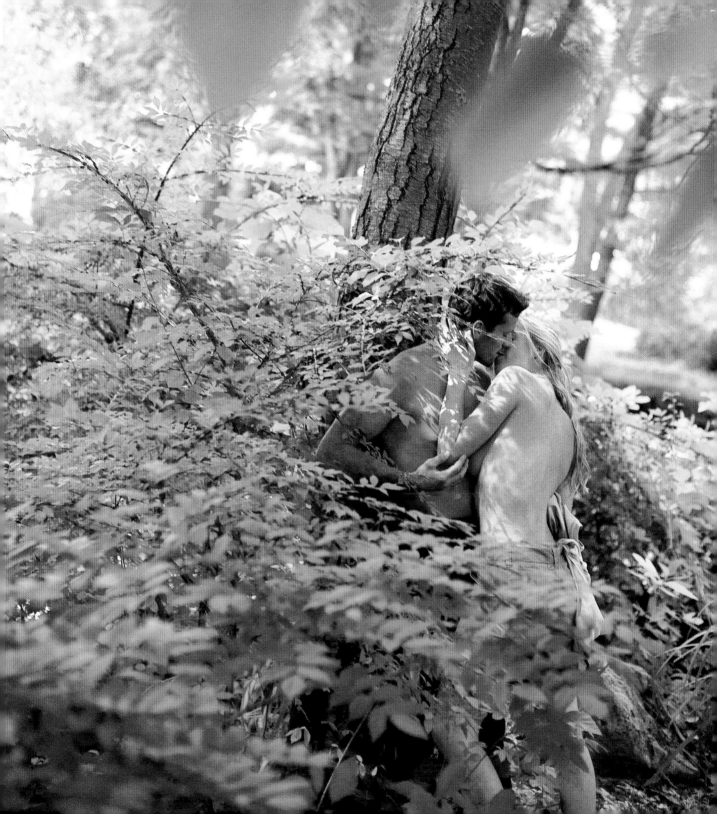

movements that bring your opponent into your range of influence is the ideal strategy for marital sparring.

"If you push hard against someone, they will push back just as hard. Aikido teaches that you must yield to win. In a marriage, backing down offers signs of appreciation for your partner's feelings. It creates a positive volley that leads to win-win," says Silvestri.

Enjoy a Quickie

As we're sure you already know, you can become aroused quickly under the right circumstances; you don't always need 10 or 20 minutes of foreplay to enjoy great sex. Believe it or not, scientific studies have documented this as well. One published in the *Journal of Sexual Medicine* found that if women ignore outside distractions (kids, TVs blaring, Blackberries humming) they can start to become aroused in just 30 seconds. So send the kids away to your sister's for the weekend and pounce on him when he least expects it (say, when he's frying eggs for breakfast or when he steps out of a shower after a workout). Quickies don't necessarily have to include intercourse. Pull him into an empty room at a party and cop a feel. Initiate a hot and heavy make out session before he goes off to work. He'll love your take-charge attitude. And quickie sex offers the added bonus of resurrecting the feelings of the early days of your courtship when you did it everywhere you had the opportunity.

Scare Your Pants Off

Take a kayaking course. Go rock climbing together. Ride a rollercoaster for better sex? Get risky then get frisky. "Trying something new or exciting before sex delivers a burst of dopamine, a chemical that activates the pleasure centers of your brain," says Gail Saltz, MD, author of *The Ripple Effect: How Better Sex Can Lead to a Better Life*. The brain chemical also influences attraction, as one study at the University of Texas at Austin demonstrated. Researchers from the Meston Sexual Psychophysiology Laboratory at the University of Texas in Austin visited a theme park and asked women there to rate the attractiveness of an average looking guy. They showed the women a photograph of the man and asked them to gauge how much they would like to kiss him or date him. Some women were questioned while standing in line for a roller coaster ride; others were questioned right after they got off the ride. It turned out that those who'd just come off the coaster, jacked on adrenaline, rated him as much more dateable and kissable than did the women who were still waiting in line.

Knead Each Other

Stand up. Look down. You will see a body part of amazing erotic ability just below waist level—your hands. Use them to massage your mate; a massage is romance you can both appreciate even if it doesn't lead to sex. Start with a good massage oil such as Neal's Yard

Remedies Ginger and Juniper Warming Oil ($15 for 1.7 fluid ounces, nealsyard-remedies.com) or Naturopathica Arnica Muscle and Joint Massage and Body Oil ($28 for 4 fluid ounces, naturopathica.com). Avoid mineral or baby oils because they are absorbed too quickly into the skin. Don't forget to rub your hands together to warm them before applying the massage oil and performing the following techniques:

1. Stroke toward the heart. That means when you're working on his legs, stroke upward. On the arms, stroke downward.

2. Ease with effleurage. The French are experts at more than retreating. They know their massage. Effleurage is a simple loosen-up stroke. Light, long, and rhythmic, it generally runs with the grain of the muscle. On the legs, for example, use your cupped palms and gently glide upward. On the back, flatten your hands and broaden your strokes.

3. Play with petrissage. This circular stroke is designed to squeeze the muscles and wring out tension from the shoulders, upper arms, legs, and buttocks. Use both hands to work the muscles in opposite directions: When stroking thighs, for example, move one palm away from you as you slide it forward, and move the other toward you.

4. Roll your thumbs. This is best for working on tension knots. Use your thumbs, one after the other, to press into the flesh, sometimes moving circularly and other times just holding pressure on one point. Lean your weight into it.

5. Be generous. Don't forget the body parts that rarely get touched, such as the backs of the arms and knees, feet, fingers, and scalp.

Watch an Erotic Film Together

Watching other people have sex—even viewing a hot scene in an R-rated flick—can trigger lusty thoughts about your partner and spice up your sex life especially when you view it together, say many sex therapists. And while more men watch porn than women do, many women do find that sexually explicit material is a way to satisfy their natural human curiosity about sex, how bodies look aroused, and what others do in bed.

A study by the University of Denver Center for Marital and Family Studies analyzed the association between viewing sexually explicit films and relationship quality in a random sample of 1,291 unmarried people in romantic relationships. While men tend to watch porn alone (77 percent), the study found that more women watch porn with their partners than by themselves (46 percent versus 32 percent). The researchers also looked at measures of communication, relationship strength, commitment, and sexual satisfaction. "We found that couples who view sexy movies together are more dedicated to each other and more sexually satisfied than those who watch them alone," says study author Amanda Maddox. The only difference between people who reported never watching erotica and those who view it only with their partners was that the porn teetotalers had lower rates of infidelity.

From a purely physiologic standpoint, women and men appear to be equally stimulated by porn. A 2006 study at McGill University found that both men and women started displaying arousal within 30 seconds of turning on the video player. But that doesn't mean cuing up *Edward Penishands* will be everyone's cup of tea. Tastes in erotica differ. And there are psychological downsides to weigh. Many men and women find porn terribly degrading to women and a huge turnoff. Some of you may feel threatened if your partner turns on a porn video (Am I not pretty enough? Am I not doing it right?). Watching porn can make both women and men feel inadequate. Remember, body image *can* have an impact on your sexual comfort level—so you have to make sure that you and your partner won't get too caught up in the body comparison and just sit back and enjoy the show.

So, before you hunt for porn websites or head to the adult video store, have a talk. Reassure him that you are happy with your relationship and sex life, but want to try something new for inspiration that you both can enjoy together. Talk about what kind of film you'd both like to see. After all, you wouldn't go to the multiplex without talking about it

first. Find videos that you both feel comfortable with. Women tend to be more aroused by films that have a good romantic plot that takes its sweet time to ease into the sex scenes, and includes a lot of foreplay. Fifty-six percent of women say seeing more regular or realistic-looking female bodies in films would make watching porn more enjoyable for them. So, look for films that use wide angles rather than genital close-ups, because full bodies (and faces in particular) help women identify with and feel like the turned-on women in the video. Those kinds of films tend to be made by women directors. Check out Pornmoviesforwomen.com for movies by Candida Royalle, Anna Span, and Annie Sprinkle. Or try Comstock Films, which features sex between actual couples. Also consider films like *The Elegant Spanking* or *Silken Sleeves* by Maria Beatty, which feature lesbian sex and look like 1920s noir films with slow, teasing sex scenes that women may find arousing.

Become a Stranger

If you're married, do you realize how different you became after you got married? Write down a list of 10 things you used to love to do before you got hitched. How many of those activities that made up your core being are you still doing? If you are like many people in long-term relationships, you've cut a big part of what made you feel vital—what attracted your partner to you in the first place—right out of your life. Why not fill up the tires on your old road bike? If you don't have the time to get back into tennis or the sense of adventure to start river running again, figure out something new to reinvent yourself. You'll immediately boost your attractiveness to your mate because the newness will tickle those areas of his brain that get off on novelty.

Men are typically better at this reinvention game than women are. That's why it's crucial for you to make an effort to explore your passions and elicit his help in accommodating your schedule.

"Women voluntarily make more sacrifices and accommodations in a marriage, especially if there are children," says Vaughan. "Eventually that can fester into resentment toward her husband, who she sees as being self-centered." The key is to make him aware of that danger, establish equitable duties in house and family, and explain that having the freedom to reinvent yourself is very important to you and your marriage.

SEX RULES!

Old Rule: The Sex Gets Better Over Time
New Rule: The Sex Gets Better Over Time—If You Help it Get Better

"As couples get to know each other's bodies, there's a reliability in sexual response," says Yvonne K. Fulbright, PhD, *Women's Health* columnist and author. Familiarity also can breed a deeper intimacy and greater willingness to explore new territory together—two things that are sure to keep you both extremely satisfied for years to come.

Employ Some Toys

Bringing a sex toy to bed with you can often crank up the heat of sex. Don't worry: most guys won't be intimidated and will find it an incredible turn on. Studies by researchers at the Center for Sexual Health Promotion at University of Indiana found that 53 percent of American women and 45 percent of men have used vibrators during sex, and that those who used them reported more positive sexual function and satisfaction.

Here are some of the most popular sex toys for women:

The classic dildo. Most women first focus these male stand-ins on their clitoris, penetrating only as climax nears, says Lisa Lawless, PhD, cofounder of the National Association for Sexual Awareness and Empowerment.

The G-spot stimulator. These instruments of pleasure target the spongy, sensitive area in the upper vaginal wall, 2 inches from the opening.

The Rabbit vibrator. With two vibrating petals shaped like a set of hare's ears, this Bugs-inspired toy rubs both sides of the clitoris.

The classic vibrator. This multispeed massager lets you focus on your most nerve-rich erogenous spot, the clitoris, while slowly increasing the intensity.

5 Common Marriage Problems Solved

Based on discussions with more than a thousand couples over the years, renowned marriage researcher John Gottman, PhD, has pinpointed the most common marriage problems. If you're married, you'll no doubt recognize many of these snags. But what may surprise you is how easily they can be untangled.

PROBLEM: In-Laws

The cause: Trouble usually originates between the wife and her husband's mother. Why? Gottman says it's usually because both women are competing for the attention of the husband.

The cure: Solidarity is essential to the success of a marriage, so you both must present a united front. Husband must side with his wife in any disagreement—even if she's wrong. Mom must understand that her son is a husband first, son second.

PROBLEM: Money

The cause: Newlyweds especially don't know how to balance the freedom and power that money brings with the security and trust that it's supposed to foster.

The cure: Plan as a financial team. Decide your goals as a couple (home, college for the kids, cars, vacation home, retirement) and review them regularly. Open a joint bank account to manage these areas and deposit 90 percent of your paycheck there. Then open individual checking accounts for the remaining 10 percent of pay. This is personal money that you can spend however the account owner wants. No questions asked.

PROBLEM: Housework

The cause: Having a husband creates an extra 7 hours a week of housework for women, while a wife saves a man an hour of housework per week, according to a University of Michigan study of a nationally representative sample of US families.

The problem lies within that disparity. Wives feel unsupported when their husbands don't pitch in with the dusting, vacuuming, dish and clothes washing— and putting away all that stuff they just washed. Men model the behavior they grew up with. If they were raised in traditional homes where the father did the hard labor and never lifted a can of Pledge, they handle garbage detail and lawn mowing and think that they've done their part.

The cure: Tell your guy how important it is to you that he pitches in around the house. Then dangle this carrot: Gottman's research shows that when husbands do their share to maintain the home, the couple reports a more satisfying sex life. We bet he makes a beeline for the Mop and Glow.

PROBLEM: Kids

The cause: Women bear the lion's share of the childcare work, which may be why 70 percent of women report being significantly less satisfied with their marriages after baby arrives.

The cure: Wake up to reality; the carefree life you used to enjoy is over. The two of you won't be going out spontaneously for happy hour Mojitos for at least 14 years. The two of you need to share the responsibility of feeding, changing, and bathing, not just the family fun time. You can flip to determine who will empty the Diaper Genie.

PROBLEM: Sex

The cause: Three months after that passionate honeymoon, you realized that your sexual desires are not as blissfully matched as you had thought. Because sex is such a difficult thing to discuss, frequent lustful advances can become annoying, unfulfilled desires perceived as rejection.

The cure: Trust is the best foreplay. It frees you to be open and honest about your feelings and desires without fear of embarrassment or hurt. Talk openly and frequently about your emotional needs and sexual desires. Make it a game: each writes five secret desires (sexual or otherwise).

A Month of Amazing Sex

LEARN HOW YOUR MENSTRUAL CYCLE CAN AFFECT YOUR LIBIDO IN INCREDIBLY HOT WAYS

Why you have sex, how often you orgasm, and how wild you are when you're tempted to get in bed all depend in part on where you are in your menstrual cycle. "When women hear the word menstrual, they tend to think of cramps and discomfort," says Gina Ogden, PhD, author of *The Return of Desire*. "But the hormones that influence your cycle—estrogen, testosterone, and progesterone—fluctuate each day and affect your sexual behavior in dramatic ways." And although every woman is different, knowing what changes your body is going through can help you plan for a month of unbelievable sex.

DAY 1

Take control during sex.
On the first day of your period you'll feel extroverted and bold, thanks to a rise in the feel-good hormones oxytocin, testosterone, and estrogen. Your libido should be amped, too, so aim for all the pleasure you can. Woman-on-top is ideal because your clitoris is extra sensitive and you can control the depth and angle while he lies back and enjoys the view. If things get messy, throw a towel on the bed or take a shower before you get busy.

DAY 2

Indulge in slow, sensual sex.
You're feeling good, because estrogen and testosterone continue to rise today. "Estrogen magnifies the five senses, so kisses feel more intense and your man looks more attractive to you, making sex a total mind-body experience," says Gabrielle Lichterman, author of *28 Days: What Your Cycle Reveals About Your Love Life, Moods, and Potential*. Light some candles, play slow tunes, and satisfy each other from head to toe.

DAY 3

Pamper him. "A surge in testosterone boosts your confidence in your union and makes any annoying habits your partner may have seem less grating," Lichterman says. So treat him to a spine-tingling massage. There's no doubt he'll return the favor.

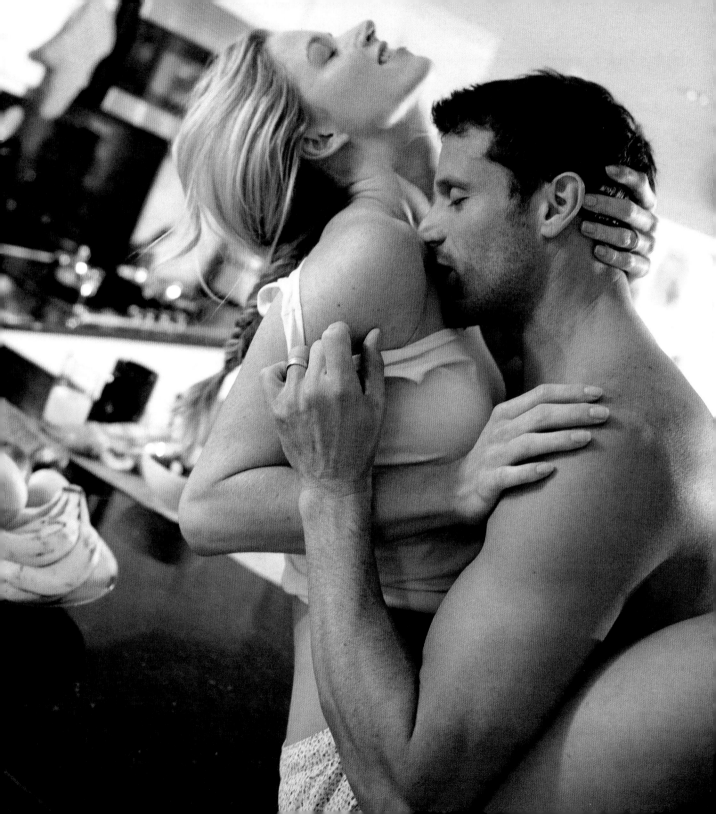

Make Lust Last | HERS

DAY 4

Think outside the box. Your right brain is famous for giving you creative ideas, and today tiny levels of rising estrogen and testosterone boost the odds you'll use this side of your mind. "You're apt to feel more imaginative when it comes to brainstorming or making decisions," Lichterman says. Your creativity will spill into the bedroom, too.

DAY 5

Get competitive. Today estrogen and testosterone will increase even more. Testosterone makes you competitive. Use that bold streak to challenge him to a naughty game, such as strip poker. If you win, so does your libido: According to a study published in the journal *Evolution and Human Behavior,* conquering a guy elevates your testosterone levels by 49 percent, making you even more amorous.

DAY 6

Bond with your guy. By now, you should be feeling calm, rational, and remarkably clear-headed. "Estrogen gets another boost, making you social and articulate," says Jed Diamond, PhD, author of *The Irritable Male Syndrome.* So take advantage of your way with words and tell your guy exactly why you love him. He'll eat it up.

DAY 7

Sync up your sex drives. You're still chatty due to elevated estrogen levels, and as an added perk, "your energy will skyrocket," Lichterman says. Since guys are often raring to go in the morning (their testosterone levels peak in the a.m.), take advantage of your extra adrenaline and hop in the shower.

Day 8

Have a quickie. Many women refrain (unnecessarily) from having sex until their periods are finished. Make up for lost time by getting busy in the middle of the afternoon, or pull him into an empty room during a party for some instant action.

DAY 9–14

Fixate on him. You'll start getting a big boost of estrogen and testosterone during these 6 days, making you especially flirty. Your voice even becomes higher pitched during this time, according to research conducted by the University of California, Los Angeles. Because back in caveman days, choices in men were limited, and once ovulation occurred, women needed a coy way to snag a man during the final push. One potential problem: You may also have a wandering eye. Scientists say women fantasize about other men 160 percent more midcycle—yet the study authors found that women initiate sex with their partners a lot more during this time, too.

DAYS 15–16

Stay connected. Welcome to Pre-PMS (think PMS but shorter and less intense). Rising levels of noradrenalin and declining levels of testosterone and estrogen may make you irritated and jealous when your guy drools over Scarlett Johansson. It's biological: During days 12 through 21, women are super catty when it comes to judging the appearances of other women. "Evolutionarily speaking, when fertile women were competing for a mate, criticizing other females may have helped catch him," says lead study author Maryanne Fisher, PhD, professor of psychology at Saint Mary's University in Halifax, Nova Scotia. Tune out other women by holing up together with takeout and a bottle of wine.

DAY 17

Have solo sex. In order to combat the dip in estrogen and testosterone and the rise in progesterone, you'll need to take matters into your own hands. "Your clitoris and nipples may be less sensitive now, and orgasms are slower to occur and weaker," Diamond says. Let him watch you masturbate: he'll get off on the visuals, and you'll be turned on by his gaze. According to Marta Meana, PhD, a professor of psychology at the University of Nevada, Las Vegas, women can become aroused when they're the object of desire.

DAY 18

Cuddle up. A boost in proges- terone still has you feeling more cuddly than carnal, so unplug your BlackBerry, snuggle down with your guy, and rent a chick flick.

DAYS 19–20

Take a break. "For these two days, your urge to nest and unwind may be stronger because progesterone levels jump, damping your desire to socialize," Lichterman says. Why is progesterone such a downer? According to Lichterman, it drains your energy, lowering the risk that you'll go out and damage your uterus in case fertiliza- tion has occurred.

DAY 21

Cook a romantic meal. You may find yourself wandering into the kitchen more than usual right now. Progesterone has caused an appetite spike, making you crave baked goods, salty treats, fats, and carbs. The reason: Your hormones want your body to be baby- ready in case you got pregnant during ovulation.

DAY 22

Tweak the usual positions. You may have to work a little harder to orgasm today because progesterone is blocking your testosterone receptors. So try this surefire way to stimulate your G-spot, says Sandor Gar- dos, PhD. "Start by straddling your guy while you face his feet. Once you're comfortable, lean back so you're lying flat on top of him." Then enjoy the ride.

DAYS 23–24

Set the mood. That inevitable time of moderate misery has come: PMS. Declining levels of progesterone and estrogen from days 23 through 28 can make you weepy—or bitchy. If you're not feeling psyched about your body right now (bloat can do that to a girl), wear your hottest lingerie, dim the lights, or do whatever it takes to

feel sexy. Just don't get a bikini wax. Researchers at the University of Michigan found that women are extra sensitive to pain at this time of the month.

DAY 25

Focus on your O. Chances are, you're feeling frisky. "One reason is that your endometrium (the lining of the uterus) is thickening, promoting blood flow to your genitals, which boosts libido," says Suzanne Gilberg-Lenz, MD, an OB-GYN based in Los Angeles. And although your orgasms should be intense, it may take longer than usual to get there because a decline in estrogen and testosterone will leave you easily distracted by your surroundings. Try a little dirty talk to stay in the moment.

DAYS 26–28

Conquer new territory. Your boobs may ache (tell your guy hands off today), but "your endometrium continues to thicken, stimulating your nerve endings down below, which in- creases your libido significantly," Lichterman says. Since creativ- ity is at an all-time high, it's the perfect time to discover new erogenous zones. Experiment with various types of touch on your favorite body parts.

80

Percentage of divorced men and women say their marriages broke up because they gradually grew apart. Only about 20 percent of couples say an extramarital affair was even partially to blame.

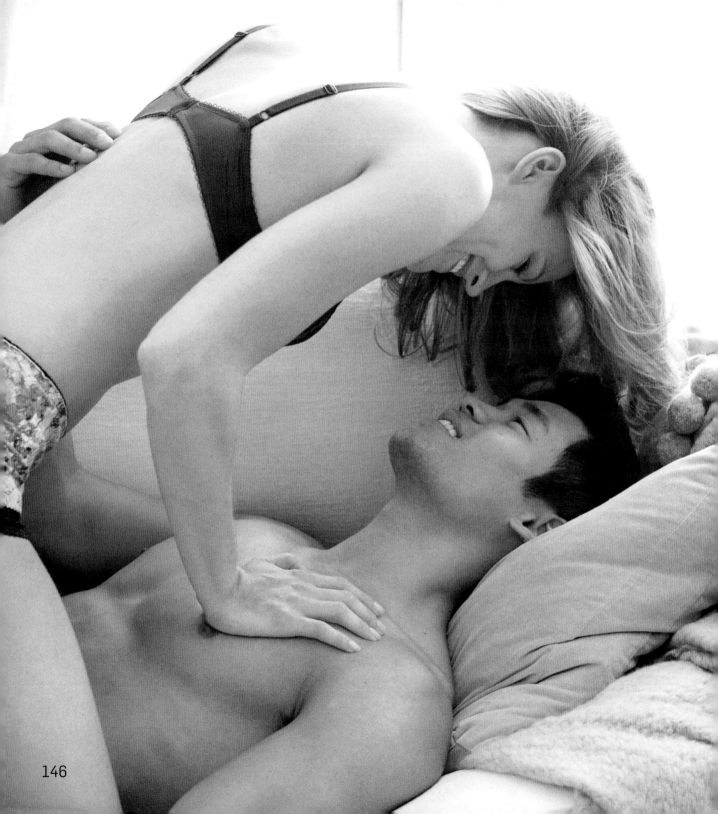

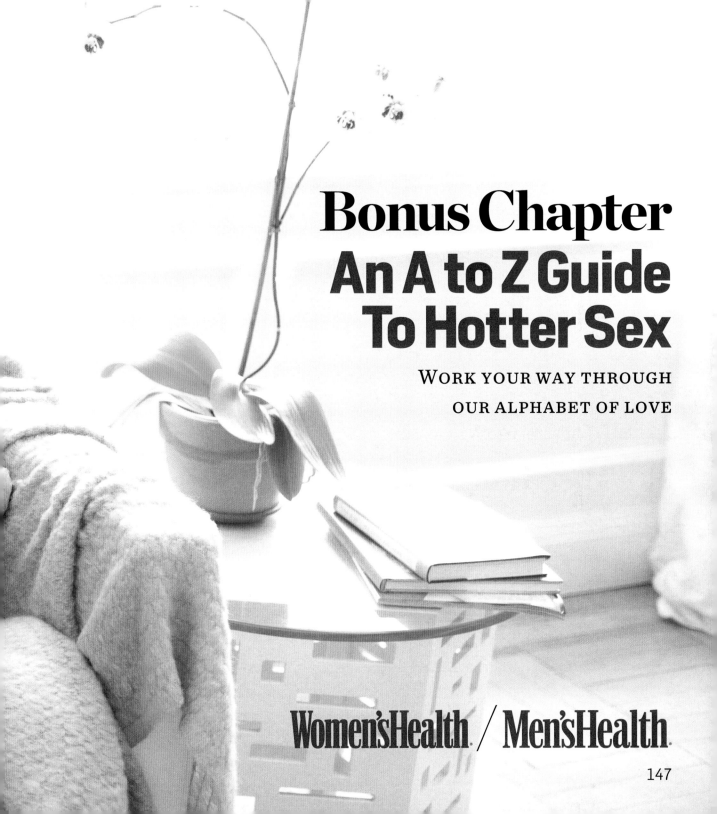

Bonus Chapter
An A to Z Guide To Hotter Sex

WORK YOUR WAY THROUGH
OUR ALPHABET OF LOVE

Women'sHealth / **Men'sHealth**

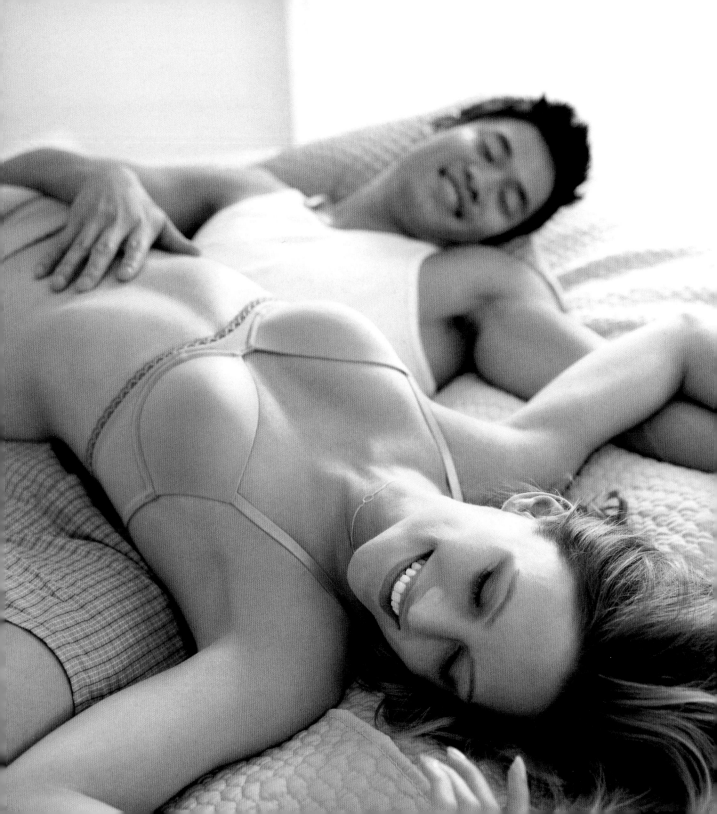

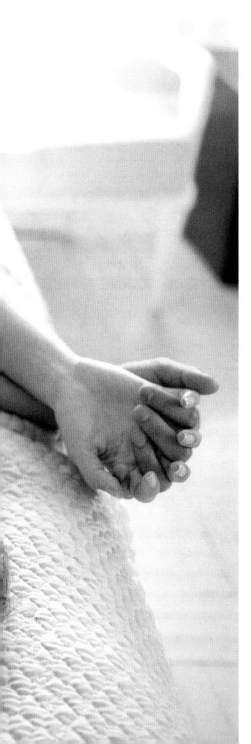

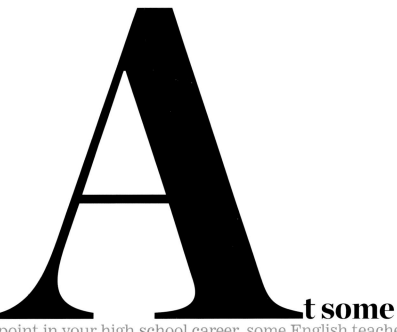

At some

point in your high school career, some English teacher probably forced you to read *The Scarlet Letter*. So you're already familiar with the concept of this chapter: that along the 26-point sequence of the alphabet there are many, many sexual touchstones, and not all of them are "XXX." In fact, once you've covered the ABCs of sex—from the part of the brain that can interfere with orgasm (it starts with A) to the essential mineral a man depletes with every climax (yep, that one starts with Z)—you may have a greater understanding of the wonders of the human body, as well as the human mind. And we guarantee the next few pages will be quite a bit easier to read than Nathaniel Hawthorne ever was!

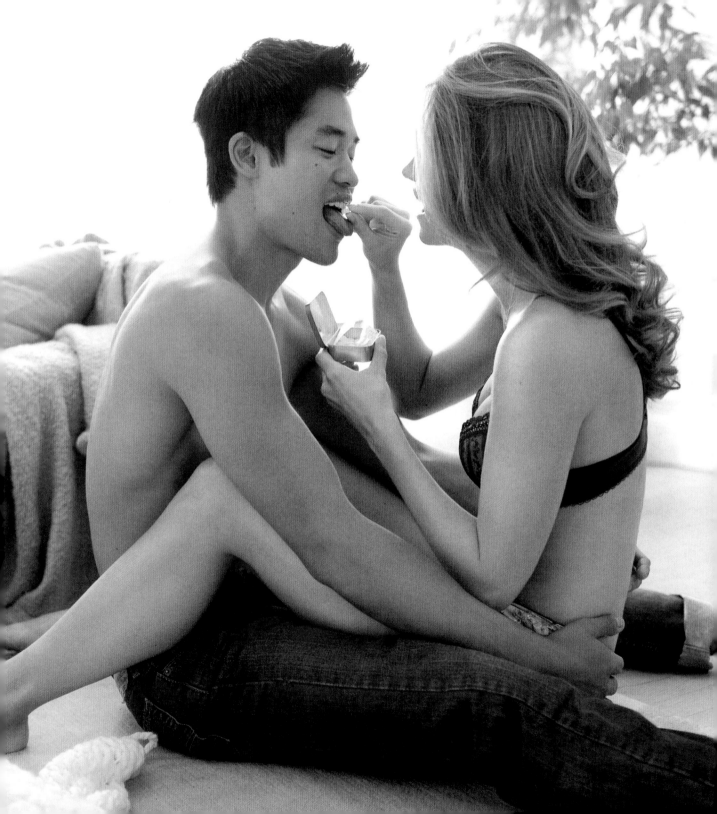

Amygdala

Almond-shaped structures deep in the brain that control the emotional processing system of fear and anxiety. In order to become aroused, you (women especially) need to power down the amygdala and relax, shelving the worries and obsessive thoughts of the day. One of the best ways to do that is to draw a steamy bath about an hour before having intercourse to calm your nerves. Listening to your favorite soothing music while in the bath helps, too. Studies have shown that hearing music you know by heart triggers a deep relaxing physiological response.

Around the World

A sex sequence in the woman-on-top position that stimulates multiple areas of his and her genitalia. She straddles him, facing him, and squeezes her PC muscles around his shaft without any up and down movement. Then she begins moving up and down the shaft for nine shallow thrusts and one deep thrust.

Next, she turns around so her back is to him and she's facing his feet, and she repeats the squeezing and thrusting sequence. Finally, she returns to facing him and squeezes while riding rhythmically up and down on his penis.

Assertiveness

Being more sexually assertive in a loving way can make your partner feel desired and needed—a big turn on for her, and especially for him—if you are normally passive about sex. "Women are traditionally more submissive, so switching to a more dominant role can break you out of a sex rut," says clinical sexologist Ian Kerner, PhD. "You don't have to don leather and wield a whip; just doing something your partner doesn't expect—like initiating sex as soon as he walks in the door—will make things hotter." Need something a bit tamer to start off with? Then try talking about sex. Recent studies have found that women who talk about sex with their partners have an easier time achieving orgasm and are more satisfied with their relationships than those who keep quiet.

A-Spot

Short for Anterior Fornix Erogenous (AFE) zone, this is a sensitive area located midway between a woman's cervix and G-spot on the front wall of the vagina. Stroking this highly sensitive spongy area causes almost immediate lubrication. To reach it, insert a lubed finger into the vagina as far as it will comfortably go. Rub gently using the length of the finger. You'll know you're there when she starts to get wet. Now triple the sensation: insert both index and middle finger and stick out your thumb. It'll pull your fingers more snugly against the vaginal walls, stimulating both A-spot and G-spot simultaneously.

Altoid

Spice up oral sex by sucking on an extra-strength mint lozenge before you stroll down below.

Anal Play

The practice of anal sex has been around for centuries, and today it is more common among heterosexuals than one might think. Many couples find it to be highly enjoyable, partly because the area near the rectum is a sensory-rich venue with loads of nerve endings close to the surface. Sexual contact can be limited to the outer area or involve penetration of the anus with the penis. The stimulation can also come from a finger, sex toy, or tongue. Most people have an opinion of anal sex, but the only one that matters is yours and your partner's. First step before entering new territory: discuss this with your partner, enjoy bathing as foreplay, and venture behind slowly and safely. Analingus can transmit hepatitis or other infections so health experts recommend using a latex barrier, such as a dental dam or a condom cut in half. Recognize that unlike the vagina, the anus doesn't self-lubricate so you'll want to use a water-based lubricant. Many health professionals urge people to put a condom over the finger, toy, or penis and add lubricant over the condom before inserting it into a partner's anus to reduce risk of cuts.

Balance Ball

That big bouncy stability ball (also called a Swiss ball) on which you do your abs exercises can be put to sexier uses. Sit on it for oral sex. Lie on it to sample different positions. Be creative.

Bed, Breakfast In

Push the raisin bran aside and serve smoked salmon, scrambled eggs, strawberries and Champagne. Why? "Salmon prolongs arousal as it's high in arginine, the amino acid the body uses to create nitric oxide," says Dr. Sara Shenker of the British Nutrition foundation. "The more NO in the body, the firmer the male organ becomes and the more lubricated the woman's organs. Alcohol (in moderation) can boost the release of dopamine, which is essential for sexual pleasure." The eggs are an excellent source of low-in-saturated-fat protein, keeping you satisfied without weighing you down. Top it off with feeding each other strawberries.

Blindfold

Blocking out one of the senses, such as sight, heightens sensitivity of the others to compensate. Plus, when you can't see what will happen next, the anticipation can be pretty exciting. Try the padded leather blindfold from MyPleasure.com. Can't wait for FedEx? Then cover his or her eyes with the shirt you were just wearing. "Your natural scent is a huge aphrodisiac," says Sharon Moalem, PhD, author of *How Sex Works*.

Body Confidence

Your sex drive and self-esteem work in tandem to bring you sexual satisfaction, according to research conducted by Tina Penhollow, PhD, a professor of exercise science and health promotion at Florida Atlantic University. "When women accept their bodies as-is, they feel more relaxed during sex, making them more willing to experiment, which paves the way for more orgasms." Boost self-assurance by:

Eating healthy food. Your body will feel better and your psyche will feel empowered by your taking control.

Exercising. Try activities that focus on fun and skill yet have a body-shaping payoff, such as swimming, cycling, or volleyball.

Taking care of details. By attending to the finer points— fresh nail polish, smooth legs, a well-fitting bra—you send the message to yourself and others that your body is worth the effort.

Body Image

Body image correlates with how inhibited people feel in bed, and that's especially true for women. Couples can improve

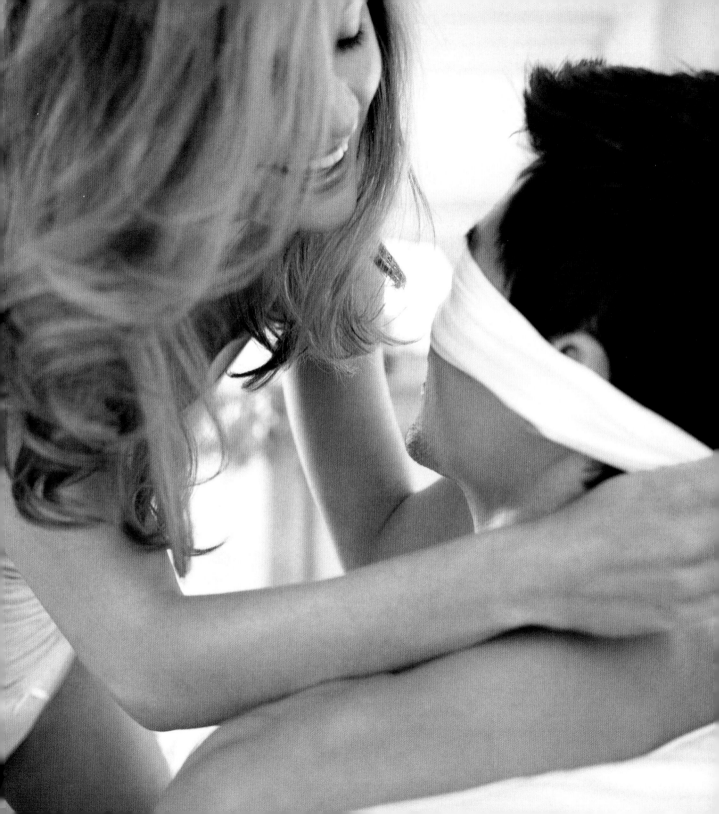

An A to Z Guide to Hotter Sex

their sex lives simply by exercising together and becoming more comfortable with how their bodies look and feel through physical activity. Men can help their partners feel more confident in their bodies by praising their partner's most guarded body parts. *The Big Book of Sex* survey found that women want to be complimented on their butt, breasts, and legs and that they felt most self-conscious about their tummies. "Women spend their lives trying to look good for men," says Rutgers University anthropologist Helen Fisher, PhD, the chief scientific advisor for Chemistry.com. "So a woman who feels she's sending the right visual signals is pleased with herself." The very best time for a "nice butt" shout-out is when there's no chance that you'll be having sex soon, like when your walking together down the street on the way to the gym. "It's a gift to compliment her outside the bedroom," says Fisher.

Booty Call

More than a one-night stand but not exactly a relationship, this low-commitment sexual relationship fills a sociological niche as a compromise between men's and women's ideal mating strategies, according

to researchers from New Mexico State University and the University of Texas at Austin. For men that means seeking numerous sexual partners with minimal investment in time and energy; for women, it's seeking longer-term relationships. The survey of undergrads found that the two top reasons for agreeing to a rendezvous were physical attractiveness and sense of timing.

Brazilian

A bikini waxing that involves the removal of a woman's pubic hair with wax. Often, a "landing strip" of hair is left in front. Women who do this receive more oral sex, according to Debby Herbenick, PhD, research scientist at Indiana University and author of *Because It Feels Good*.

"It may be that women who crave oral sex groom themselves in anticipation of it," she says. "Many feel more comfortable receiving oral sex when there is little or no hair to get in the way." But pubic hair can actually make the area more sensitive to the touch. "Some people find that having a bit of hair to gently tug on feels very sensual and enhances sensation."

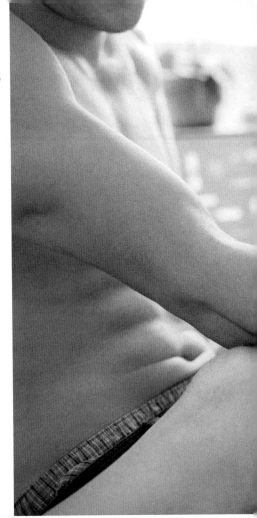

Clitoral Complex

Not that new office park in Bethesda, it's a new spot of vaginal pleasure recently identified by the scientists who look into these things. You know about the G-spot, a couple of inches

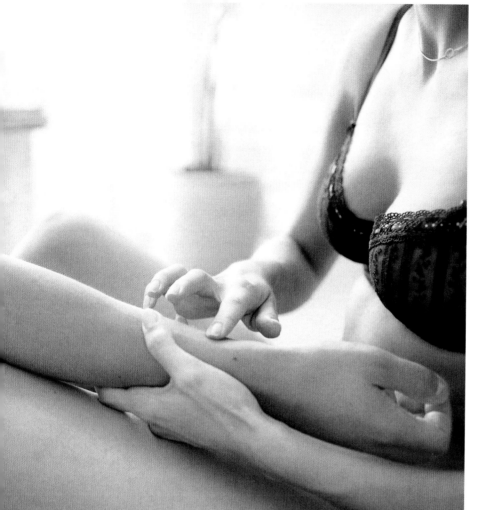

a second—they send signals to the limbic system, an area of the brain associated with trust and affection.

Churning

Refers to a number of variations on a thrusting technique in which he holds the base of his penis and turns it in circles inside her vagina as if churning butter. Another version involves holding the shaft of his penis and rubbing his glands over her clitoris until she is on the verge of orgasm. Just before her point of no return, he penetrates her.

Cock Ring

Also known as a constriction device, it's usually made of an elastic material that acts as a mild tourniquet to slow blood flow out of the penis and help men achieve a wider, stronger, and longer erection—which then intensifies orgasm. It can be worn around the base of the penis or stretched over the testicles to rest between the scrotum and the body. A word of caution: testicle cuffs and cock rings should be removed within 20 minutes or so. Falling asleep while wearing one can cause numbness, priaprism, or even penile gangrene.

inside the front of the vagina? Well, French researchers may have found out why touching that spot feels so darn good: you may actually be stimulating the root of the clitoris through the vaginal wall. Reporting in the *Journal of Sexual Medicine,* the scientists say ultrasound tests revealed that the clitoris is really a "clitoral complex," not just the small bud you can see. It also extends along the sides of the vulva, which explains why exterior stimulation can be so arousing.

C-Tactile Nerve Fibers

The body is brimming with these pleasurable nerves, especially on the forearms. British researchers say that when these nerves are stroked just right—with the light pressure of a painter's brushstroke, at 1 to 10 centimeters

Condoms, the Best

Sex researchers at the Kinsey Institute asked 30 couples to test a slew of different condoms. Their results can help you find the right one for you and your partner.

Best all-around
TROJAN ULTRA RIBBED ECSTASY

More than a third of participants rated it as their favorite. It's shaped like a baseball bat (to allow more movement inside), lubricated inside and out, and has two sets of ribs. Testers said it flexed well, the lube was long-lasting, and the women loved the ribs.
Rated high for: comfort, fun
Rated low for: natural feel

Best for her pleasure
TROJAN HER PLEASURE ECSTASY

It's shaped like a slim light bulb, ribbed at the base, and covered in lube—all designed, Trojan says, for enhancing female pleasure. The condom's roominess made some guys worry it had fallen off. But the women said it felt great.
Rated high for: her pleasure
Rated low for: natural feel, increased sensation

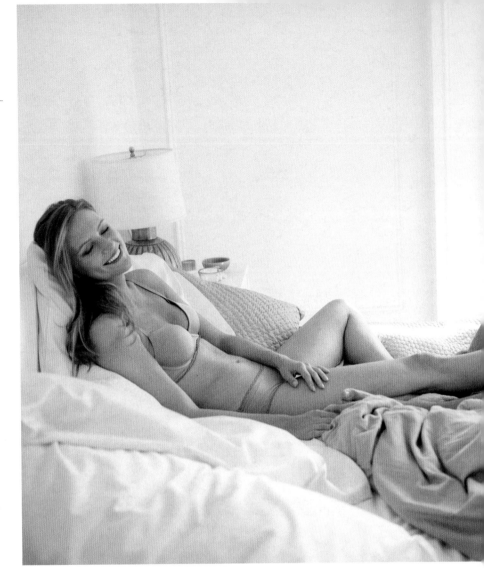

Best for his pleasure
LIFESTYLES X2

It's lubed inside and out and contains L-arginine, a natural supplement the company says heightens sensation during sex.
Rated high for: increased sensation, comfort
Rated low for: lasting longer, natural feel

Most comfortable
LIFESTYLES SKYN

It's made from polyisoprene, which is marketed as softer and more flexible than latex.
Rated high for: comfort, natural feel
Rated low for: increased pleasure, lasting longer

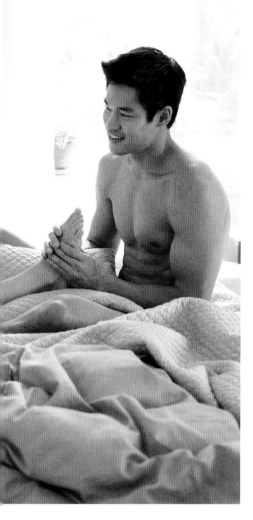

for both feeling natural and helping to maintain an erection.
Rated high for: comfort
Rated low for: her pleasure

Most surprising
INSPIRAL

Its large, spiral-shaped head twists and turns during sex, creating friction. Testers said it's a "corkscrewlike action" that "felt like a completely different experience."
Rated high for: fun
Rated low for: ability to maintain an erection, natural feel

Cunnilingus

At most, only 43 percent of women can climax through intercourse alone; most also need direct clitoral stimulation, as evidenced by the fact that it takes women an average of only four to six minutes to climax when they masturbate and 10 to 20 during intercourse. Assure your partner that going down on her turns you on, and consider the virtue of the flat, still tongue, which she can move against to climax.

Most natural feel
DUREX EXTRA SENSITIVE

The company describes it as "super thin" and says it's shaped to be sleek and feel less like a condom. Testers confirmed it: "It felt very close to sex without a condom," one wrote. It was also the only condom testers said was best

Double Protection

Using two forms of birth control may make sex twice as good. The Kinsey Institute found that women who use a hormonal contraceptive plus condoms report higher overall sexual satisfaction. Researchers believe that when women are less worried about pregnancy and STIs, they can relax and enjoy themselves more.

Emotional Intelligence

Women who are in touch with their feelings as well as sensitive to others are two and a half times as likely to orgasm as women who aren't as emotionally intelligent.

Erotic Literature

Sneak over to the erotica section of the bookstore. Purchase a few copies and reenact some particularly literary scenes. Check out *Heat Wave: Sizzling Sex Stories* by Alison Tyler, *The Black Lace Series* by Kerri Sharp, *Seducing the Highlander* by Emma Wildes, and *Do Not Disturb: Hotel Sex Stories* edited by Rachel Kramer Bussel.

Fantasizing

Surveys suggest that men fantasize about sexual encounters about twice as often as women do. But it can be one of the most effective ways for women to tune in to a sexual experience, says Kerner, because it helps "turn off the parts of [the] brain associated with stress and anxiety." (See amygdala.) In fact, fantasizing is powerful enough to trigger orgasms in some women. In a study, Beverly Whipple, PhD, co-author of *The Science of Orgasm,* along with colleagues Gena Ogden, PhD and Barry Komisaruk, PhD, monitored the blood pressure, heart rate, pupil diameters, and pain tolerance of 10 women who claimed they could think their

way to climax. As the subjects fantasized in a lab, seven exhibited the exact physical responses caused by hands-on stimulation. Encouraging your partner to fantasize may be difficult; a study by the University of Vermont shows that nearly 25 percent of people feel guilty about their fantasies. One way to plant the idea of fantasizing in his or her mind is to tell your partner you had a wild dream about him or her, then play coy. Make your partner pry it out of you. You may spark some interest and learn that he or she has had fantasies, too. Presenting your fantasies as a dream avoids making your partner feel as if he or she isn't satisfying you.

Foot Rub

When you massage the arches of his or her feet, you stimulate about 30 inches due north. "The foot-sensation area of the brain is right next door to the clitoral and penile region," says Daniel G. Amen, MD, author of *The Brain in Love.*

How To Give Good Foot:

1. Place a pillow on your lap and cover it with a hand towel. Rest his or her right foot on the pillow. Slide your palm under and support the heel with one hand. Use your other hand to gently rotate her foot, three times clockwise and three times counterclockwise. This increases flexibility and blood flow, says certified massage therapist Michelle Ebbin.

2. Return the foot to your lap. Now put a dollop of moisturizer (unscented Lubriderm works great) on each of your thumbs before placing them at the center of the arch. Apply light pressure and rub silver-dollar-sized circles with your right thumb moving clockwise and your left counterclockwise. Do this for 30 seconds.

3. Move on to the toes. Use your thumb and index finger to lightly squeeze each toe beginning with the big one and ending with the pinkie toe. Then use just your thumb to make small clockwise circles beneath each toe for 10 seconds moving from pinky up to big toe.

4. Starting at the ball of the foot, make circles with your thumbs (right clockwise, left counterclockwise) and move down, adding pressure as you near the heel. Finish up by using your thumb and middle finger to gently squeeze the hollow area below the ankle for about 10 seconds. This is the ultimate erogenous zone, says Ebbin. Repeat all the steps with the left foot.

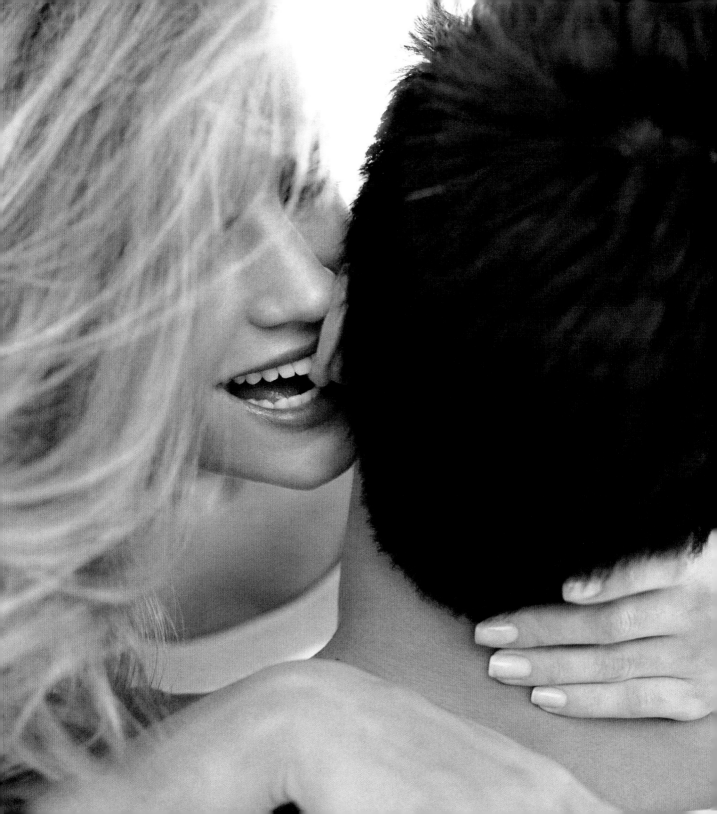

Flibanserin
(the so-called female Viagra drug)

A drug originally designed as an antidepressant that some small studies showed may help some premenopausal women suffering from low sexual desire or hypo-active sexual desire disorder (HSDD). An FDA panel of experts decided that the benefits of the pill, from German pharmaceutical company Boehringer Ingelheim, did not outweigh the side effects, which included fatigue, depression, and fainting spells.

Forefinger

While he's inside you, insert one of your forefingers alongside his penis. This will help you achieve that fuller feeling you're after. And he will enjoy the extra texture to rub against.

Fleshlight

A masturbation sleeve for men shaped like one of those Maglites mall security guards carry around. Instead of a bulb, it's fitted with a rubbery pink "skin" that resembles the lips of a vagina.

Flirt

Just like you did when you first met. "Pretending you don't know each other well at a crowded party ups the excitement factor,"

says Yvonne K. Fulbright, PhD, author of *Touch Me There! A Hands-On Guide to Your Orgasmic Hot Spots*. Here's proof: A study at the University of Chicago found that when pairs exchanged flirty banter for just 5 minutes, the men got a 30 percent boost in testosterone, making them feel more amorous.

Games

Most sex games are cheesier than a Kraft Foods convention. But, with the right attitude, you might find that makes them all the more fun.

Classic: Bumps and Grinds. Drinking and stripping board game for two to six players, circa 1967.

Free: Check out Adultsexygames.com for free downloadable games that you can play with your partner. Try Romantic Dares, where you take turns flipping over virtual cards on screen with sex tasks for you to complete.

Couples: Hearts are Wild (available from tootimid.com): a love adventure game for two that comes with game board, card decks, cinnamon massage oil, blindfold, and feather tickler. Secret Agent (available from babeland.com): you write down a sex secret and lock it in a box. If your partner wants to know it, he or she uses ribbons and satin to "torture" you with light bondage until you give in.

Hand-Job

Stimulating a man to orgasm using only your hand is a pleasure that only seems to happen at the beginning of a relationship before couples get to the penetration stage. Why not bring the hand-job back as part of foreplay or as the main event? Some ideas on how to give a guy a hand from Tracey Cox, author of *Secrets of a Supersexpert* (remember to lube first!):

The Blow-Up Doll: Interlock your fingers like a basket leaving a hole between your thumbs and fingers like a tight vagina. Keeping a firm grip on his penis inside, move your hand up and down.

The Big Squeeze: Clasp one hand firmly around his hard erection at the top of the shaft. Your fingers should be nudged up against the corona of the head. Squeeze firmly for a second, then release and repeat. It'll give him a completely different sensation than the typical sliding-hand technique.

The Boy Scout: Build a fire by friction! Just as a Scout rolls a stick between his hands to start a fire without a match in the woods, place your palms on either side of your partner's penis and use a rolling motion. Start at the bottom and slide up the shaft, then down again as you roll, keeping a consistent rhythm. Start slowly, then increase speed and pressure as he nears climax.

Hummer

A mouth move in which she puts his testicles in her mouth and hums like a human vibrator.

IUD

Only 2 percent of American women use an intrauterine device for birth control, but of those 99 percent report being satisfied. A recent poll of OB-GYNs suggests that it's their birth control method of choice. Among the reasons: it's more foolproof than the pill, with a failure rate of less than 1 percent. The pill is only 92 to 95 percent effective with typical, not perfect, use.

Joy of Sex, The

First published in 1972 by British gerontologist Alex Comfort, MD, PhD, *The Joy of Sex: A Gourmet Guide to Lovemaking,* is a landmark sex book known for its erotic sketches of sexual positions.

Kama Sutra

Probably the oldest and most widely read sex book, the *Kama Sutra* was written sometime around the fifth century by the Indian slave Vatsyayana. Kama refers to the ancient responsibilities of men in their roles as heads of households: pleasure and love. Sutra, loosely translated, means teachings. Old though it may be, the *Kama Sutra* is far from dated—with a few notable exceptions. One is the advice for men on how to keep women from going astray: Sprinkle a potion made of monkey dung on her head. The most famous part of the book, however, the extensive collection of sexual positions, is still right on point. Here's one example: The Tight Position: The woman lifts her legs up and crosses them while he is inside her, causing her vagina to squeeze around his penis. You and your partner might want to pick up a copy to sample some ancient Indian lovin' techniques.

Kissing, Advanced

Add novelty. Lightly suck and nibble her lower lip while she softly kisses your upper lip, then switch. It's a move William Cane calls "lip-o-suction" in his book *The Art of Kissing.*

Balm's away. Swipe mint lip balm on your kisser before planting one on him. "Menthol triggers the body's cold receptors, and when that's combined with your warm breath, you'll feel a tingly sensation from your lips straight down to your genitals," says sexologist Ava Cadell.

Play vampire. Kiss the throat. The neck is one of the most ticklish spots on the body, so exploring different degrees of sensation can be tantalizing. And softly kissing and licking it will feel like erotic torture.

Sweeten the deal. Eat a strawberry before making out. The sugar activates the sweetness receptors in your mouth, so when you kiss your sense of taste will go into overdrive, says Krista Bloom, PhD, author of *The Ultimate Compatibility Quiz.*

Try facial intercourse. This smooch mimics sex from foreplay to penetration, beginning with a tongue exploration inside the mouth. "Rub your tongues together in small and large circles, then dart them in and out of your mouths as if you were having intercourse," says Cadell.

Kegel Exercises

Named after doctor Arnold Kegel, these exercises target your pubococcygeus or PC muscle. These are the same muscles men and women tighten to stop the flow of urine. Exercising them can improve sexual function and enhance orgasm. To learn how, see pages 21 and 61.

K-Y Jelly

The grandmamma of sex lubricants, it was originally designed to ease entry of your doctor's finger for prostate and gynecological exams. It's available in drugstores and supermarkets, and since it's water soluble, it won't break down a condom like petroleum-based lubes do. (See lubricants.) The granddaughter of K-Y J might be K-Y Intense Arousal Gel For Her. Its pleasing warm sensation increases blood flow and skin sensitivity down there.

Loyalty

Loyalty to your partner is crucial to a solid relationship. If there are conflicting loyalties to parents, siblings, or children you'll begin to weaken your bond as a couple and tread the slippery slope of side-taking. Experts in marriage and step-family counseling agree that creating the most stable marriage requires putting the needs of your partner and relationship above those of your kids and step-kids.

Lubricants

Thanks to good marketing, personal lubricants have finally shed their medicinal reputation and are now considered a sex kit essential. They can help make intercourse more comfortable for a woman and reduce friction for a man, helping him to last longer. *Women's Health* contributors tested a box of popular brands and chose these favorites:

Best for sex toys
HYDRA SMOOTH
Creamy, water-based formula won't damage silicone sex toys. Compatible with condoms, unlike oil-based lubes. Glycerin-free to avoid irritation.

Best for marathon sessions
PINK LUBE
Silicone formula lasts as long as you do and never gets sticky, unlike water-based lubes. The hand-blown, Italian glass bottle hides its naughty side.

Best for speedy arousal
DUREX PLAY O AND K-Y INTENSE
These lubes encourage blood flow to the clitoris, which results in warming and tingling sensations.

Best for oral sex
ID JUICY LUBE COOL MINT
Its minty freshness stimulates nerve endings and hides latex taste. Comes in 12 water-based flavors. Passion fruit, mmmm.

Best for watery play
UBERLUBE
Silicone-based lube won't wash away in the bathtub or shower. And the flavorless formula won't shock anyone's tastebuds. Use liberally with its easy-access pump dispenser.

Best for masturbation
GOOD LUBRICATIONS CREAM LUBRICANT
Its thick, creamy texture keeps things slick.

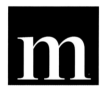

Masturbation
The more often people masturbate, the more often they have sex. "It's a surprising correlation," says Rutgers University anthropologist Helen Fisher, PhD, author of *Why We Love*. "It's probably because sexual arousal elevates testosterone and dopamine, and that can lead to more sex."

Other experts believe that people who masturbate regularly are likely to be better lovers because they know what pleases them most. Surveys suggest that 20 percent of women and 40 percent of men masturbate once a week. *The Big Book of Sex* survey found that 69 percent of female respondents reported masturbating one or more times a week (26 percent said "several times a week"), while 89 percent of men said they masturbate one or more times a week (46 percent said "several times a week").

Ménage a Trois
A French phrase that translates into "household of three," and describes a living arrangement between a married couple and an extra man or woman who has a sexual relationship with one of the spouses. But it more commonly refers to a threesome, which has become a favorite fantasy of many men and women and has also become a pop-culture cliché. But it's more often talked about than acted out. The Kinsey Institute says only about 3 percent of married men and 1 percent of married women have had sex with another partner while with the spouse. And most of those people said they only did it

once. If you're thinking of proposing a ménage a trios to your partner, consider his or her potential response. It could make your partner think, "What's wrong with me? Am I not good enough on my own?" Or, "You selfish creep." Tread carefully in this emotional space and have serious discussions before acting to avoid any morning-after regrets.

Mirrors
Double your viewing pleasure during sex by strategically placing a large mirror near the bed to catch the flickers of candlelight and your bodies in motion. Seeing yourselves engaged in the act will heighten your arousal. Another move to reflect upon: Place a full-length mirror in front of the bed and have him sit on the edge of the bed facing it. Straddle him from behind, wrapping your legs over his and pressing your mound into his butt and your breasts against his back. Now reach around with a lubed hand and stroke his erection. You'll enjoy the unexpected view of his intense orgasm.

Outercourse

This is sex without penetration, and it can be incredibly hot. In fact, many women find that because the focus of the friction is on the clitoris, they can orgasm quicker and more often through outercourse than intercourse.

How-to: Apply a water-based lubricant liberally to the head and shaft of the penis and the labia and clitoris. In one popular version, the woman lies on her back and keeps her legs together, spreading her well-lubed inner thighs just enough for her partner, on top, to slide his erect penis between them and her lips. She can now squeeze her lips to tighten her grip on his penis as he thrusts and stimulates her clitoris with his moving shaft. From this position, try various circular motions, and grinding thrusts to create a massage for the clitoris and head of the penis. If there's ejaculation, sperm may still be able to enter the vagina, so protection is needed. By the same token, avoid STIs by practicing safe sex.

Pillows

Missionary, from behind, spoon, almost any position can be enhanced with a few strategically placed pillows. By elevating your hips with a pillow or two, you can alter the angle of his penetration and hit a good spot he may not otherwise reach. You might also try angling pillows like the Liberator (liberator.com) and other types of sex furniture. They'll make your moves easier and more comfortable.

Prostate

The prostate is a male reproductive organ that produces the white liquid that becomes part of semen. About the size and shape of a walnut, the prostate wraps around the urethra and is found in front of the rectum, just under the bladder. When a man is sexually excited, the prostate responds to stimulation; it's similar to the G-spot in women. Many men find prostate massage via the anus with a lubed finger extremely pleasurable. You can put a condom gently over your finger, lube up, and insert it about two inches into his anus, curving the finger toward the belly to reach the prostate. If you're not ready for anal play, gently push up against his perineum with your hand. This is a non-insertive way to arouse his prostate.

Positive Statements

There's power in being positive about your relationship. When discussing problems, couples in a happy marriage make at least five times as many positive statements to and about each other as negative statements, according to research by John Gottman, PhD, founder of the Gottman Institute. Other research shows that couples who use positive words like "happy" and "great" in text messaging are more likely to stay together longer than partners who use sarcasm and downer words. Also, future-oriented phrases like "Looking forward to tonight" or "Can't wait to see you" help partners feel connected and valued.

Pumpkin Pie

Put one in the oven. The scent of it baking can be arousing to men. Likewise for lavendar, according to studies at the Smell and Taste Treatment and Research Foundation in Chicago. Researchers say the combo of scents increased blood flow to the penis by 40 percent in one study.

Risky Sex

Having sex at the risk of being observed or getting caught is very exciting for couples that have a touch of exhibitionism in them. If it doesn't harm anyone physically or emotionally, we don't see anything wrong with what you're doing. (Just be discreet when there are kids around.) The problem is that many other risky sexual behaviors can and do hurt people. At the risk of stating the obvious, when it comes to sex, we hope you will enjoy yourself, respect one another's wishes, and do no harm.

Role Playing

"Part of enjoying tantalizing sex is experiencing a level of escape," says Scott Haltzman, MD, an assistant professor of psychiatry at Brown University and the author of *The Secrets of Happily Married Men.* "Role playing interweaves well with the natural tendency to dissociate from the daily demands of life." It can help both partners experience more liberation between the sheets because you can put yourselves mentally in a different, more

exciting place. In an online poll, *Men's Health* asked 4,000 women and men what role-playing scenarios they'd consider trying. Top play-acting pairs included: employee and female boss; athlete and cheerleader; strangers in a bar; and rich man and French maid. If dressing up like a French maid and a baron is too hilarious for your taste, start off slowly, and give yourself permission to laugh. Many couples find the meeting-at-a-bar scenario easy enough and still exciting. First, agree that neither of you will be offended by anything you do or say while in character. Then, go to a bar or nightclub, entering 15 minutes apart. Mingle and find each other, acting out the pickup scene as complete strangers each in a new persona. You might agree on a code word to signal when it's time to end the game. Or just say, "Okay, that's enough." If role playing comes from a place of love and trust, there are few downsides, say sex therapists. Adopting an alter ego for a night can be a comfortable way for couples to explore their sexuality from behind masks. Often the roles people enjoy most are the ones that are most different from their normal lives.

Rough Sex

Being dominated is a common female fantasy. "That doesn't mean rape, but it does involve the man using a certain amount of force," says Brian Zamboni, PhD, a clinical psychologist and sex therapist at the University of Minnesota Medical School. In a caring relationship founded on communication and trust, couples can be free to explore such fantasies safely. Zamboni suggests combining assertiveness with tenderness and having a mutual understanding of expectations. During more aggressive sex, have a code word that means, "Stop. Too much."

Sensate Touch

A series of exercises designed to increase trust and arousal without touching each other's genitals. **How-to:** get naked, then take 10-minute turns playing giver and receiver. The giver applies stimulation—rubs, light touches, kisses—everywhere but the genitals. Try to focus on how you feel touching him or her. Then switch positions and have your partner touch you. Sensate touch can help you to slow down sex and teach total-body foreplay.

Shower Sex

Think safe sex first: make sure to use a bath mat for grip so you won't slip. Have him step into the shower first to make sure the water temperature is just right. Soap yourself up, then reach around and give him a genital massage. Press your body against his and massage your mound on his buns. Then turn him around and bring his hands to your sudsy breasts if he hasn't beaten you to it. Then turn around and brace yourself against the tiles as you bend forward to offer him rear entry. He can hold onto your waist for balance (bend your knees so you don't strain your legs). Splish, splash. Warm water may wash away your natural lubrication so you may want to bring a silicone-based lubricant into the shower with you.

Sox, Sexy Love

These socks are a cheat sheet for an erotic foot massage. Slip them on your partner's feet and follow the tips printed on the undersides, which show pressure points and pictures of the erogenous zones they stimulate. Find them sexylovesox.com.

Spanking

A love tap on the butt can increase the bond between couples, according to researchers at Northern Illinois University. Plus, women get a jolt of testosterone when they are on the receiving end, but men don't, according to researchers at the University of Pisa in Italy. In *The Big Book of Sex* survey, 77 percent of women respondents and 40 percent of men said they'd enjoy a couple of butt slaps on occasion.

Sports

Physical, competitive sports can boost testosterone levels in women as well as men. The male hormone is associated with sex drive in both genders, but because women have less of it, they actually get a bigger lift than men do from competition, according to researchers from Penn State University.

Sweat

After your workout, skip the shower and attack your man. Don't worry about your sweaty skin and scent. Most men will find it all highly arousing. Have your way with him. He won't complain.

Tahitian Method

An oral sex technique in which he lies perpendicular to her body, and moves his tongue back and forth over the hood of her clitoris, stimulating both sides of the clit. By resting a finger on her perineum, just below her vagina, he can feel involuntary contractions that'll offer clues when he's doing the tongue work properly.

Talking Dirty

Surveys show that more than half of Americans believe that a bit of raunchy sex talk during intercourse or leading up to it is a stimulating practice for a healthy sexual relationship. Most people who haven't tried it before say they are shy about it and think they'll sound silly. If you're hesitant, you may want to experiment with a suggestive email to your partner or some dirty talk over the phone. Removing the face-to-face aspect makes it easier for some people to open up. Sex experts also suggest that partners write two side-by-side lists naming sexual parts and sex acts, one clinically proper, the other using dirty words. Exchange lists and discuss which are uncomfortable and which are mutually arousing.

Tantric Sex

Tantra is a 2,000-year-old Hindu spiritual doctrine that has developed worldwide into a modern system whose followers practice sexual exercises to gain a spiritual connection and deeper sexual satisfaction with their partner. Sex as a spiritual act was popularized in the West in recent years by singer Sting, who claimed in an interview to have used the tantric sex techniques to have sex for 6 hours. Practitioners of tantric sex don't allow themselves to climax, believing that the semen they reserve gives them greater energy and increased sexual vitality. One sexual practice of tantra that you and you partner can sample is simply using a ratio of nine shallow thrusts for one deep penetration during sex.

Testicles

Their primary duty is to pump out sperm cells, but they also produce the male hormone testosterone. Many men enjoy having them caressed gently. The seam (that dark line down the center of the scrotum) is rich in sensitive nerves.

Thumbs Up

Gentlemen, bring your thumb into foreplay with your index finger. Insert your index into her vagina, then press your thumb against her frenulum, the area just below the clitoral head, and massage. Next, rotate your thumb to the six o'clock position and lightly touch her perineum, the area below her vagina and just above her anus, to "oohs" and "ahhs" of delight.

V Technique

This is a good move for adding clitoral stimulation during masturbation or intercourse. Either one of you can perform it. Form a V with your index and middle fingers and slide them, fingertips pointing down, over the outer labia. As you draw your fingers up and down to stimulate the inner clitoris you'll be drawing the clitoral hood lightly up and down as well, which will also stimulate the outside clitoris, says Tracey Cox.

Vacation Sex

"Couples tend to have more explosive sex on vacation, because without the stressors of the daily grind—a major libido killer—they can really focus on their relationship," says Gilda Carle, PhD, author of *99 Prescriptions for Fidelity*. "After all that undivided attention, you'll feel closer because you'll remember why you fell in love in the first place." Can't get away for the weekend because family is visiting? Then let them stay at your place and you take the hotel room.

Vaginal Squeeze

This is just a variation of the Kegel using a finger or dildo for resistance. Lie on you back or sit on the edge of a chair and insert two lubricated fingers or a dildo into your vagina. Squeeze your PC muscle. You'll feel a contraction of the walls of your vagina about an inch from the opening. Do as many as you can. Now, if using fingers, spread them into a peace sign and see if you can force your fingers together by contracting your PC muscle.

An A to Z Guide to Hotter Sex

Vibrators, the Best

Women who use vibrators are more likely to report higher levels of desire, arousal, lubrication, and orgasm than those who don't, according to a recent study. Men who use vibrators during sex also reported better sexual functioning. Of those women who use vibrators, 46 percent use them during masturbation, 41 for foreplay, and 37 percent during intercourse. These are some top-performing models worth taking for a spin:

Best mini
NEA
Petite but powerful, this vibrator's sleek curves hug all the essential girl parts. Just three inches long, it has a rechargeable ion battery that delivers seven hours of bliss ($89, lelo.com).

Best maxi
DOC JOHNSON LUCID DREAM VIBRATOR: NO.14
Control the buzz level with a quick turn of the dial; no wires to get tangled up in. Made of bendy jelly rubber, it provides Mary Lou Retton-esque flexibility to target every hot spot ($29.99, drugstore.com).

Best ring
THE ICONIC RING
Disposable vibrating cock rings—for hand-free vibration—have become very popular. This battery-operated one is reusable, offers dual vibration modes, is waterproof, and is backed by a 1-year warranty ($35, jimmyjane.com).

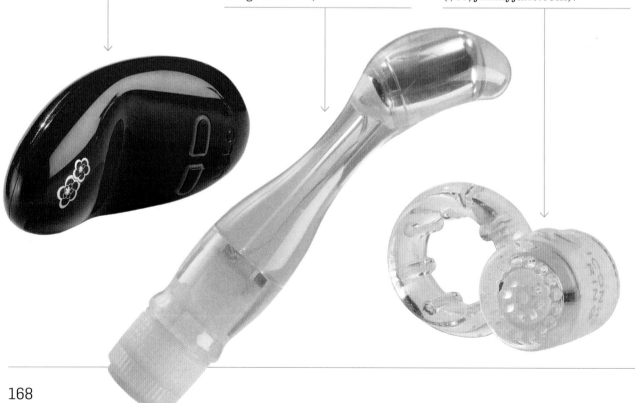

Best bath toy
THE SCREAMING OCTOPUS
This device has textured tentacle tips that vibrate with moderate intensity for under-water arousal (three for $16.96, thescreamingo.com).

Quietest
LITTLE GOLD
Whisper-quiet so you won't tip off those in the adjoining room, this 24K gold vibrator delivers a sophisticated and elegant buzz. Made of dishwasher-safe medical-grade stainless steel, it can be used in the bath or shower. The Little Gold is 5.25 inches long and 0.67 inches in diameter. Its motor is replaceable should you happen to burn it out with use ($325, jimmyjane.com).

Most accurate
FORM 3
This palm-fitting vibrator has a small touch pad for directing the vibrations with finger point precision. It follows the Form 2, which won a design award for its cool look and dual vibrating "ears" ($145 and $135, respectively, jimmyjane.com).

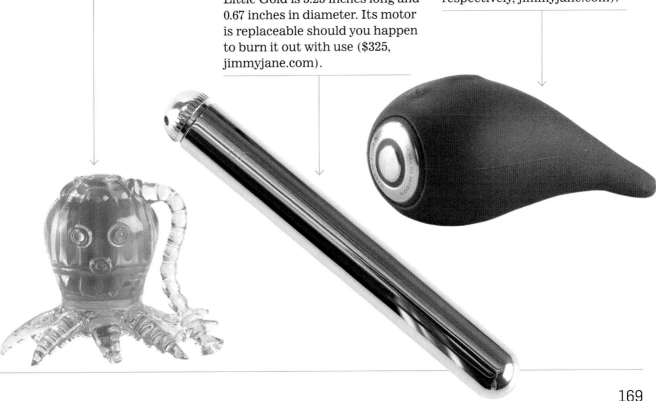

An A to Z Guide to Hotter Sex | OURS

We-Vibe II

The first vibrator that can be used during intercourse. Inserted into the vagina, the U-shaped device stimulates her clitoris and G-spot simultaneously—and is narrow enough to allow her partner in ($99, babeland.com).

Xandria Collection

One of the oldest adult product catalogs offering vibrators, exotic lotions and lubricants, massage products, books, and videos (Xandria.com). Other top online catalogs for sex toys include Babeland (babeland.com), Good Vibrations (goodvibes.com), Jimmyjane (jimmyjane.com), Eve's Garden (evesgarden.com), and MyPleasure.com.

Yab-Yum

Not a new candy, but a tantric position. She faces you sitting on your lap with a pillow under her bottom for easier penetration. The position affords constant penis-clitoris contact, but she controls the pressure. Move slowly. The emotional connection created makes Yab-Yum intense, says Lou Paget, a sex educator and author in Los Angeles. (See Tantric Sex.)

Yohimbine

A pharmaceutical that some clinical studies have shown helps improve erections in up to a third of men suffering from ED. It is derived from the African yohimbe tree whose bark has been used for centuries in tea form as a love potion for its erection-enhancing benefits. Yohimbine supplements are available in nutrition and health food stories in many different potencies. A word of caution: These supplements are not regulated by the U.S. Food and Drug Administration and it is still unclear if the stuff works or how it does so when it is effective. Because yohimbine produces stimulant effects and may boost blood pressure and heart rate, it is not recommended for people with heart problems, hypertension, or diabetes. To be safe, ask your doctor about yohimbine hydochloride. He or she will be able to adjust the dosage and monitor your progress and any side effects you may experience.

Zinc

Healthy levels of this mineral boost sex drive and support good sexual function. Make sure your multivitamin is fortified with zinc. Also, eat zinc-rich foods such as oysters, crab, wheat germ, chickpeas, and steak.

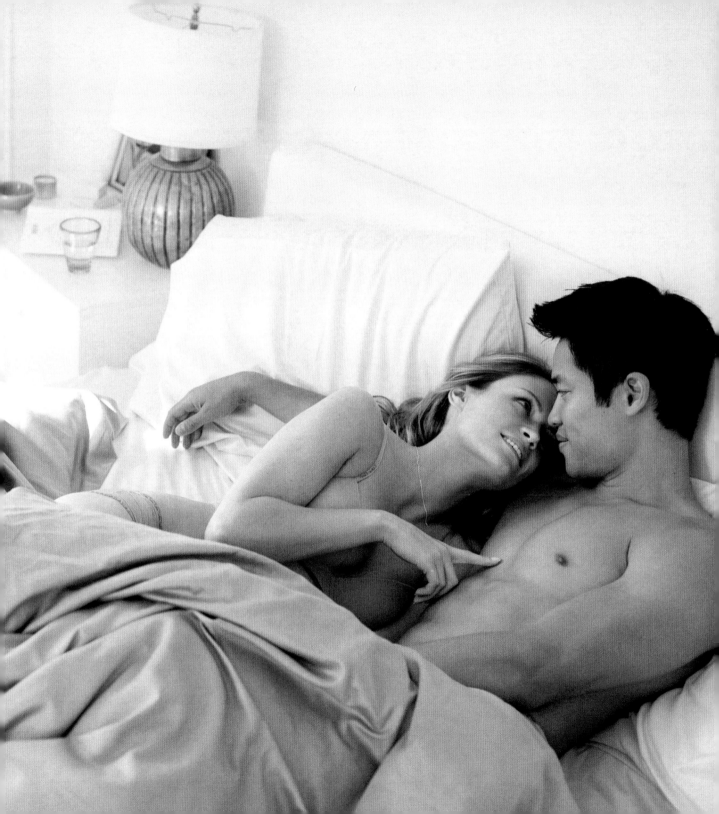

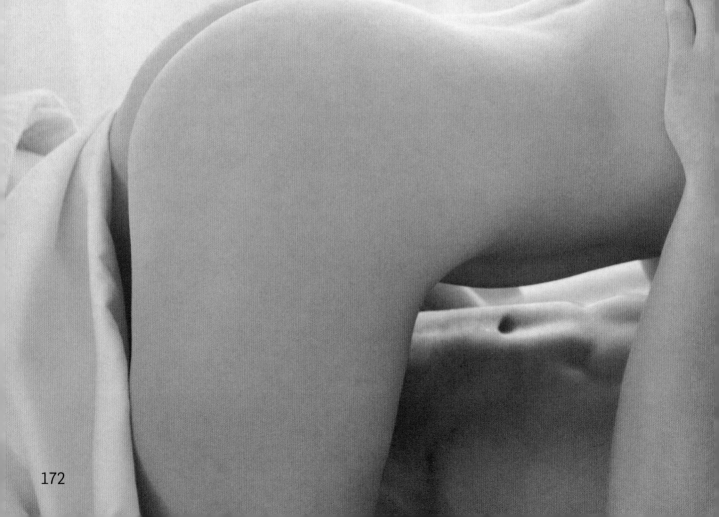

Chapter 8
The Big Book of Sex Positions Sampler

SOME EXCITING TWISTS (AND SHOUTS) ON OLD STANDBYS

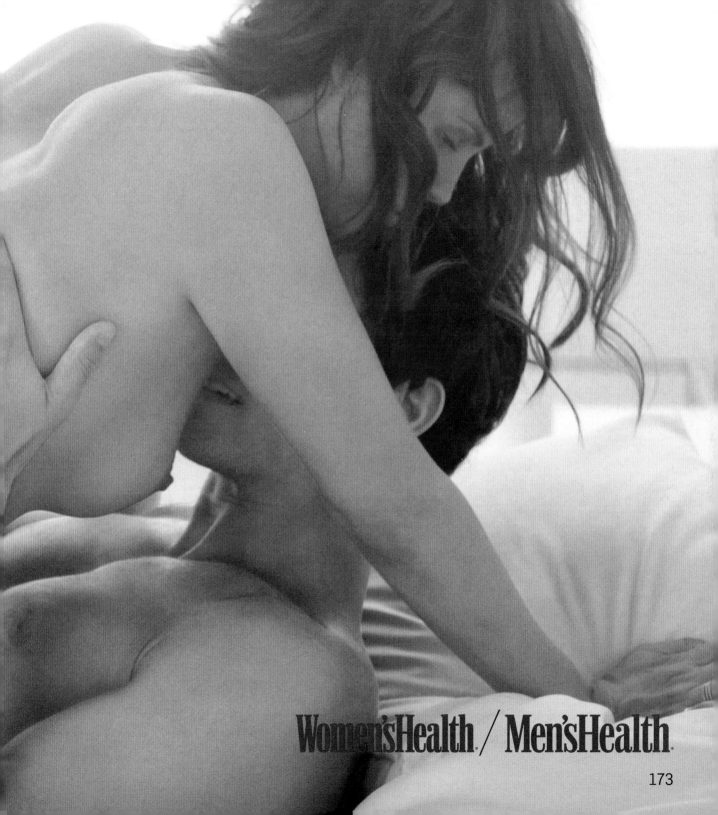

Women'sHealth / Men'sHealth

When you

feel a strong sexual connection with someone, it's tempting to tear off their clothes and go at it. But taking time to savor the experience has a big pleasure payoff. "When you engage your body and mind in bed, you'll feel more relaxed, connected to your partner, and aroused—all of which result in better sex," says Logan Levkoff, PhD, a certified sexuality educator. By taking your time and being creative, you'll also avoid the danger of making sex routine—with the same foreplay sequence, same position, same result. This chapter is designed to give you some ideas to play around with in the bedroom, new positions you may not have tried, and slight tweaks and touches that'll result in

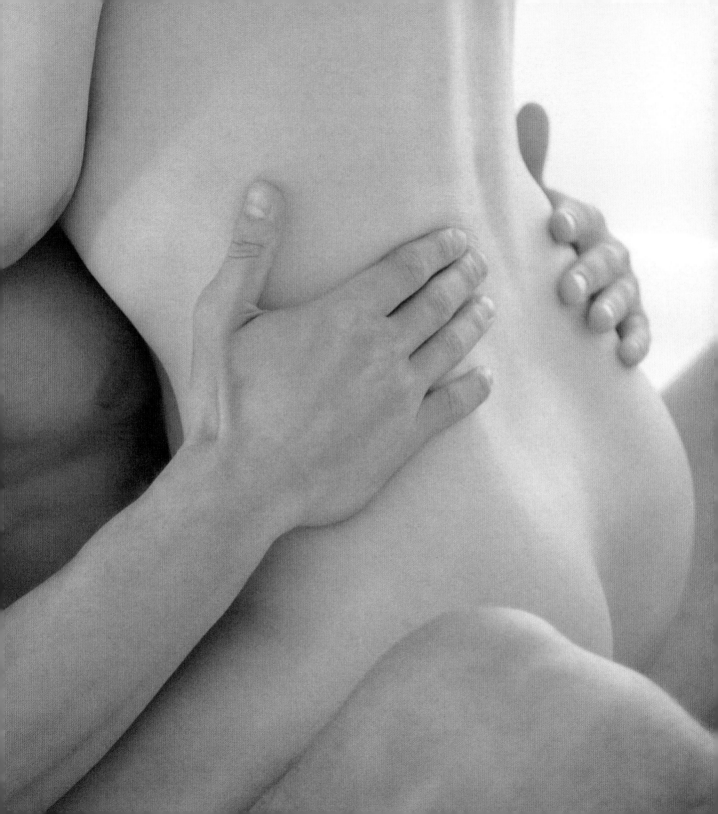

greater pleasures. But new positions won't guarantee great sex. To make tonight amazing, start using these tips to bring more mindfulness to lovemaking.

Before Sex

In the morning, shoot him a sexy text: "What are you going to do to me later?" or "I can't wait to get you out of your work clothes." (Just make sure you don't write anything too graphic—you never know who might end up reading it.) According to Ian Kerner, PhD, "The act of writing stimulates the imagination in ways that other sensory media does not. Writing compels you to fill in the blanks and create your own visuals. The combination of the writer's words and the receiver's interpretation is actually a form of sex in and of itself." Plus, telling him what you're planning to do to him that evening will keep you on his mind all day.

To become aroused, you need to switch off your amygdala, the portion of your brain that controls fear and anxiety. So, about an hour before you plan to get busy, draw yourself a steamy bath to calm your mind and awaken your nerve endings; the hot temperature of the water will bring blood to your skin's surface, making your whole body more sensitive to touch.

During Sex

Foreplay is an important part of slow sex. Prolong it by stopping in the middle to make out, share a sexual fantasy, or exchange massages. Start things off with sensate touch—a series of exercises designed to increase trust and arousal without touching each other's genitals. "The goal of it is to relax and build intimacy," says licensed psychologist and sex therapist Arlene Goldman, PhD, coauthor of *Secrets of Sexual Ecstasy*.

Ready for intercourse? Choose a position that encourages you to stare into each other's eyes, such as missionary or women-on-top, with him sitting up and facing you. Sample the 15 hot moves on the following pages; you'll find another 15 by turning the book over. "Positions that give you a full view of each other's naked bodies can build arousal too quickly, while ones that lend themselves to eye contact increase intimacy and tend to build arousal more gradually," says Levkoff. Start moving slowly in random, circular patterns rather than fast thrusting—it will feel good for both of you without building that steady momentum that leads to immediate orgasm. And try switching positions for variety—the short break will prolong lovemaking. But here's the important thing to know about trying new sex positions: "People can twist themselves into the most creative sexual positions, but if they're not feeling relaxed, open to pleasure or present in the moment, they are unlikely to find that sex feels good," says Debbie Herbenick, PhD. In fact, if not done smoothly, switching positions can break your momentum toward orgasm even in the midst of having one.

32

Percentage of women responding to *The Big Book of Sex* survey who said they wish they had sex at least once a day. Nearly 31 percent said they'd like it every other day and 29 percent a couple of times a week.

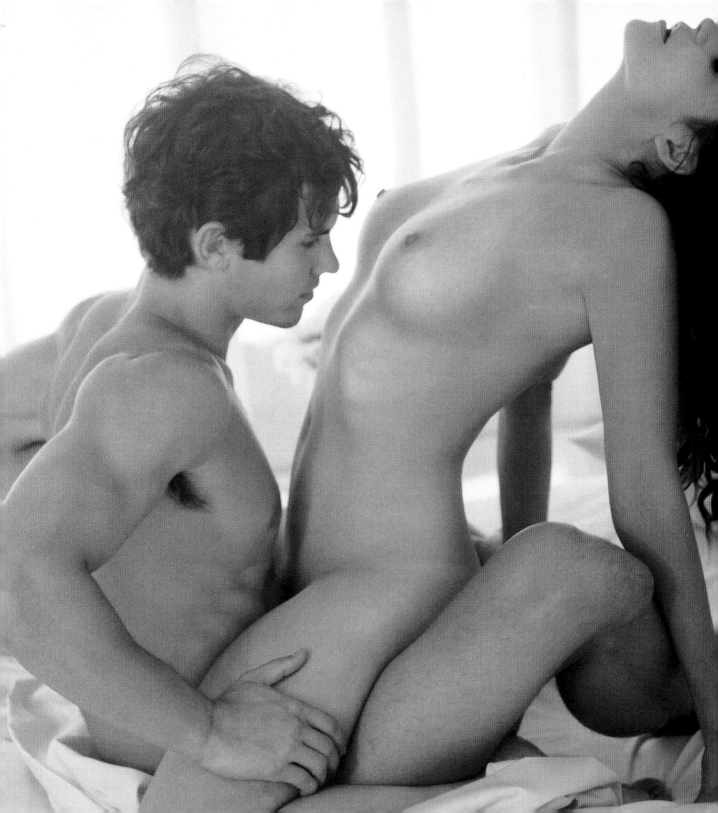

Woman on Top

The Cowgirl

a.k.a. My Turn, Woman On Top
Heat Index: ★★★
Benefits: Puts you in control. Great for G-spot stimulation.

The woman-on-top position allows for a variety of interesting sights and sensations, and offers you the psychological advantage of taking charge of pace and depth of penetration. Alternate between shallow and deep thrusts. "Shallow will stimulate the front third of the vagina, which is the most sensitive," says sex therapist Rebecca Rosenblat, author of *Seducing Your Man*.

Now try this: Lie chest to chest on him, stretching your legs out on top of his. Brace your feet on the tops of his and push off to create a rocking motion that will rub your vulva and clitorial area against his pubic bone for greater pleasure.

Hot Tip—Hers

Give yourself a hand with the V stroke: Make a V with the index and ring finger of one hand and place the fingers on either side of your clitoris with his penis in between. Push your fingers down in a rocking motion.

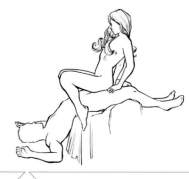

YOUR NEXT MOVE

Waterfall (a.k.a. Head Rush)

Move to the edge of the bed and have him lie back with his head and shoulders on the floor. The blood will rush to his head creating mind-blowing sensations as he climaxes.

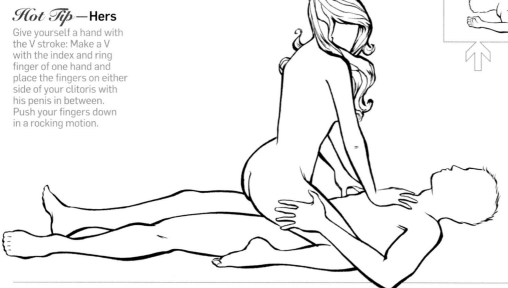

Hot Tip—His

It will be easier for her to climax if you stimulate her manually and orally until she is extremely aroused. From the woman-on-top position, have her squat over your face where you can orally stimulate her.

Reverse Cowgirl

a.k.a. Rodeo Drive, Half Way Around the World
Heat Index: ★★★★★
Benefits: With a pillow under his head, he gets an awesome view of your backside. You can control depth of penetration and pace.

Have him lie on his back with his legs outstretched. Kneel next to him, then turn and spread your legs, straddling his hips and facing his feet. Kneeling, lower yourself onto his penis and begin riding him up and down.
Now try this: Lean forward or back to change the angle of his penis inside you for greater stimulation.

Hot Tip—**Hers**
From this position, you can easily reach down to stimulate yourself or direct his penis to where it feels best.

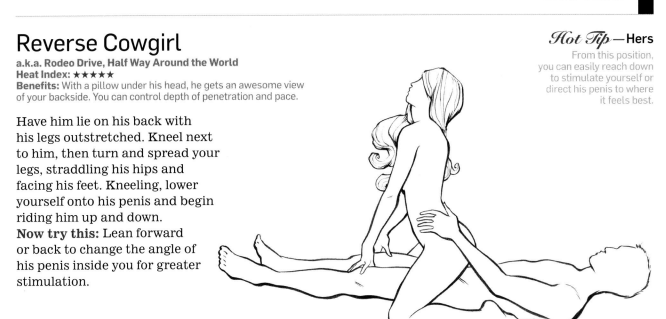

Pole Position

a.k.a. Thighmaster
Heat Index: ★★★★★
Benefits: Dual stimulation for you; a great view of your rear and his penis entering you for him.

Have your guy lie on his back and bend one of his legs, keeping the other outstretched. Straddle the raised leg with a thigh on either side and lower yourself onto his member so that your back is facing him. Hold his knee and use it for support as you rock up and down.
Now try this: Press your vulva hard against his upper thigh rubbing as the feeling dictates until you reach orgasm.

Hot Tip—**Hers**
From Pole position, you can massage his raised leg during the action. Or reach down and touch his perineum. Glance backward to watch him enjoying your erotic movements.

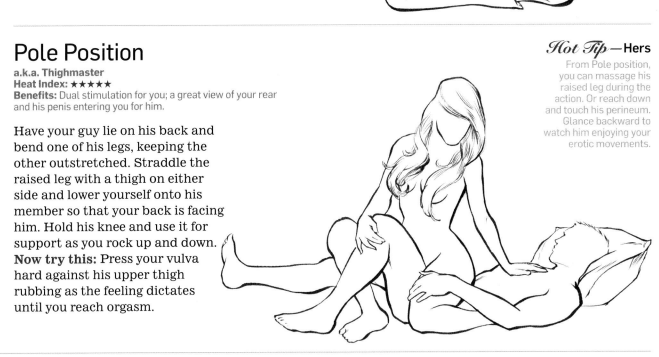

Seated

The Hot Seat

a.k.a. The Love Seat, The Man Chair
Heat Index: ★★
Benefits: Good G-spot stimulation.

Ask him to sit on the edge of the bed or on a chair with his feet on the floor. Turn away from him and back up onto him, sitting between his legs. You can ride back and forth by pushing off the chair arms or pressing up with your feet. Control the angle of entry by arching your back and pressing your buttocks into his groin. While doggy-style is about his dominance, The Hot Seat puts you in the driver's seat.

Now try this: Reach under with your hand and stimulate the base of his penis, scrotum, and perineum. Meanwhile, ask him to reach around and stimulate your nipples.

Hot Tip — **Hers**
Best way to help him get interested in sex when you can tell it's the farthest thing from his mind: undress in front of him.

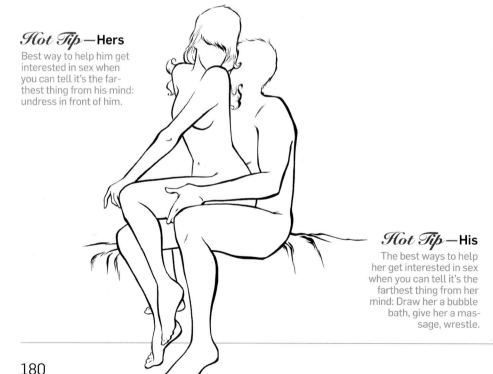

Hot Tip — **His**
The best ways to help her get interested in sex when you can tell it's the farthest thing from her mind: Draw her a bubble bath, give her a massage, wrestle.

Take It Out of the Bedroom

VARIATION #1
Swiss Ball Blitz
Have a ball in your workout room: Use a stability ball to add some bounce to The Hot Seat.

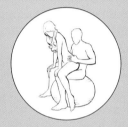

VARIATION #2
Spin Cycle
Plant yourselves on top of a washing machine set at the highest agitator cycle.

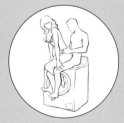

VARIATION #3
Stairway to Heaven
Stairs offer good seating possibilities and a hand rail for extra support and lifting leverage.

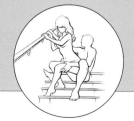

Face Off

a.k.a. The Lap Dance
Heat Index: ★★★
Benefits: Allows for face-to-face intimacy; cozy for long sessions.

Ask him to sit on a chair or the edge of the bed. Facing him, wrap your arms around his back, climb on top of him, and sit on his lap. Once in the saddle, you can can ride up and down on his penis by pressing with your legs or knees. Want to go faster? Ask him to assist by grabbing your buttocks and lifting and bouncing.
Now try this: Sit astride facing him on a rocking chair. Old wooden rockers on hardwood or stone floors provide the greatest variety of good vibes.

Hot Tip—Hers

Ask him to lick your nipples and let his hands roam. There's lots of room for creativity in this position for stimulating erogenous areas of the upper body, head, neck, and face.

The Lazy Man

a.k.a. The Squat Thrust
Heat Index: ★★★★
Benefits: Puts you in control; maintains intimacy.

Place pillows behind his back and have him sit on the bed with legs outstretched. Now straddle his waist, feet on the bed. Bend your knees to lower yourself onto him, using one hand to direct his penis in. Just by pressing on the balls of your feet and releasing, you can raise and lower yourself on his shaft as slowly or quickly as you please.
Now try this: From this position, you both can lie back into the Spider position (page 184) or its more challenging variation The X (page 185).

Hot Tip—Hers

Think of his penis as a masturbatory tool, something to rub and stimulate your clitoris with and against.
–Tracey Cox, author of
Tracey Cox Kama Sutra

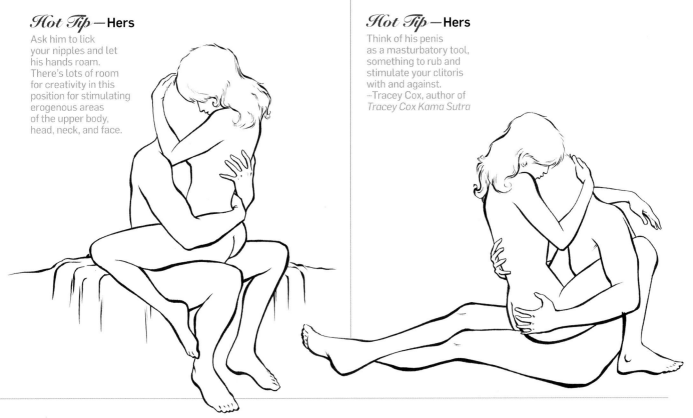

Side By Side

Spoon, Facing

a.k.a. Sidewinder
Heat Index: ★★
Benefits: A very intimate face-to-face position that encourages hugging and kissing.

This is an ideal position if you are pregnant or either one of you had a knee injury because it keeps weight off the body. To get into the position, begin by lying on your sides and facing one another. Spread your legs slightly to allow him to enter you, then close your legs so the part of his shaft that's outside of you can press against your clitoris. It's easy to kiss from this intimate face-to-face position. **Now try this:** Because thrusting is more difficult in this position, use different techniques such as grinding, circular, and up-and-down motions for added stimulation.

Hot Tip —**Hers**

Hug each other for 20 seconds before getting busy. Hugging raises your levels of oxytocin, a bonding hormone your body produces naturally, and that will enhance your connection. Awww . . .

YOUR NEXT MOVE
Gift Wrapped

Both of you lie on your sides facing one another. Bend and spread your legs, and angle your vagina toward him. He will lift his legs between yours to enter you. Wrap your legs around his back.

Now try this: *Use your legs and feet to pull him close during thrusts for deeper penetration.*

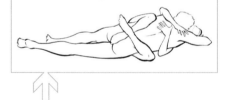

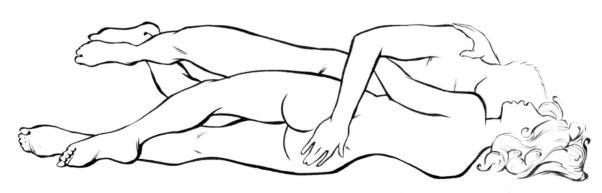

Spork

a.k.a. Spoon and Fork Combo, Scissoring
Heat Index: ★★★
Benefits: Offers a natural bridge to more creative positions.

While you lie on your back, raise your right leg so he can position himself between your legs at a 90-degree angle and enter you. Your legs will form the tines of a spork, a spoon-and-fork utensil. You can do this with him facing you or facing your back.
Now try this: If you are limber, lift your left leg up to increase the depth of penetration.

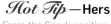

Hot Tip—**Hers**

From the Spork position, you can lift your top leg and support it by resting it on his shoulder. From here, you can easily stimulate your clitoris using your fingers while he is inside you.

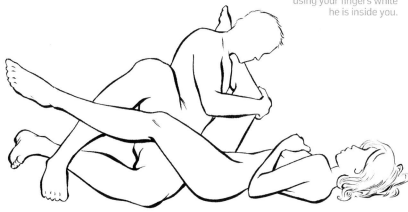

Spoon

a.k.a. The Sleeper Hold
Heat Index: ★★
Benefits: Comfortable position if you are pregnant or if he is heavy. Also ideal for long lovemaking. Good one for falling asleep afterward.

You both lie on your sides facing the same direction, him behind you. Bend your knees and push your rear back toward him for easier access to your vagina. Adjusting the lean of your bodies will vary the angle of entry and help with rocking and thrusting.
Now try this: Synchronize your breathing. One of you takes the lead and the other follows so that you inhale and exhale together. The coordinated rhythm opens an unspoken dialogue of intimacy.

Hot Tip—**His**

To give her the sensation of greater width inside her, from the Spoon position have her bend and lift her top leg to her breasts. Adjust your position so you are more on top of her top hip than behind her.

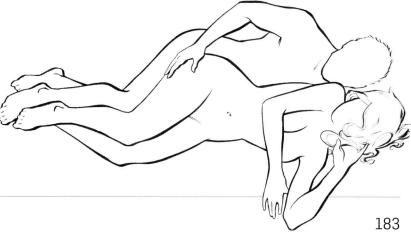

Head to Toe

The Spider
a.k.a. The Crab Walk
Heat Index: ★★★★
Benefits: You can still maintain eye contact while viewing the action at center stage.

Both of you are seated on the bed with legs toward one another, arms back to support yourselves. Now move together and onto his penis. Your hips will be between his spread legs, your knees bent and feet outside of his hips and flat on the bed. Now rock back and forth.

Now try this: Grab his hands and pull yourself up into a squatting position while he lies back. Or he can remain seated upright and pull you against his chest into the Lazy Man position (page 181).

YOUR NEXT MOVE
The Fusion
From The Spider, you can lift your legs onto his shoulders, which increases the muscular tension that advances the orgasm sequence. By elevating your butt off the bed, it'll be easier to thrust and grind in circles.

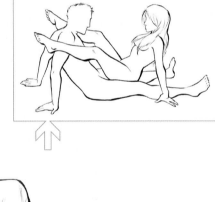

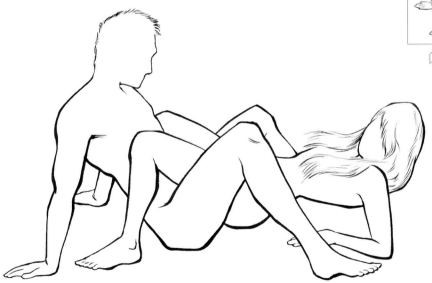

Hot Tip — **Hers**
Help him turn you on while he's giving you a massage. Have him straddle your bottom and massage your back. While he's busy with his hands, wiggle, grind, and move your mons pubis in a circular motion against the sheets to stimulate your clitoris.

Snow Angel

a.k.a. Bottom's Up
Heat Index: ★★★★
Benefits: You get a prime view of his derriere.

This is challenging: Lie on your back and have him straddle you facing away. Lift your legs and wrap them around his back to elevate your pelvis so he can enter you. Grab his butt to help him slide up and back. Add a little massage action to your grip.
Now try this: Have him spin around into missionary style to face you while trying to stay inserted. Then switch positions, this time with you on top and facing away.

Hot Tip —**Hers**
From this position, you have easy access to fondle his testicles. Lightly run your finger between his testicles and anus to simulate his perineum.

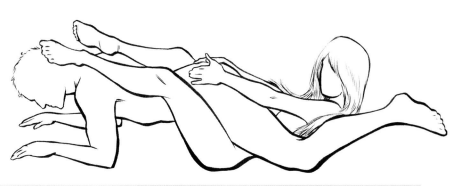

The X Position

a.k.a. Crisscross
Heat Index: ★★★★
Benefits: Prolonged slow sex to build your arousal. Shallow thrusts stimulate the nerve endings in the head of his penis.

Sit on the bed facing each other with legs forward. Lift his right leg over your left and lift your right leg over his left. Come together so he can enter you. Now both of you lie back, your legs forming an X. Slow, leisurely gyrations replace thrusting.
Now try this: Reach out and hold hands to pull together for pelvic thrusting. Also, take turns alternatively sitting up and lying back without changing the rhythm.

Hot Tip —**Hers**
Clear your mind of the day's worries by fantasizing about pleasurable feelings. During masturbation or foreplay, imagine an erotic encounter with your partner or someone else. Don't censor your thoughts. Be completely open to awakening your libido and arousal.

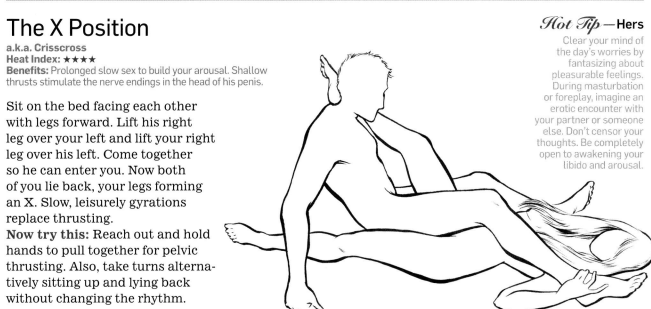

Oral

The Elevator

a.k.a. The Bees Knees
Heat Index: ★★★★
Benefits: Great for out-of-bedroom fellatio.

Kneel in front of him. Cover your teeth with your lips and encircle his glans with your mouth. Slowly piston your lips up and down on his shaft, alternating speeds. Occasionally glance up at him. Showing your enthusiasm and enjoyment are enormous factors in his pleasure. Stop to move your tongue over and around his head. Be careful of your teeth, although occasional light nibbling on the less sensitive shaft is enjoyable for many men. **Now try this:** Lean a dressing mirror against a wall to the side of his body so he can enjoy the view of you going down on him from the side versus top down.

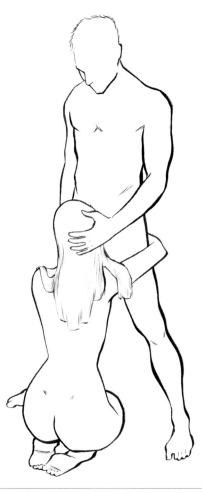

Hot Tip —Hers

Don't ignore his pals. For a variation he'll find extremely erotic, take one of his testicles into your mouth as you stroke his shaft with your hand.

YOUR NEXT MOVE

The Face Sitter

A comfortable position for you. An erotic one for him. Rest a pillow behind your head, then have him straddle your shoulders. He can support himself by holding the bed's headboard or the wall.

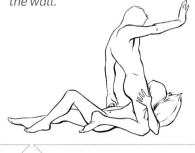

Hot Tip —Hers

If your mouth becomes dry after awhile, add some mint- or fruit-flavored lube to his shaft. Many women don't like the taste and texture of semen. To keep from gagging when he erupts, you may want to place his penis between your breasts as he nears climax and move it in and out of your cleavage, allowing him to ejaculate over your chest.

Cowgirl 69

a.k.a. Inverted 69, Over and Under
Heat Index: ★★★★
Benefits: Simultaneous oral pleasure.

When you are on top in 69, you can control the intensity of oral stimulation on your clitoris by lifting or pressing your pelvis. From this position it's easy to work your finger magic on his perineum, the sensitive area just below his testicles. Also try the him-on-top position.

Now try this: Roll over onto your sides in the 69 position. Then massage each other's butts as you lick away.

Hot Tip —**Hers**
Place a cup of warm tea and an ice cube on the nightstand near the bed. When you give him oral sex, alternate placing the ice cube then the tea in your mouth.

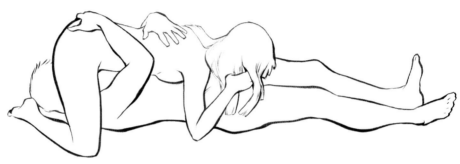

Hovering Butterfly

a.k.a. The Face Sitter
Heat Index: ★★★★
Benefits: You can direct the position of his tongue and the pressure against you by rising up or pressing down.

Straddle him by placing your knees at his ears. Hold onto a wall or headboard for support. While he's doing his thing, use your fingers to graze your nipples or rub the top of your vulva.

Now try this: Have him hold his tongue firm as you gyrate your hips, pressing your clitoris against it.

Hot Tip —**Hers**
Women often worry about how they smell down there, even though most guys love your scent. Ease your mind with a rinse in the bathroom before getting busy.

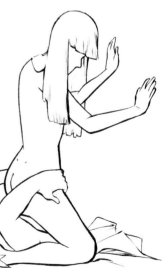

187

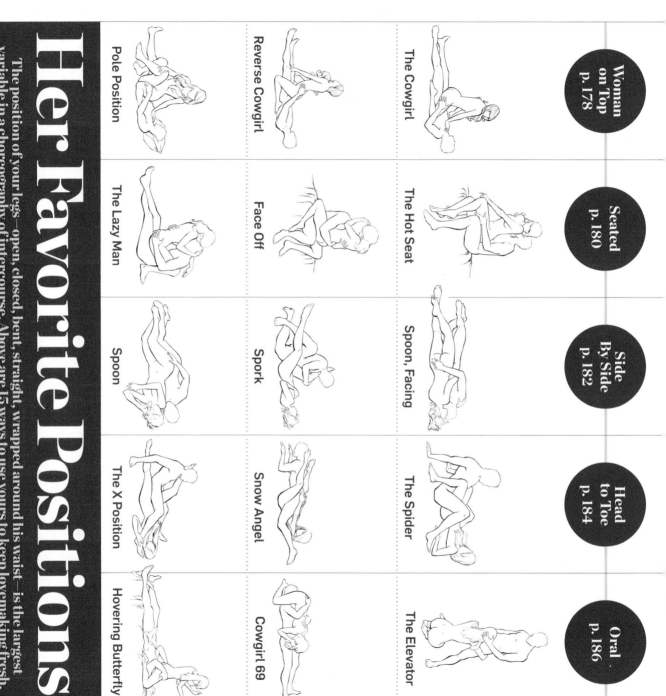

Her Favorite Positions

The position of your legs—open, closed, bent, straight, wrapped around his waist—is the largest variable in a choreography of intercourse. Above are 15 ways to use yours to keep lovemaking fresh.

Woman on Top p. 178	Seated p. 180	Side By Side p. 182	Head to Toe p. 184	Oral p. 186
The Cowgirl	The Hot Seat	Spoon, Facing	The Spider	The Elevator
Reverse Cowgirl	Face Off	Spork	Snow Angel	Cowgirl 69
Pole Position	The Lazy Man	Spoon	The X Position	Hovering Butterfly

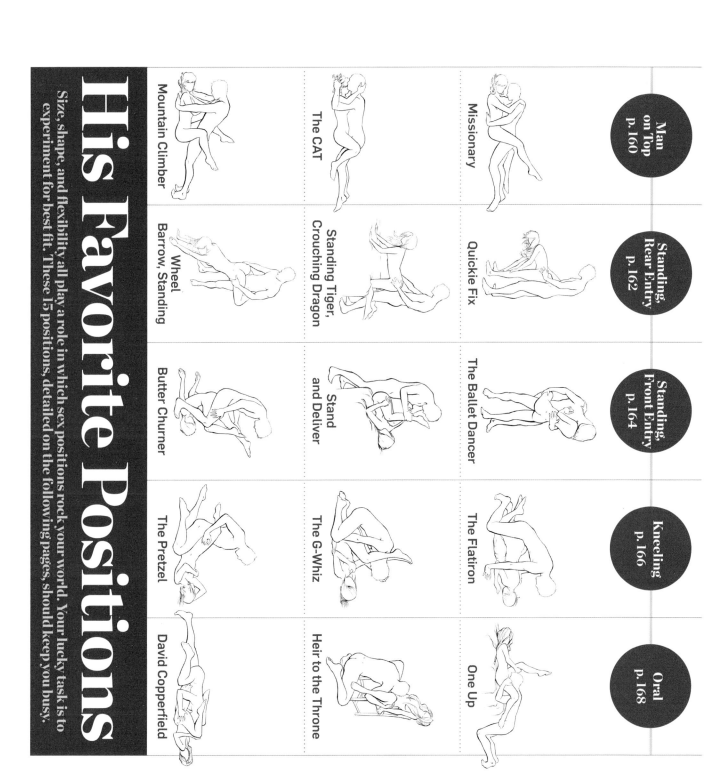

His Favorite Positions

Size, shape, and flexibility all play a role in which sex positions rock your world. Your lucky task is to experiment for best fit. These 15 positions, detailed on the following pages, should keep you busy.

Man on Top p. 160	Standing, Rear Entry p. 162	Standing, Front Entry p. 164	Kneeling p. 166	Oral p. 168
Missionary	Quickie Fix	The Ballet Dancer	The Flatiron	One Up
The CAT	Standing Tiger, Crouching Dragon	Stand and Deliver	The G-Whiz	Heir to the Throne
Mountain Climber	Wheel Barrow, Standing	Butter Churner	The Pretzel	David Copperfield

THE Men's Health

and Women's Health

BIG
BOOK
of SEX

RODALE

THE Men'sHealth
BIG
BOOK
of SEX

RODALE

SEX AND VALUES AT RODALE
We believe that an active and healthy sex life, based on mutual consent and respect between partners, is an important component of physical and mental well-being. We also respect that sex is a private matter and that each person has a different opinion of what sexual practices or levels of discourse are appropriate. Rodale is committed to offering responsible, practical advice about sexual matters, supported by accredited professionals and legitimate scientific research. Our goal—for sex and all other topics—is to publish information that empowers people's lives.
Mention of specific companies, organizations, or authorities in this book does not imply endorsement by the author or publisher, nor does mention of specific companies, organizations, or authorities imply that they endorse this book, its author, or the publisher.
Internet addresses and telephone numbers given in this book were accurate at the time it went to press.

© 2011 by Rodale Inc.

All rights reserved. No part of this publication may be reproduced or transmitted in any form or by any means, electronic or mechanical, including photocopying, recording, or any other information storage and retrieval system, without the written permission of the publisher.

Rodale books may be purchased for business or promotional use or for special sales.
For information, please write to:
Special Markets Department, Rodale, Inc.,
733 Third Avenue, New York, NY 10017

Men's Health and *Women's Health* are registered trademarks of Rodale Inc.

Printed in the United States of America
Rodale Inc. makes every effort to use acid-free ♾, recycled paper ♻.
Credits appear on p. iv of *Women's Health* section

Book design by George Karabotsos, design director of Men's Health and Women's Health Books
and Courtney Eltringham,
with Mark Michaelson, Elizabeth Neal, and Laura White
Photo director: Lila Garnett

Library of Congress Cataloging-in-Publication Data is on file with publisher.
ISBN-13: 978-1-60529-303-5
Distributed to the trade by Macmillan

2   4   6   8   10   9   7   5   3   1   paperback

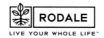

We inspire and enable people to improve their lives and the world around them

Contents

Acknowledgments

In Bed With 10,000 Sexperts

G ood lovin' is a multidisciplinary pleasure.

As primal and intuitive as sexual intercourse is, on another level it's highly complex. Amazing sex and the healthiest of relationships are products of numerous scientific and academic disciplines: cardiology, exercise physiology, psychology, psychiatry, urology, nutrition and weight loss, behavioral therapy, sexology, religion, and more.

Nobody owns the last word on sex.

That's why *Women's Health* and *Men's Health* (and our readers) are so fortunate to be able to tap the brains of the most knowledgeable and influential experts in each of those fields every month. And we've done it for years. *The Big Book of Sex* is a result of hundreds of interviews with the most notable doctors and researchers in the world—as well has many more thousands of hours spent reviewing reams of scholarly journal articles and studies.

There are many experts to thank for help on this project, but none more so than our readers—the thousands of men and women who responded to *The Big Book of Sex* online survey, and whose attitudes and opinions helped inform these pages.

We also want to extend our deep appreciation for the help and guidance of our esteemed *Men's Health* and *Women's Health* advisory board members (you'll find them highlighted in the front of our magazines), and especially those experts whose research and wisdom features prominently throughout this book, including:

Jennifer R. Berman, MD, director of The Berman Women's Wellness Center in Los Angeles; Laura Berman, PhD, president and director of Chicago's Berman Center; Louann Brizendine, MD, professor of clinical psychiatry at the University of California; evolutionary psychologist David M. Buss, PhD, coauthor with Cindy M. Meston, PhD, of *Why Women Have Sex;* anthropologist Helen Fisher, PhD, research professor, Rutgers University, and scientific advisor to Chemistry.com; Debbie Herbenick, PhD, associate director of the Center for Sexual Health Promotion at Indiana University and *Men's Health* relationship advisor; John Gottman, PhD, founder of The Gottman Institute; sexologist Ian Kerner, PhD; Barry Komisaruk, PhD, adjunct psychology professor at Rutgers University; Steven Lamm, MD, assistant professor at NYU School of Medicine; *Men's Health* urology advisor Larry I. Lipshultz, MD, chief of the division of male reproductive medicine at Baylor College of Medicine; Cindy M. Meston, PhD, director of the Meston Sexual Psychophysiology Laboratory at University of Texas at Austin; Ridwan Shabsigh, MD, president of the International Society of Men's Health; Beverly Whipple, PhD, renowned sex researcher and professor emeritus, Rutgers University.

Thanks also to: Bianca Acevedo, PhD; Suman Abwani, PhD; Daniel G. Amen, MD; Arthur Aron, PhD; Craig Ballantyne; Linda Banner, PhD; Rosemary Basson, MD; Jeff Bell; Martin Binks, PhD; Jeffrey Blumberg, PhD; Karen Boyle, MD; Lucy Brown, PhD; Rachel Cosgrove; Tracey Cox; Joy Davidson, PhD; Harry Fisch, MD; Yvonne K. Fulbright, PhD; Sandor Gardos, PhD; Marc Goldstein, MD; Dean Graham; Susan Hall, PhD; Scott Haltzman, MD; Lisa Lawless, PhD; Marta Meana, PhD; Lou Paget; Amy Reiley; Gail Saltz, MD; Pepper Schwartz, PhD; Tara Stiles; Peggy Vaughan; and Vivian Zayas, PhD.

And finally, *The Big Book of Sex* would not exist without the fine work of the following contributing writers, editors, and designers: Lisa Bain; Matt Bean; Adam Campbell; Sara Cox; Jeff Csatari; Courtney Eltringham; Jason Feifer; Lila Garnett; Jennifer Giandomenico; George Karabotsos; Carolyn Kylstra; Chris Krogermeier; Mark Michaelson; Debbie McHugh; Elizabeth Neal; Elise Nersesian; Hugh O'Neill; Stephen Perrine; Michele Promaulayko; Karen Rinaldi; Lesley Rotchford; Sean Sabo; Bill Stieg; Erin Williams; David Zinczenko.

Here's to your physical, emotional, and sexual health!

The Editors

Index

Boldface page references indicate illustrations. Underscored references indicate boxed text.

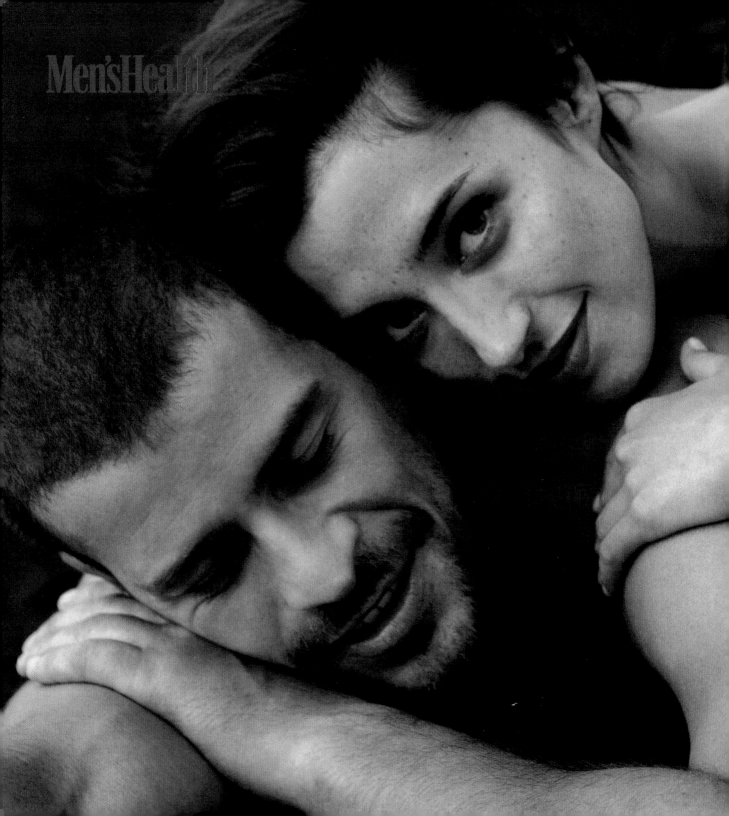

Men'sHealth

Chapter 1
Better Sex Starts Here

FOR OUTSTANDING PERFORMANCE AND EVEN
MORE FUN BETWEEN THE SHEETS, NOTHING BEATS
A FIT AND HEALTHY BODY AND MIND

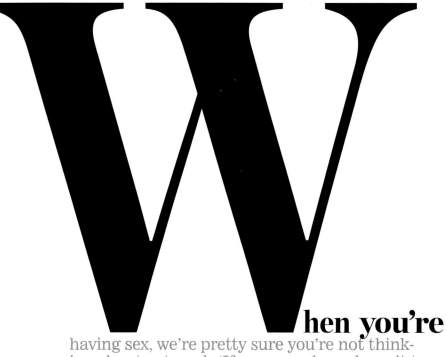

When you're

having sex, we're pretty sure you're not thinking about oatmeal. (If you are, please keep it to yourself.) Your cholesterol numbers are the furthest things from your mind. You're probably not consumed with thoughts of how the single-leg stability ball jackknife or squat thrusts might improve your performance. And we'd bet you're not pondering the chemical and psychological mysteries of her libido at … this … very … moment.

One of the many very nice things about sex is that you don't have to do a lot of thinking. But with sex, as with anything you wish to be skilled at and enjoy more, a little additional knowledge—authoritative, intensely researched, cutting-edge knowledge—can make the difference between "good" and "great."

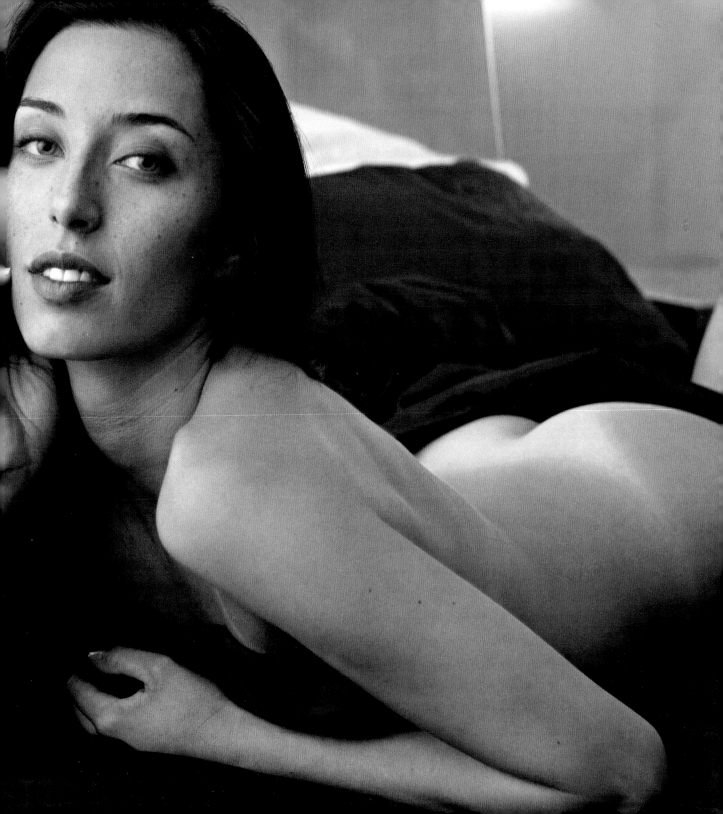

Better Sex Starts Here |

You probably picked up this book because you are familiar with the *Men's Health* brand and what it stands for: practical, authoritative information that inspires and enables you to improve your life. And it's likely that you are one of those men who is confident enough to admit that there are still things to learn about women and sex that Dad or Penthouse Forum never covered.

When your iPad puzzles you, you run to the closest Genius Bar. When you need the proper drywall screws, you visit Harvey's Hardware. But when she seems to have suddenly lost interest in sex or when you feel a strange twinge in your most private parts, who are you going to consult? The guys on your rugby team?

You can see our point: When it comes to sex, there are few comfortable places to go for useful information you can trust. That's where *Men's Health* magazine comes in. We tackle the tough questions and give you exclusive access to the world's top sexual health experts who share important revelations and wisdom like:

- The typical penis does not behave like those you see in porn movies.
- The typical woman is just fine with that fact, even relieved.
- Girth matters more to women than length, and a particularly skillful tongue is better still.
- Women are turned on by men's hands. Keep them clean and groomed.
- The real secrets to amazing sex are honesty, trust, and communication.

While advice is never a substitute for experience, good advice can make the experience gathering much less dangerous. *The Big Book of Sex* is loaded with sophisticated sex advice to make any man a better lover, husband, and friend. For starters, you'll discover how closely great sex and a strong body, nutritious diet, and healthy mind are linked. *The Big Book of Sex* will show you how improving those parts of your life will lead to firmer erections, lasting longer during sex, forging a deeper, more satisfying relationship with your partner, finding ways to have more sex and more pleasure, including rocket-fueled, total-body orgasms. Sound good? Let's dig a little deeper into what *The Big Book of Sex* has to offer YOU:

Firmer Erections and Better Endurance

Sex, at its best, is an athletic event. Like football, tennis, and Greco-Roman wrestling, amazing sex is a head-to-toe activity that calls on all your faculties—the muscles, cardiovascular system, and brain. A rock-her-world performance takes stamina—both staying power and aerobic endurance. It requires upper-body, lower-body, and core strength for lifting her up and thrusting, and flexibility for smooth position changes.

If you're not fit? Being out of shape and overweight can completely sack your sex life by stealing the lead out of your pencil. Men who are obese are five times more likely to suffer from erectile dysfunction (ED) or impotence

7,200
Number of times the average man will ejaculate in his lifetime.

78
Percentage of men who wish they could delay the inevitable.

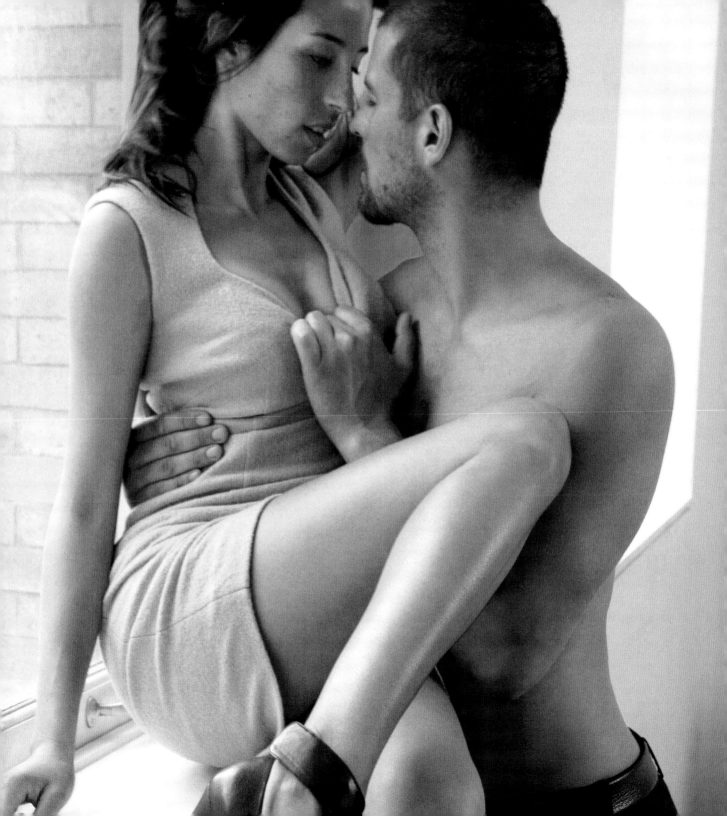

than men who are of normal weight and health. That's serious.

The expert advice, workouts, and dietary plans in this book will help any man avoid that fate in his thirties, forties, fifties, even his eighties. Sex is much too important to a healthy mind and body to allow ED to complicate things, even in this age of little blue helper pills.

A Blueprint for Building a Stronger, Sexier Relationship

Physical fitness is just one part of total-body training for sex. There's the more complex and challenging emotional side of the game, where most men need extra drilling. This is where understanding how the whole female works—from mind to vagina—can give a man an advantage in arousing a woman's interest.

Amazing sex requires connecting with your partner on a deeper level. And you get there with special care and feeding. A football team cannot win if the receivers aren't communicating with their quarterback. Likewise loving partners need to foster intimate connections that have nothing to do with their genitals but everything to do with their eyes, ears, mouths, and cerebellums. Communication is an important foundation of great sex. More on that later.

Lift Here for Sweatier Sex

The medical literature is rich with studies showing how exercise makes sex more breathtaking. Here are eight inspiring reasons to dust off your dumbbells and throw on those sexy running shorts.

Your erections will be harder and more reliable. Good sex requires good cardiovascular and respiratory health. Your heart's job is to pump blood to all the limbs and organs in your body, including your brain and the one between your legs. A strong heart and healthy lungs team up to bring oxygen-rich blood to your muscles so you can have the desire and the energy to sustain you through a long night of lovemaking. Exercise strengthens both systems.

Exercise boosts blood flow. Exercise also opens the floodgates that allow blood to enter the penis for strong erections. Physical activity keeps arteries flexible so they can easily dilate, especially those tiny ones in the genitals that need to respond when the time is right.

Research reported at the 2010 meeting of the American Urological Association shows the powerful link between exercise and erections. Scientists surveyed 178 healthy men at Durham VA Medical Center in North Carolina about their exercise habits, frequency and quality of erections, and overall sexual satisfaction. It turned out that men who exercised moderately had substantially higher scores on the sex survey than men who were sedentary. The men who reported exercise of at least 9 METs per week were 65 percent less likely to report sexual problems

SAVE YOUR BACK IN THE SACK

Sex is great for your back. It's probably the single best exercise for releasing muscular constriction, toning back muscles, and relaxing the nervous system. It has been scientifically demonstrated that orgasm has 10 times the anxiety/muscle spasm-reducing effect of Valium.

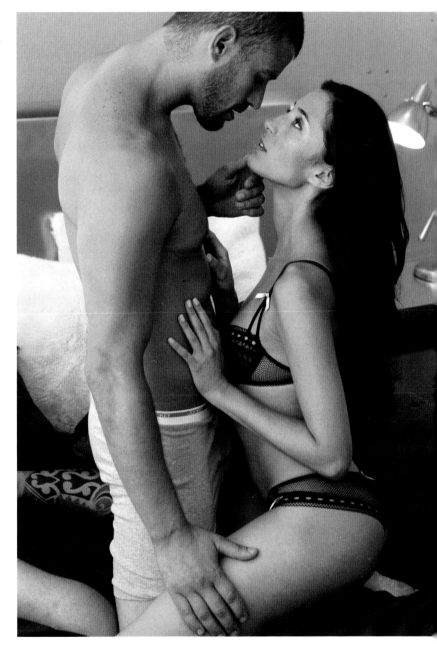

than men who did no exercise. (MET, by the way, is short for metabolic equivalent task, a system used to gauge exercise intensity based on oxygen use. Brisk walking for 30 minutes a day, 4 days a week is roughly equal to those 9 METs.) In the study, sexual function scores rose even higher in men who were more active and exercised at intensities beyond 9 METs. But the point of the study was clear: it doesn't take much effort to maintain good wood. "If men won't exercise for the cardiovascular health, well, maybe this will convince them to exercise to have better sex," says researcher Erin R. McNamara, MD, of the Duke University Medical Center.

Exercise raises good cholesterol.
LDL, commonly known as the "bad" cholesterol, is the waxy stuff that clogs arteries and, more critically, causes the arterial inflammation that leads to most heart attacks. It doesn't just gunk up the coronary arteries; cholesterol deposits show up first in the tiny arteries leading to and within the penis, effectively blocking blood flow like a jack-knifed tractor trailer stalls traffic on the interstate. Fortunately, moderate to intense exercise raises the HDL or "good" cholesterol, which acts like arterial drain cleaner, picking up excess cholesterol from artery walls and carting it to the liver for removal from the body. In one experiment at Auburn University, men ages 35 to 50 who exercised for 30 to 45 minutes for 4 consecutive days saw their HDL levels rise by 4 to 6 points.

Better Sex Starts Here | HIS

GIDDY UP AGAIN, AND AGAIN

How to have a round 2, 3, or more:

1. Don't masturbate for several days. The more you ejaculate, the longer your refractory periods will be.

2. Skip the post-romp cigarette. Nicotine kills erections.

3. Trade post-sex massages. Releasing muscle tension eases anxiety, a factor in subsequent erections.

4. Have a sip of wine. Alcohol in low doses increases the arousal signals from your brain to your penile tissue.

5. Stand up and move around. Improving blood circulation will help.

6. Change the stimuli. Move into another room, watch an erotic movie, whip out a sex toy, or try a sexy new position.

That's important because changing the ratio between LDL and HDL cholesterol reduces plaque build-up on arteries that affect erections.

You'll be happier and hornier. Exercise is a terrific mood and libido booster. Going for a run outside on a beautiful day triggers your brain to release endorphins, feel-good neurochemicals that elevate mood and take your mind off of work, so you can focus on more pleasurable pursuits. Numerous studies show that exercise can even fight clinical depression, which is a prime destroyer of sexual desire and performance. Psychiatrists at the University of Texas Southwestern's Mood Disorders Research Program and Clinic found that patients suffering from depression who did moderately intense aerobics for 35 minutes a day experienced a nearly 50 percent decline in depression symptoms, which is comparable to the effect of antidepressant medication like Prozac or Zoloft, but without the negative sexual side effects. Exercise also provides opportunity for social interaction, which elevates mood and may help you meet an equally happy member of the opposite sex on your next run.

Your penis will act younger. A Harvard University study of 160 male and female swimmers in their 40s and 60s showed a positive relationship between regular physical activity and the frequency and enjoyment of sexual intercourse. The research showed that swimmers in their 60s reported sex lives comparable

to people in the general population who were 20 years younger.

You'll feel sexier. Getting back in shape can make you feel pretty good about yourself, and that self-confidence can be very attractive to women. In a survey of 450 college students, University of Arkansas researchers investigated correlations between physical activity and sexual desirability. For the males in the study, the researchers found that fitness made them feel a lot hotter looking. Over 90 percent of the men who claimed above average physical fitness also rated themselves as above average in sexual desirability. All of the men who reported exercising 6 days a week rated themselves as excellent mate material and damn good in bed.

You'll knock out stress. Easy to understand why a caveman would lose all interest in procreating when he's being chased by a sabertooth tiger. Priorities, you know. Well, today's priorities—work pressures, deadlines, and worry about illness, jobs, family matters—trigger the same sort of biological fight-or-flight response that hungry tigers did back in the day. When that happens, blood flow is directed away from the genitals to the muscles where it's needed to address a different kind of action. Stress can stifle libido in men. When you're anxious, it's difficult to be in the moment, connect with your partner, and become aroused. But exercise is the fast fix for stress. It provides an instant release for that survival-mode energy and it floods the body with calming brain chemicals. And when you exercise regularly, you train your body to handle stress better all the time. Texas A&M University researchers found that men who are fit have lower levels of stress hormones in their blood than unfit people do, which means that their bodies are better prepared for sex when the moment is right, or stress when it strikes.

You'll sleep sounder and have erotic dreams. Exhausting your muscles will help you get to sleep faster and sleep deeper, according to National Sleep Foundation scientists. One study found that sleep-lab patients who exercised three times a week for 8 weeks improved their quality of sleep by nearly 25 percent. Deep restful sleep is important to good sexual function, too. When you have rejuvenating sleep, you produce norepinephrine and dopamine, two neurotransmitters that play a role in desire and arousal. And a full night's sleep, 7 to 8 hours, ensures that you'll experience REM, or dream, sleep. That's when your eyes twitch rapidly under your lids and you experience nocturnal penile tumescence, erections that bring nourishing blood to your member in slumber.

The Big Book of Sex Will Help You Lose Weight

Surveys show that overweight people are 14 percent less attractive to the opposite sex, and 43 percent less attractive if they are obese. While it may seem shallow, looks count in partner hunting. But being overweight can even depress the sex lives of people already in solid relationships. A survey of 1,210 people of different weights and sizes conducted by researchers at Duke University Medical Center showed that obese people were 25 times as likely to report dissatisfaction with sex as normal weight people. The fantastic news is that good sex can be achieved with minimal improvement in body composition. Several studies have shown that people report much greater enjoyment of sexual activity following a weight loss of just 10 percent, says Martin Binks, PhD, clinical director of Binks Behavioral Health and an assistant consulting professor at Duke University Medical Center. "It's important to realize that these folks did not get to some ideal weight, but rather that just moderate improvements that we know benefit overall health also helped in the bedroom," he says.

Some other ways taking off pounds can lift your love life:

You'll boost testosterone. Testosterone is the hormone responsible for fueling your sex drive. Women have it, too, but not as much as men. When testosterone dips below normal levels, as it typically does with age, desire and sexual function may suffer. A recent study suggests that age may not be the only thing that stifles T levels. In that epidemiological study of 1,822 men in the Boston area, scientists from the New England Research Institutes found that the size

35
Percent increase in your chance of getting sick if you have an unhappy marriage. Bad lovin' also can shorten your life by 4 years.

of a man's waist strongly correlated with low testosterone levels and other male hormones. A waist circumference of 41 inches or greater was a stronger predictor of low testosterone than any other risk factors including weight. This is good news because body size is a risk factor people can improve themselves through exercise and diet, says epidemiology researcher Susan Hall, PhD. In fact, one effective way to lose belly fat and keep testosterone levels normal is to build muscle. Lifting weights can burn just as many calories as fairly intense aerobic exercise does, but scientists have found that resistance exercise fries a greater percentage of calories from fat.

You'll make your member look bigger.
Blubber hanging over a man's waistband puts the penis at a distinct disadvantage. Just as even a tall man looks diminutive next to an NBA player, your penis will appear smaller than it actually is when overshadowed by a big gut. We're talking about perspective here. But there's a physical cover-up going on, too. Excess fat around the pubic bone itself will cover the base of the penis, obscuring some of your endowment. But losing 10 to 20 pounds of abdominal fat, will visually add up to a half an inch to penis size.

You'll avoid the big sex killer: diabetes.
Studies show that men with diabetes are four times more likely to suffer from erectile dysfunction than healthy men. What's more, erection problems start as much as a decade earlier in these guys. Type 2 diabetes, or adult onset diabetes, occurs when your body becomes resistant to insulin over time because you've flooded your system with massive amounts of glucose through overeating. When your pancreas doesn't produce insulin effectively enough to do its job, the glucose starts to do damage, including to your sex life. Over time, high blood sugar causes damage to nerves and blood vessels, which affects erections and reduces testosterone. But by losing belly fat through diet and exercise, you can improve your sensitivity to insulin and actually reverse type 2 diabetes. In one Austrian study, people with type 2 diabetes on a 4-month-long strength-training program significantly lowered their blood sugar levels and vastly improved control over their diabetes.

Eat This, Stay Hard
Adding a smart eating plan to a workout regimen works better for weight loss than just exercise alone. Consider a study from the Human Performance Laboratory at the University of Connecticut. In an experiment, two groups of men were put on a diet and weight lifting program. One group of men trimmed carbohydrates from their meals, the other trimmed dietary fat. After 12 weeks, both groups lost weight, but the low-carb lifters dropped an average of 17 pounds of fat, twice as much as low-fat lifters. The researchers believe the disparity is because restricting carbohydrates forces

TURN HER ON WITH ATTENTION

1. **Get off the Internet.**

2. **Listen to what she's saying.**

3. **Repeat what she's just said.**

4. **Tell her what she's said makes sense to you.**

5. **Grasp her hand when an attractive woman walks by.**

the body to burn fat instead of sugar. So, the foods you choose to eat have a strong bearing on your body composition and how well your body functions.

You'll increase your sex drive. High-fat meats, other saturated fats, and trans fats in processed foods decrease testosterone levels and lower libido. By replacing the fatty-foods in your diet with fresh vegetables and fruits, whole grains, and lean proteins, you'll increase your desire to have sex and your stamina.

You'll pave the way to more responsive erections. As we mentioned above, high cholesterol disrupts the pathways that feed blood to the penis. Studies have shown a direct correlation between blood cholesterol levels and erection problems. Men with total cholesterol levels over 250 milligrams per deciliter nearly double their risk of ED. Boosting your dietary fiber intake can open the floodgates to stiff, reliable erections.

You'll boost your chances of achieving immortality. If you want to be a dad some day, put down that fried corn dog and grab a handful of pumpkin seeds. How you eat directly affects your ability to produce your own healthy seed. Foods rich in antioxidant vitamins and important minerals are crucial to the production of sperm and boosting sperm motility (their swimming ability). Zinc in particular, found in seeds, nuts, and beans, is an important component in sperm production.

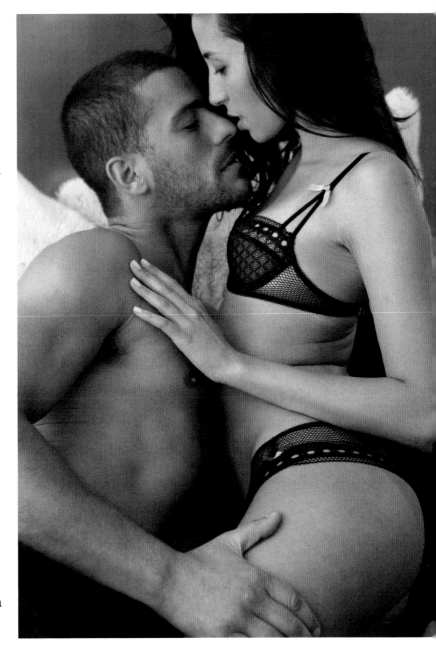

10 Ways Having More Sex Can Improve Your Health

LEAVE THIS PAGE OPEN ON YOUR NIGHTSTAND

Sex may protect your heart.

A study in the *American Journal of Cardiology* suggests that men who have sex twice a week have a lower risk of cardiovascular disease (CVD) than men who have less frequent sex. And this was true even after researchers adjusted for erectile dysfunction. Analyzing the health records of 1,165 men who were monitored for 16 years as part of the Massachusetts Male Aging Study, epidemiologists at the New England Research Institutes found that men who had sexual activity once a month or less were at 50 percent greater risk of cardiovascular disease than the men who had sex more than once a week.

"Our research found that a low frequency of sexual activity predicted new cardiovascular events," says Susan Hall, PhD. Hall says a number of possible factors could have contributed to the study's finding: The psychical capacity to have sex might be a marker for overall health, or the physical exercise from sex might directly protect against CVD. Or it might be that men who have regular sex enjoy improved health through stress reduction from a supportive relationship. Whatever the reason, it appears that sex is good for your ticker.

Doing it burns calories.

Due to its brevity, having an orgasm fries only two or three calories. But the prelude can burn quite a bit more, depending on your weight and the length and vigor of the lovemaking session. For example, a raucous romp uses about 5 METs (metabolic equivalents), a system for gauging the intensity of physical activity. (Sitting quietly, for comparison, is equal to 1 MET.) So, a 190-pound man would burn 413 calories in an hour of vigorous sexual activity. But since the average lovemaking session is about 20 minutes, you're talking about only around 150 calories. Still, that's more than double the caloric expenditure of sitting alone on the couch.

Sex, the natural sleeping pill.

As women know all too well, orgasm is a rather effective sleep aid for most men.

Sex stifles stress.

Research at the University of the West of Scotland shows that sex, like exercise, releases anxiety, lowers stress hormones, and can help people cope with mental pressure for at least a week. In the study, 46 men and women were put in a stressful situation involving speaking and working math problems in front of a tough audience. Participants were also asked to keep a diary of their sexual activity for two weeks prior to the test. Those who had sex were the least stressed out, and their blood pressures returned to normal faster after the public speaking test. "People who had penile-vaginal intercourse did twice as well as people who only masturbated or had no sex at all," says psychologist and lead researcher Stuart Brody.

A roll in the hay keeps the doctor away.

People who have sex once or twice weekly have stronger immune systems than people who have sex less than once a week, according to a study at Wilkes University in Pennsylvania by psychologists Carl J. Charnetski, PhD, and Francis X. Brennan Jr., PhD. In their book, *Feeling Good is Good for You: How Pleasure Can Boost Your Immune System and Lengthen Your Life,* they describe their study in which they took saliva samples from 111 college students and asked them about their frequency of sex over the course of a month. Analysis showed that the saliva of the students who had sex once or twice a week had 30 percent more of the antigen immunoglobulin A (IgA) than the saliva of students who had sex less often. "IgA is the body's first line of defense against colds and flu," says Charnetski.

Other studies show that happy relationships are good for health. In one experiment reported in the *New England Journal of Medicine,* University of Pittsburgh scientists shot live cold viruses up the noses of volunteers. Those who reported having strong ties with lovers, friends, and family were the least likely to catch a cold.

Good love is better than a bandage.

Researchers at Ohio State University Medical Center inflicted minor blister wounds on the arms of 45 married couples during 24-hour visits on two different occasions. On the first visit, the couples were prompted to engage in a positive, supportive discussion. Two months later they returned and new wounds were administered, the couples were prompted to argue. Results showed that wounds healed nearly two times faster after the positive interaction.

More sex may turn back the clock.

Can having sex keep wrinkles away? British neuropsychologist David Weeks, MD, of Royal Edinburgh Hospital believes so. In a 10-year-long study, he interviewed 3,500 adults in England and the United States, and found that people who reported having sex four times a week looked about 10 years younger than they actually were. Pleasure derived from having loving sex releases hormones, including human growth hormone, that are crucial in preserving youth, he says.

Frequent orgasms may protect against cancer.

Several studies have suggested that frequent ejaculation over many years may decrease risk of prostate cancer. In one US study, 29,000 men, ages 46 to 81, were asked their history of sexual intercourse and masturbation between the ages of 20 and 49. Researchers at the National Cancer Institute analyzed the data and determined that the group of men who reported 21 orgasms per month was much less likely to have prostate cancer than men who averaged seven or fewer ejaculations per month. The researchers speculated that several protective factors may contribute: ejaculation may clear the prostate of carcinogenic secretions and the stress-reduction benefit from orgasm may limit potential harmful substances that could trigger cancer.

Love longer, live longer.

An Irish study published in the *British Medical Journal* in 1997 tracked the mortality of 1,000 middle-aged men over the course of a decade and concluded that sexual activity may have a protective effect on health. By comparing men according to age and health, researchers found that men who had the highest frequency of orgasms had a death rate 50-percent lower than men who did not ejaculate frequently.

Men who have more sex are— surprise—happier!

An Australian survey of 5,000 people showed that married men are 135 percent more likely to report happiness than single men, while only 52 percent of married women are happier than unmarried women. Could it have something to do with the fact that sex is easier for cohabiting couples? According to a national sex survey conducted by the University of Chicago, sexual activity is 25 percent to 300 percent greater for married couples compared to non-married people, depending on age.

Men'sHealth.

Chapter 2
The Penis:
An Owner's Manual

OPERATING INSTRUCTIONS

FOR YOUR FAVORITE TOOL

You may think

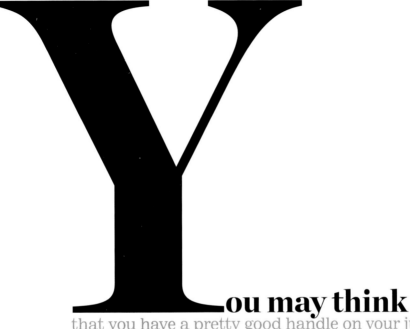

that you have a pretty good handle on your junk. After all it has been a focus of your attention long before it became a focus of airport screeners'. Heck, you had erections in utero, you stud! Many proud dad's have seen them poking through the grainy image of the obstetric ultrasound. What's not so surprising is that after birth male infants discover their penises and testicles three months earlier than female babies find their vaginas. With your genitals flopping around for such easy inspection, contemplation, and entertainment for so many years, it's kind of surprising that men are much more ignorant of their bat and balls than women are about their home plate.

"Men are completely clueless about what's going on down there," says urologist Harry Fisch, MD, a professor of clinical urology at Weill Cornell Medical College/New York-Presbyterian Hospital.

The Penis: An Owner's Manual

RISE AND SHINE

Male hormones peak between 5 a.m. and 9 a.m., maximizing both performance and pleasure.

"Men are in denial. They ignore problems because they are afraid or they want to appear invincible. Well, men should pay attention to their testicles. The testicles are headquarters for a man's health."

When Socrates advised us to "know thyself" he wasn't talking penises and testicles, but he wouldn't have been wrong if he had been. Some general genital knowledge can keep you out of a heap of trouble.

Think of it this way: You wouldn't operate a Chicago Pneumatic 857 Heavy Duty Angle Grinder without first reading the user manual, would you? Men benefit from becoming better acquainted with their own equipment. The more you know about your body, the healthier it will likely be and the more pleasure you will derive from it.

Now turn your head and cough.

The Parts

We'll pass over the penis for the moment and skip to the undercarriage, the twin testicles (or testes), where your genital tract begins. Each testicle contains millions of tiny angel hair spaghetti-like tubes that are tightly compressed in a strong casing. Each is a little bigger than a ping-pong ball, a little smaller than a hardboiled egg. (Get to know how healthy testes should feel by learning the testicular cancer self test on page 23.)

Your testicles hang beneath the big guy in a gnarly hacky sack called the scrotum. They swing there away from the body for good reason: to keep cool.

Optimal sperm production requires testes temperature to be a few degrees cooler than the body, ideally 94.6 degrees. Too warm and sperm-making begins to suffer, something to keep in mind if you're trying to become a father. German researchers studying testicular temperatures found that heated car seats can hinder a man's fertility. In their experiments, men who spent an hour planted in a hot seat experienced a significant jump in testicular temperature, to 99.14 degrees. Turn the seat heater off. You can also avoid roasting your nuts by wearing boxer shorts. Use those bikini briefs as rags for detailing your car.

By the way, you've probably noticed that one of your testicles hangs a bit lower than its brother. Rarely are both identical. The left is low ball in 85 percent of cases. (Now there's some cocktail party fodder for you!) As you've no doubt experienced, testicles retreat to the warmth of your body when you jump in a chilly lake or pool. That's due to muscles in the scrotum that automatically contract when cold or when your neighbor's rottweiler surprises you. It's a survival tactic.

Catching a baseball with your crotch will drop you to the ground in agony. This happens because there's no protective muscle or bone down there. A blow to the testicles triggers immediate swelling, presses on the testicular casing, and infuriates millions of nerve endings, which, in turn, send angry complaints to nerves throughout

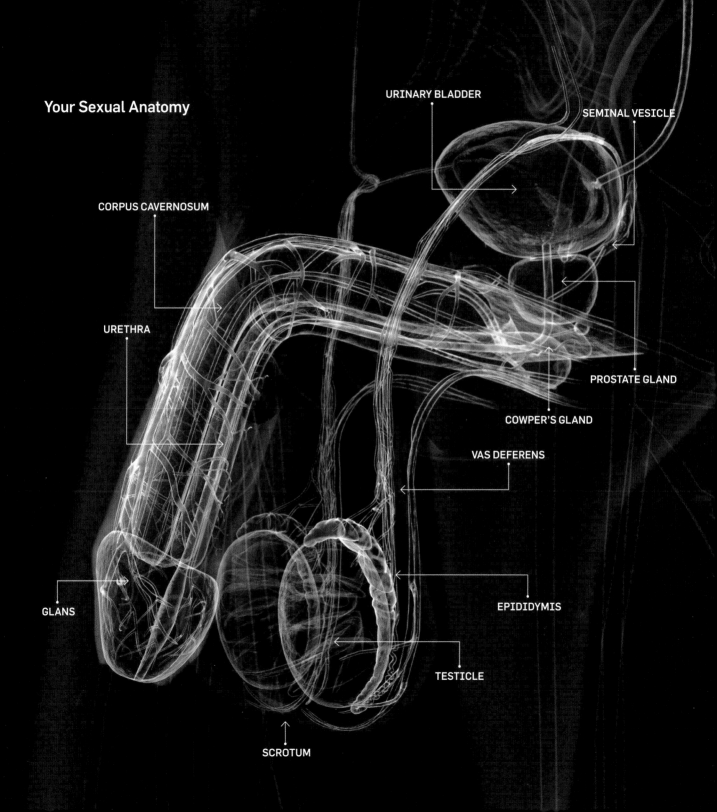

Your Sexual Anatomy

URINARY BLADDER

SEMINAL VESICLE

CORPUS CAVERNOSUM

URETHRA

PROSTATE GLAND

COWPER'S GLAND

VAS DEFERENS

GLANS

EPIDIDYMIS

TESTICLE

SCROTUM

The Penis: An Owner's Manual | HIS

HIS

BUY A WIDER BIKE SEAT

Bicycling is great cardio exercise, but it has a downside. When a rider rests his weight on the narrow protruding nose of a bicycle saddle, the nerves and arteries can be compressed against the pelvic bone, compromising blood flow to the genitals and causing numbness and tingling in the penis, according to Irwin Goldstein, MD, editor-in-chief of the *Journal of Sexual Medicine.* A study of 1,700 men in their 40s to 70s that included recreational cyclists, exercisers on stationary bikes and serious cyclists, demonstrated a correlation between cycling at least 3 hours per week and long-term damage. If you're a cyclist, you can reduce your risk by replacing your narrow saddle with a wider seat that transfers pressure onto your "sit bones" and muscle of the buttocks. In a 2008 study, 90 bicycling police officers replaced their traditional saddles with noseless bicycle saddles. After 6 months, the number of men reporting no penile numbness from riding rose from 27 percent to 82 percent.

the abdomen. Fire in the belly! You know how it feels. First aid: Wrap an ice pack or a bag of frozen peas in a dishtowel and cradle your testicles for 20-minute intervals with a 10-minute break in between. The skin's thin there, so never apply ice directly. Next time you play aggressive sports wear a cup.

Why They're There

The testicles do two jobs: produce sperm and generate testosterone, which is linked to your sex drive. At puberty, the testicles pump large amounts of testosterone into the bloodstream to fuel the maturation of genitals; sprout chest, pubic and facial hair, boost bone and muscle size and strength; and trigger the desire in young lads to hump everything with a pulse. It's a myth that testosterone fuels obnoxious male behavior, stupidity, and rage. In fact scientists are finding that testosterone makes men friendly, easygoing, and energetic. And, yes, women have some testosterone, just as men have some estrogen. By the time men hit middle age, testosterone levels decline by about a third, which tempers the insatiable sex drive of youth. (For information on testosterone deficiency and its affect on desire, see Chapter 5: The Sexual Diagnostic.)

The testicles begin manufacturing sperm during puberty to the tune of 50,000 sperm per minute every day and, barring complications, will continue to do so well into old age. Sperm mature in a holding site in the back of each testicle, a coiled tube called the epididymis.

Then they travel up and out of the scrotum through another pair of tubes, the vasa deferentia, or vas deferens, when speaking about just one. By the way, these are the tubes that are severed, tied, and cauterized during vasectomy surgery. Both tubes must get snipped for sterilization to occur. Each vas deferens passes through glands called the seminal vesicles where sperm is stored and mixed with yellowish seminal fluid that nourishes them on their journey. From there, the sperm continue through the vasa deferentia into the prostate—a walnut-sized gland under the bladder—where both tubes merge with the urethra. The prostate's main task is to produce the bulk of the fluid that comprises semen. Secondarily, it controls a cut-off valve that keeps urine from passing through when you have an erection. This is why only semen enters the penis even if you're having sex with a full bladder.

With age the prostate typically grows larger and can squeeze the urethra making urinating painful and sporadic, a problem known as benign prostatic hyperplasia (BPH). This isn't prostate cancer. It's a benign condition in which common symptoms include feeling an urge to urinate often, most disruptively at night, and feeling like you have to go some more to no avail. Far more serious is prostate cancer, which affects about 12 percent of men, mostly over the age of 65. If you are 40 or older, your doctor may recommend a digital rectal exam (in which he inserts a gloved, lubed finger in your rectum to feel the prostate for abnormalities) and a blood test called prostate-specific antigen (PSA), which may help detect prostate cancer early. But before having these tests, learn about the possibility of false positive tests and the risks involved in the various treatments of prostate cancer. There has been much new thinking on prostate cancer diagnosis and treatment, and you'll read more about it in Chapter 5.

Some men enjoy having the prostate gland stimulated by their partner's lubed finger inserted in the anus. Full of nerves, this muscular tissue has been nicknamed the male G-spot for its sensitivity and difficult access. In fact, the prostate and female G-spot are thought to originate from the same embryonic tissue.

The Big Kahuna

We've all measured it. And are we any less obsessed with our size after that little experiment? You've heard this before: The average flaccid penis is 2.4 to 3.5 inches in length, which is a fairly useless statistic since it has nothing to do with the ultimate size of an erection. Studies show that the smaller the limp penis, the larger in length and girth it grows during an erection. As for the erection size, one study found that 76 percent of penises measured from $4^5/_8$ to $6^1/_4$ inches, with an average of about 5.1 inches and a diameter of about 1.6 inches. Porn actors notwithstanding, most women are happy with

a medium-sized penis. In fact, most prefer a little more girth to length, or a particularly talented tongue.

More good news: Your penis is actually bigger than it looks when you peer down between your legs because you're viewing it from a foreshortened perspective. When you catch a glance of another guy's member as he comes out of the gym shower, he'll often look slightly better endowed. It's the angle, son. Relax. You're fine, size-wise. Focus on making better use of it during sexual intercourse.

Your penis is amazing—well, not yours specifically—but penises in general. You'll appreciate yours all the more if you understand how it operates. First of all, your penis is probably twice as long as you can see because half of the shaft is hidden inside you. This is what helps give the erect penis foundation and structure for doing its sexual duty. The remarkable penis is made up of smooth and highly elastic muscle tissue surrounding three spongy tubes, two called the corpora cavernosa and a third called the corpus spongiosum, which surrounds the urethra. At the end of the shaft is the glans, or head, which resembles a mushroom top. At birth, the head is covered by a sheath of skin called the foreskin that retracts with help of the frenulum when the penis becomes erect. Many males have a circumcision shortly after birth, in which this fold of skin is surgically removed. There's no medical reason to do this, except in cases when

THE ANGLE OF THE DANGLE

The erect penis at age . . .

135 to 120 degrees.
Everything is hunky-dory.

120 to 100 degrees.
Watching your partner undress may not trigger as firm an erection as it once did. You may need foreplay just as she does. Refractory period starts to increase.

100 to 80 degrees
Nerves in the penis begin to lose sensitivity. It may take some men longer to ejaculate.

80 to 90 degrees.
Slower arterial flow of blood to the penis affects erection strength. Volume and velocity of the ejaculate decreases. Your refractory period may last 3 days.

The Penis: An Owner's Manual | HIS

MY BALONEY HAS A FIRST NAME

American men have never been comfortable saying "penis." Maybe it's because the word sounds teeny weenie. Maybe that's why they've come up with such creative euphemisms. Some common monikers for penis:

- Godzilla
- Thor
- Buddy and the Sidewinders
- Big Jim and the Twins
- Any name preceded by Mr. as in Bo Dangles
- Big Red
- Big Daddy
- Big Fred
- The Big Hardee Combo
- Happy, Sneezy, or any of the other seven dwarfs
- Hugo
- Dr. Schwantz
- Little Elvis
- Herman the One-Eyed German
- Russell the Love Muscle
- Willy (Free him, please!)

the foreskin doesn't retract properly. It's typically done for reasons of hygiene, since dirt and bacteria can accumulate under the folds of skin. The frenulum, a V-shaped structure underneath the head of the glans, is highly sensitive to manual or oral stimulation.

Your penis has just three things to do in life:

1. Pass urine. Since it's flexible, this hose can be directed to aim at flies on urinals at sporting events. Your pubococcygeal (PC) muscles are what you squeeze to keep from peeing yourself on long car rides and to rid yourself of those last few drops that tend to hesitate at the urethral opening (a.k.a the meatus) until you zip up.

2. Become erect in order to penetrate a vagina during sexual intercourse. When sexually stimulated, nerve cells in the penis release nitric oxide, which causes the blood vessels of the corpora carvernosa and corpus spongiosum to relax and fill up the caveranous spaces with blood. The penis expands into an erection and the blood is trapped there to maintain it.

3. Deposit semen into the vagina during ejaculation. As arousal heightens, the vas deferentia contract to squeeze sperm toward the base of the penis while the prostate and seminal vesicles release their liquid to form semen. Upon arousal, when the penis is fully erect, you'll often notice a clear secretion from the tip of your glans. This isn't semen but a fluid contributed by the Cowper's glands (a.k.a. bulboure-

thral glands), two tiny peas just below the prostate and connected to the urethra. Named for the English surgeon William Cowper, who discovered them, Cowper's glands emit this fluid to neutralize the natural acidity of the urethra to protect sperm while passing through. They may also contribute some lubrication to the vagina.

Anatomy of Your Orgasm

In 1953 Alfred Kinsey described orgasm as "the expulsive discharge of neuromuscular tensions at the peak of sexual response." Sex researchers William Masters and Virginia Johnson called it "a brief episode of physical release from the vasocongestion and myotonic increment developed in response to sexual stimuli."

Sounds erotic enough to make you lose an erection.

Masters and Johnson identified the four phases of male sexual response in the early 1960s.

Excitement: muscles tense, heart rate increases, blood vessels in the penis relax and become engorged.

Plateau: arousal intensifies; muscles at the base of the penis begin contracting.

Orgasm: involuntary muscle contractions and ejaculation of semen.

Resolution: heart rate, blood pressure and muscle contraction return to normal.

Scientists still aren't very sure how the ejaculation really happens—what exactly triggers it—though it's pretty clear it has something to do with muscles, the neurological system, and the spine.

Let's take a look at the process from a mechanical perspective, based on the reigning theory described in *The Science of Orgasm* by Rutgers University scientists Barry Komisaruk, Beverly Whipple, and Carlos Beyer-Flores.

1. When aroused and nearing ejaculation, your testicles pull in toward your pelvis. Contractions in the smooth muscle in the testicles, inside the ducts of the epididymis and vas deferens, seminal vesicles, and prostate begin to propel semen forward into your ejaculatory duct system. Right about then, the area of your brain that registers pleasure fires up, and sends signals triggering more blood flow to your penis.

2. Pressure builds up behind a closed internal sphincter valve, unique to males, that creates a sort of pressure chamber in your urethra. A different valve, the prostatic sphincter, keeps the seminal fluid from back flowing into the bladder.

The chamber is filled; you're locked and loaded. This is probably the point of ejaculatory inevitability, when even the thought of your granny's jammies couldn't halt what is about to commence.

3. Something triggers a sudden opening of the sphincter valve that releases the seminal fluid. Simultaneously, your pelvic muscles including your penis begin rhythmic, involuntary contractions that help spurt semen out of the urethra and the tip of your penis. Immediately, the sphincter valve closes as the ducts fill up again.

4. Ditto #3. Another spurt of ejaculate. And so on. The process repeats rapidly about five to seven times about once every 0.8 seconds.

Again, what triggers this firing isn't quite clear, but you can feel the sensation from your head to your toes, and not just from semen shooting through your penis. But that feels amazing, too.

Erector Sets AN EXERCISE FOR BETTER ORGASMS

Kegels. You've heard of these, named after gynecologist Arnold Kegel who prescribed the pelvic floor strengthening exercises to patients to remedy incontinence. But they may also be useful for improving ejaculatory control and enhancing sexual pleasure. You do them by flexing the pubococcygeus (PC) muscle—the one you use to stop the flow of urine. Without using your butt muscles, contract those pee-stopping muscles for 15 seconds, then release. Do three sets of 10 reps. Over time, work up to longer holds, 30 seconds or a minute. The nice thing about these exercises is that nobody can tell you're doing them. So you can tap the Kegel anytime—during meetings, while driving, or watching TV. Or make it a game for two. After your penis becomes erect, flex your PC muscle. You'll notice that Jack jumps slightly. Have your partner hold a finger about an inch above the tip of your penis; try to flex hard enough to touch it 10 times. Be creative. Make your penis jump and tap her nipples, clitoris, or tongue. Drape a hand towel over it to add resistance. Yachtsmen can attach a small flag and practice their semaphore. Later, when your ship's docked, you and your partner can practice your Kegels together—the ultimate in synchronized schwinging!

How to Keep Your Private Parts Healthy

ROUTINE MAINTENANCE ENSURES OPTIMUM PERFORMANCE

"All health issues have effects on your penis," says Steven Lamm, MD, an assistant professor at the New York University School of Medicine and the author of *The Hardness Factor: How to Achieve Your Best Health and Sexual Fitness at Any Age.* "A 50-year-old man who is healthy is probably performing as well sexually as an out-of-shape 30-year-old who smokes and drinks."

While healthy blood flow is essential to rock-hard erections, other physical and mental health factors play a role in good penis functionality. If you are stressed out from work or poor relationships, suffering from depression, addicted to alcohol or drugs, or woefully overweight and out of shape, that miraculous mechanical wonder between your legs won't work as well as it could. Fortunately, there's much you can do to keep your member in good standing so you can still have sex well into your eighties and maybe even beyond. How's that for incentive to shape up? Do your private parts a favor.

Lose the belly.

Eat a healthy diet and exercise regularly to achieve ideal body weight and eliminate the fat around your gut. Abdominal fat blocks the testosterone that should be available to you, which in turn affects sexual functioning. A fat gut is a bad marker for overall health—including your sexual health. Your penis is a barometer for your heart and artery health or a "canary in the coal mine" that can warn you of impending trouble. That's because a penile artery is quite a bit narrower than a coronary artery. If plaque and artery hardening is starting to occur, it'll often show up first by affecting your erection.

Quit smoking.

"Smoking just clenches down on your blood vessels and prevents them from being reactive," says Lamm. Nicotine restricts penile blood flow and weakens erections. It contributes to plaque buildup in the arteries, making smokers twice as likely to experience erectile dysfunction.

Take a walk every day.

When you exercise, blood flow increases—blood rushes through the endothelial cells (the lining of the blood vessels) and stimulates them to make more nitric oxide, a key chemical involved in producing erections. "The healthier a man is, the more nitric oxide he produces, and the harder his erection is," says Lamm. Also exercise has been shown to be as effective as medication in reducing symptoms of mild depression, another downer for penis performance.

Do a ball check.

Testicular cancer strikes nearly 8,000 men a year, mostly young men between the ages of 15 and 40. When caught early enough, testicular cancer can be cured more than 95 percent of the time. Left undetected, though, it can spread to other parts of the body—in Lance Armstrong's case, to the lungs and brain. Check in with your boys once a month. Here's the play-by-play from *Men's Health* urology advisor Larry I. Lipshultz, MD, chief of the division of male reproductive medicine at Baylor College of Medicine.

Step 1. Take a hot bath or shower. Warm water relaxes the muscles that pull the testicles up into your scrotum, allowing you to handle them more easily.

Step 2. Cup your scrotum. Feel both testicles at once. They may not be identical, but there shouldn't be any dramatic difference in size.

Step 3. Gently examine each testicle individually with both hands. Place your index and middle fingers underneath and your thumbs on top of a testicle. Roll the testicle between your fingers around the entire surface for about 30 seconds using light pressure. Feel for lumps or bumps. Each testicle should feel smooth like a peeled hardboiled egg. If you think you felt something, don't panic. A lot of men mistake the epididymis, a soft tube located in the back of each testicle, for a bump. If you're unsure or if you feel any other bumps, consult your doctor.

Go to bed earlier.

Testosterone levels peak in the morning for men. So irregular sleep patterns, or getting fewer than 7 hours of sleep, can affect the quality of your sleep and your sexual health. Poor sleep is also associated with many health issues that contribute to sexual problems including high blood pressure, sleep apnea, and diabetes. Sleepiness is a national problem. A study of 8,000 adults by researchers from Stanford University found that 1 in 5 Americans suffers from chronic excessive sleepiness.

Eat more fish.

The omega-3 fatty acids DHA and EPA are good for heart and penis health. But toxins like PCBs and dioxins in some fish can hit you below the belt by reducing your sperm count and lowering testosterone. Try to avoid large bluefish, striped bass, and farmed salmon. PCBs and dioxins accumulate in the fatty tissues of those fish more so than in younger, smaller fish or species such as wild salmon, skipjack tuna, or sea bass.

Pop supplemental insurance.

If you aren't eating two to three servings of fatty fish per week, take two omega-3 fatty-acid supplements daily, totaling at least 300 milligrams (mg) of DHA and 400 mg of EPA as a kind of insurance policy. And consider taking the antioxidants pycnogenol (80 mg) and L-arginine (3 grams) daily. They'll shield your endothelium from harm and facilitate the use of nitric oxide.

Drink moderately.

A glass of red wine may fuel the libido, but a full bottle may screw with your penis-brain circuitry and eliminate any chance of getting an erection. Clinical studies have shown that alcohol acts as a depressant in the brain, dulling anxiety and inhibitions about sex, but larger amounts can have the opposite effect. In one study, men with a blood alcohol concentration (BAC) of 0.06 and 0.09 had trouble ejaculating while masturbating. Another study measured penile swelling in response to erotic stimulation. Those men who had three or more mixed drinks within 2 hours couldn't get it up. Over time, chronic use of alcohol can cause hormonal and brain chemical changes that stifle sexual functioning. Alcoholism has also been linked to gyneocomastia and shrinkage of the penis and testicles.

Relax and unwind.

In men especially, stress can trigger the fight-or-flight response. When that happens, your nervous system floods your body with stress hormones like adrenaline. Adrenaline spurs the heart to beat faster and your blood vessels to constrict so that blood is directed to where it's needed most to deal with the crisis—your muscles, not your penis. It doesn't have to be an urgent stress to cause problems. Chronic low-level stress, like a difficult boss, looming deadlines, and fear of financial ruin can interfere with erections and sex drive. Fortunately, exercise, sleep, and a healthy diet can help to ease the stress response.

Hard Facts

Bad to the Bone *Most reported cases of penile fracture happen when the woman is on top of the man or when the woman is sitting on a desk and the man is facing her and suddenly pushes his penis into the desk by mistake.*

55

Percentage of men who are happy with the size of their penises

5.1"

Average length of a penis when erect

1

Average number of teaspoons of semen in each ejaculation

Roll With It Only 20 percent of men do a testicular self exam monthly; 43 percent rarely or never check their balls for bumps or varicoceles.

2.6
Average number
of minutes from
stimulation
to ejaculation

28
Average airspeed
(in MPH) of
ejaculate

12"
Size of longest medically
recorded erection

14
Percentage
of men who
stress about
timing a
simultaneous
orgasm

4.8"
Average
circumference
of an erect penis

LOW BALL
*The left testicle
hangs lower than
the right in
85 percent of men*

22
Percentage of men who
describe their member
as "large"

Bumping Uglies
43 percent of women
find male genitalia
visually appealing only
when erect

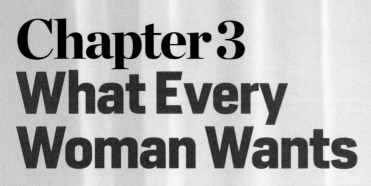

Chapter 3
What Every Woman Wants

Fulfill her most secret desires and
become her best lover, ever

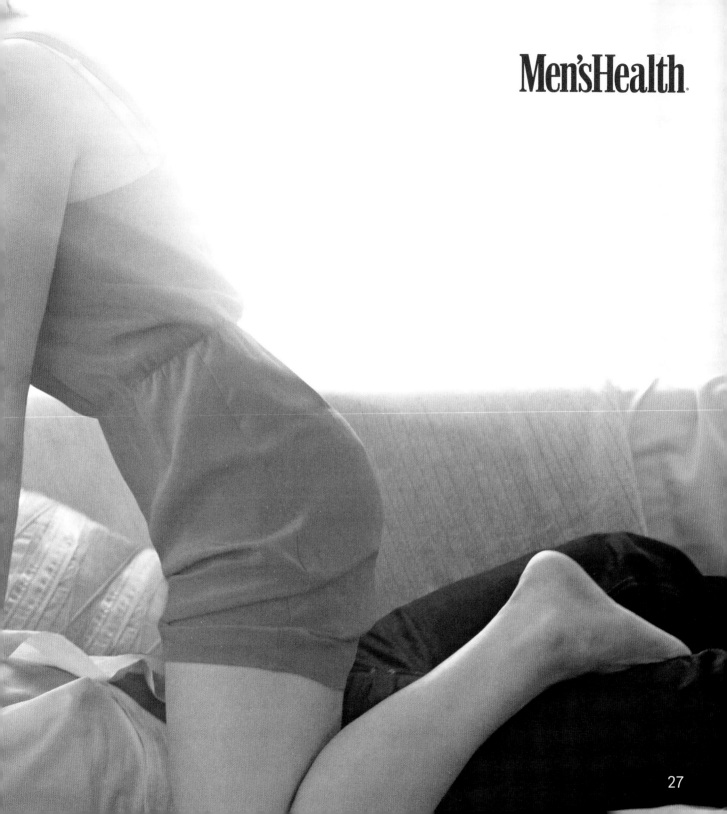

Men'sHealth.

W

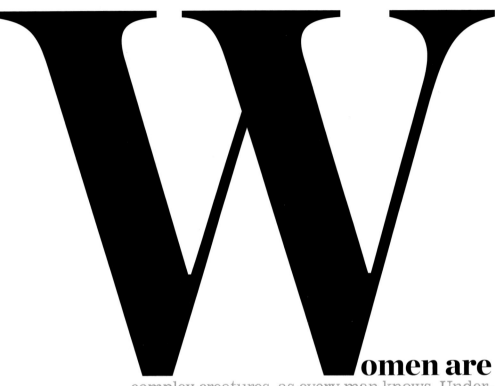

omen are

complex creatures, as every man knows. Understanding how their brains are wired differently from yours will make all the difference in the world in figuring them out and turning them on.

One of the most important things to understand about women is that the female's brain does not have a 24/7 appetite for sex like yours does. The area of the hypothalamus responsible for sexual pursuit is 2.5 times larger in your head than it is in hers, explains neuropsychiatrist Louann Brizendine, MD, author of the books *The Male Brain* and *The Female Brain*. "Evolution biologically hard-wired a man to be ready for sex at every opportunity," she says. "Mother nature made it so a man is consumed with sexual fantasies about

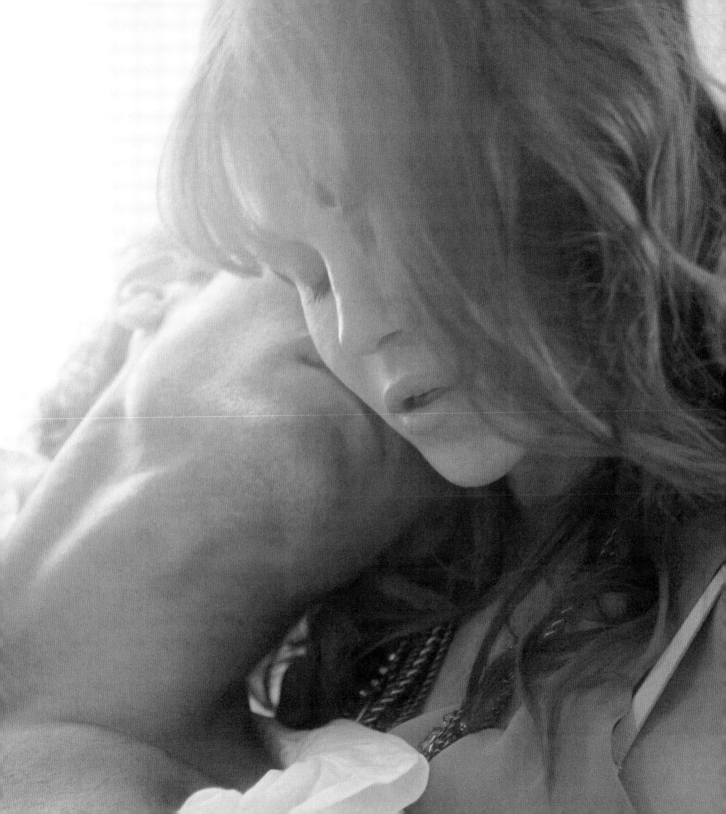

What Every Woman Wants | HIS

female body parts." So, while you are a big-eyed dog drooling over every curvy female who walks by as if she was a juicy pork chop with breasts, her brain is working quite differently, quite a bit more intelligently. She's sizing you up in a far different way—by talking, getting to know you, assessing if she feels comfortable with you, or determining that you're a creep—for a different purpose. Because pregnancy and nursing are such dangerous, painful, and time-consuming undertakings, women have evolved to be far more thoughtful about whom they'll agree to talk with at a bar and ultimately have sex with. (Do I risk having a baby with the unemployed hunk on the motorcycle or the nice man in khakis with the degree from Dartmouth?) The area of her brain that analyzes risk—is he safe or an axe murderer?—the anterior cingulate cortex, or ACC, is much larger than it is in men. "Her prefrontal cortex—essentially the brain's nanny, which tries to prevent her from making a fool of herself—is bigger than a man's, too," says Brizendine. These differences help her to evaluate guys for the likelihood that they will become devoted mates who will protect and provide for their children, which naturally makes her more cerebral when it comes to sex.

"This contrast in our evolutionary goals, etched deep in our brains, continues to cause no end to conflict between the sexes," says Brizendine.

If it helps, think of our differences regarding sex in these most basic ways: she needs to feel safety and intimacy in order to desire sex; you need sex in order to feel intimacy. To the female brain, talking with you on the couch is as essential to your relationship as sex in the hammock is to your Neanderthal brain. But a meeting of these two disparate minds is possible, even highly likely, when you make an effort to understand a woman's special needs, realize that they are not just like yours, and focus on fulfilling those deep-seated desires. Start here:

Make a good first impression.

If getting anywhere with a woman sexually starts with talking, talking starts with letting her know you exist. That's treacherous ground as anyone who has encountered barstool rejection knows all too well, and it's why meeting women is always easier in the context of some activity or pursuit other than meeting women, like at a sailing class or volunteering in your community, which present ample opportunities for non-threatening talk.

But if you must attempt the risky approach, be funny. Women love funny, and they generally find stories more humorous than one-liners or sarcasm. So be funny with anecdotes. That's how women share and bond. Stories bring the teller and listener closer. If you can't be funny, be natural and sincere. Don't try too hard, though, or be sappy. Women like to see confidence in men. One of the best ways to snag a woman's attention and disarm her is by showing

WHAT'S SEXY TO HER

"Be the man in the fairy tale—chase the girl. If you can't, don't wonder why you're not attracting women."
—Singer/songwriter Joss Stone

30

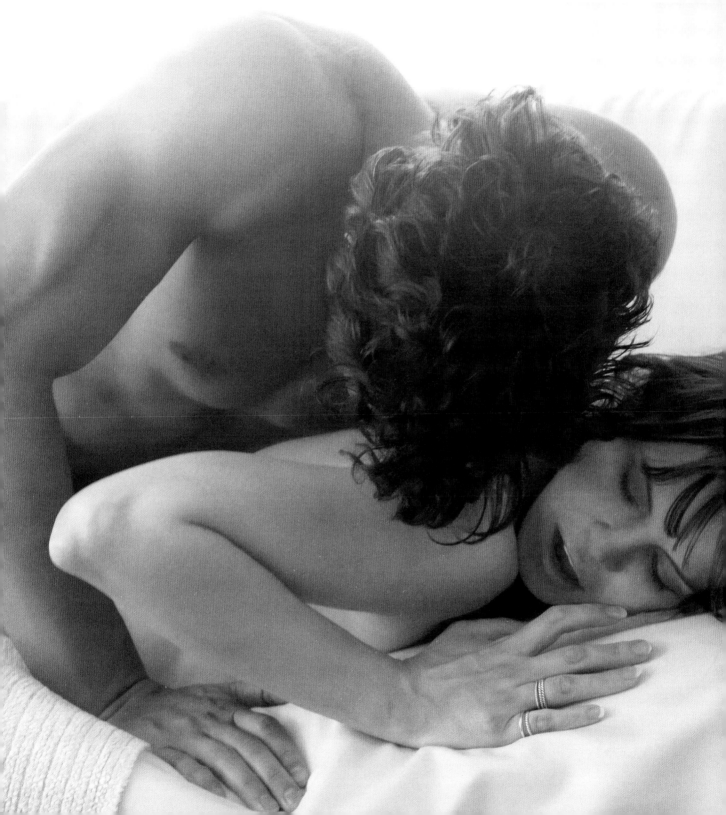

kindness and generosity. If you can find an opportunity to display your willingness to help someone in front of the woman of your interest, you'll gain major points and break down her guard. (That's why volunteer opportunities are such great places to meet women to date.) So at a supermarket checkout, let the person with two items go ahead of you. It can be as simple as offering your chair or seat on a bus to someone. Unconditional selflessness may be an evolutionary signal of intelligence and resourcefulness, according to a study in the *Journal of Research in Personality*. Showing off your willingness to do for others suggests intelligence, problem-solving ability, higher creativity, higher social status, and demonstrates that you have resources to spare and, perhaps more income opportunities, says study author Mark Prokosch, PhD.

Be intimate without an erection.

Unlike men, women feel sexual as a result of intimacy that begins outside of the bedroom. This is the greatest lesson you can learn about how to satisfy a woman emotionally, physically, and sexually. "To a man, foreplay is just the three minutes before insertion," says Brizendine. "But for a woman foreplay is everything that happens 24 hours before sex." So, getting her into the right frame of mind for great sex takes all-day-long communication, sending frequent signals that say "I'm thinking about you," and

"I want to get close to you." Little things you can do to and for your partner will encourage her to think of you in a positive, romantic way that can trigger desire on a hormonal level. And most of them require very little effort and have nothing to do with sex and everything to do with sex at the same time. The big, important ones are talking, touching, listening, paying attention to her needs, and making her feel that you appreciate and value her very much.

In his book, *If Only He Knew: What No Woman Can Resist*, author Gary Smalley says praise is the one thing that no woman can resist. And it can be the easiest and most important thing a man can do for the woman in his life. "Men should realize their need, because we, too, want to know that we are valued to other people," says Smalley. However, our preoccupation with our own needs, vocations, and activities often prevents us from expressing praise and appreciation. It takes intentional effort to change, but the results can be dramatic. Sex educator and psychotherapist Laura Berman, PhD, says that every woman has a treasure chest, a secret part of her that she cherishes, that men need to find in order to target their praise most effectively.

"Typically, it's a non-body trait like her intellectual curiosity, her sense of humor, her outlandishness," Berman says. "But it could be the color of her eyes or even her laugh. It's when a man discovers this, when he comes to appreciate and love that part of her, that he really gets the girl both emotionally and

72

Percentage of women who say it turns them on when a man helps around the house.

sexually. That's when she feels she's being loved as a complete person." If you have no clue what's inside your woman's treasure chest, listen closely the next time she's with her father. Dads are usually the ones who instill these gems in their little girls. Note what he compliments about her and what makes her sparkle. For now, any praise that is genuine and honest will be appreciated more than you know.

She likes the sound of your voice.

Plan a night for just the two of you. Light candles, cue up some Diana Krall, hold hands across the table while gazing deeply into each other's eyes, and discuss the merits of Berber versus plush carpet. Talk about anything. Just converse, you know, take turns talking. Be careful to avoid making statements, like you are debating, and dominating the air space. In other words, talk less, listen more. And talk more like women talk. Women use language to bond, while men use it like a hammer drill. "Men are literal communicators," says Audrey Nelson, PhD, a gender communications expert. "It serves them well in the business world but often causes them trouble with women." If you can learn to share your feelings, spend do-nothing time together, and use talk as a social exercise rather than a means to a specific goal, you will automatically connect with your partner in ways she understands. And that can elevate her interest in having sex with you.

Studies by researchers Gurit Birnbaum, PhD, at the Interdisciplinary Center Herzliya in Israel, and Harry Reis, PhD, at the University of Rochester show a strong correlation between a man's nonsexual responsiveness to his partner and her increased sexual fantasizing and heightened interest in having sex with him. Translation: Talk about carpet and she may start thinking about creative uses for it. "Being responsive to your partner's non-sexual needs is so important because it signals that you are really concerned with her welfare," says Birnbaum. "One of the best ways you can make your wife or girlfriend feel special and desired is to pay attention and really listen without interrupting or prejudging. Sexual desire thrives on this rising intimacy; it's better than any pyrotechnic sex."

She's addicted to oxytocin.

Start her day with a 20-second embrace. A long hug releases the hormone oxytocin, which produces feelings of trust and attachment. Holding hands triggers it, too. Neuroscientist James A. Coan, PhD, and his colleagues at the University of Virginia found that non-sexual touch, such as holding hands, has a significant impact on the brain and that who is doing the touching is critical to the effect. In a study, they put 16 married women inside an MRI machine (no, not all at once!) and told them to expect to receive mild electric shocks. This obviously made the women pretty

38

Percentage of women who admit to having "poached" a man in a relationship so that they could have a short-term fling.

anxious, which showed up brilliantly on the MRI machine. But when husbands held their wives' hands during the test, the MRI scans showed a significant decrease in stress response, much lower than, say, when a stranger (or no one) held the women's hands. One reason humans form relationships, Coan believes, is to spread problem solving across brains; when someone is helping us cope, our brains don't have to work as hard. Understandably, Coan's study found that women in the strongest marriages had the lowest activation of these brain circuits when their husbands held their hands. "The effect was comparable to taking an analgesic," says Coan. So, after that morning hug, make a point of touching some part of her each time you pass by her throughout the day—and see if she doesn't notice.

She wants to hear you laugh at yourself.

To most women, a guy who takes himself too seriously is about as interesting as tofu. Women are attracted to men who smile, laugh, joke, tease, and know how to have a good time. In a survey of more than 1,000 women conducted by *Men's Health*, 77 percent said a sense of humor was the most important personality trait they look for in a man, followed by intelligence, passion, confidence, and generosity. Being able to make women laugh—and being able to laugh at yourself—tells them that you are confident and that you can handle

life's many difficulties with the right attitude. What's more, laughter is healthy, both physically and emotionally. Couples who share a love of laughter and tell kind, light-hearted jokes to defuse tension tend to have stronger, happier marriages, according to psychologist John Gottman, PhD, of the Gottman Institute, a relationship counseling center in Seattle. And since 90 percent of laughs involve deep exhalations, laughing has an immediate effect on reducing heart rate and blood pressure and decreasing stress hormones.

Go ahead, kiss her in public.

Better yet, kiss her in front of her friends or co-workers. She'll enjoy the public attention, but so much more importantly, she will revel in seeing her friends notice your outward expression of love for her. They'll think you're having sizzling sex every night. A hug, hand hold, arm around the waist, any public display of affection fulfills one of a woman's deepest desires: acknowledgment that you want her, love her, need her outside of the bedroom, and aren't timid about demonstrating this before others.

She thrives on your kindness and support.

There's a reason why it's so common for marriage ceremonies to incorporate this passage from the Bible, 1 Corinthians 13:4: "Love is patient, love is kind, and is not jealous … love is not arrogant.…" It is, perhaps, the perfect litany for how to make a woman feel loved and free of

GIGGLE HER INTO BED

Men who can laugh at themselves are seen as sexy, according to a University of New Mexico study in which women listened to men tell self-depreciating jokes. "It makes you more approachable to women when you use humor to show a little weakness," says study author Gill Greengross, PhD, whose research focuses on the evolutionary roots of laughter and humor.

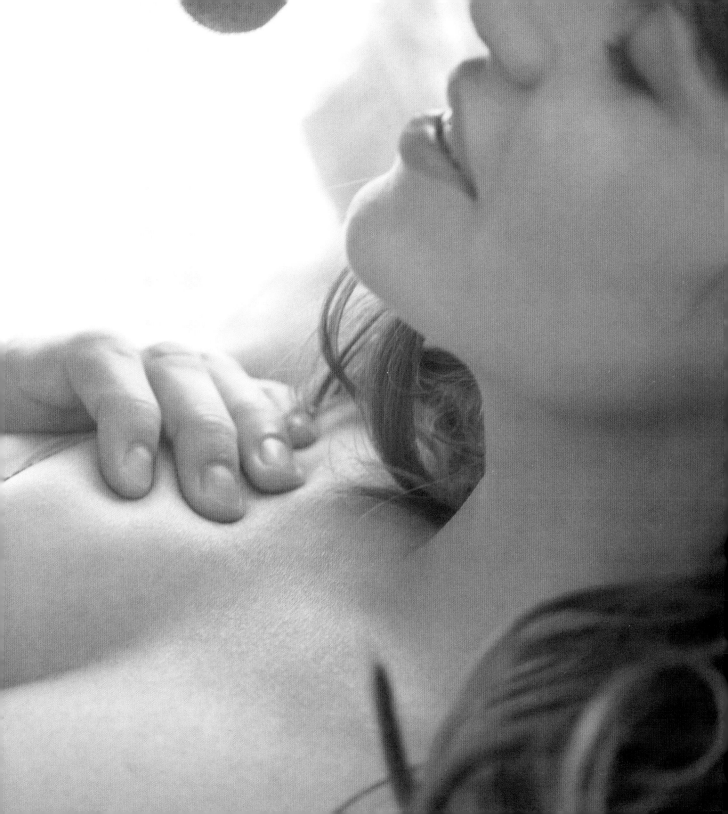

WHAT SHE'S WORRIED ABOUT DURING SEX

26% Her weight

20% She won't reach orgasm

17% Other parts of her body

14% You're not enjoying it

9% Someone might walk in

5% Pregnancy

9% Other (STIs, you're using her, you don't respect her, you might not orgasm)

anxiety. Acceptance counts. And the flip side, rejection, can wield a significant blow to woman's psyche very quickly. How quickly? In just 250 milliseconds. That's all it takes for the hint of rejection to trigger a cascade of brain processes that may turn the tide of her mood.

We know this because of experiments by Vivian Zayas, PhD, who heads the Personality, Attachment, and Control Lab at Cornell University. She outfitted women with bathing caps studded with electrodes to measure brain cortex activity. Through headphones, the women listened to a voice making statements like, "If I am upset and turn to my partner for support, he will be..." and concluding with either "comforting" or "distant." Neurons fired at the cold slap of rejection. By contrast, an accepting response produced very little brain activity. The findings show how dramatically and quickly—within a quarter of a second—women begin trying to make sense of perceived rejection.

"Before she's even aware of how she is feeling, in the blink of an eye, a lot has already happened in her mind," explains Zayas. She didn't study men, but believes that women may be more sensitive to and respond more strongly to these interpersonal cues than men would. If men understand this about women—that some women can process rejection quickly without the awareness that they're doing so—then maybe men can help women regulate their emotions, Zayas believes, by trying to provide clear communication.

"Relationships provide a lot of our happiness," she says, "but they also have the potential to really hurt us." And in the case of sexual arousal, even something you may feel is inconsequential—like an innocent ribbing or a comment about her sensitivity—can spoil her concentration and immediately break the mood. Remember that women's senses—touch, hearing, smell, taste, and vision—are more finely tuned than yours. This is one reason women are more socially intelligent and adept at interpersonal sensitivity or what neuroscientists call "executive cognition." They are good at reading people, and they can detect the tiniest signals that you are sending with your voice, choice of words, even the slightest of facial expressions. This also may be why women are more likely than men to become distracted by sounds, images, and thoughts during sex. When her concentration is broken, she needs to refocus and rebuild her sexual arousal. Again, very different from a guy who has no trouble staying focused on his thrusting.

Keep in mind that arousal and orgasm are essentially a conversation between her clitoris and her nervous system. And you can begin to stimulate her pleasure center—without even touching her—with kindness, patience, and your calming, attentive presence.

Her neck is her most surprising erogenous zone.

The vast majority of women who responded to *The Big Book of Sex* survey described their necks as their most unexpected pleasure zone. Considering what we learned earlier that makes perfect sense. Brain scans have shown that women can achieve orgasm more easily if their brain's stress centers are switched off. "Many women need a transition period between dealing with the stress of everyday life and feeling sexual," says Ian Kerner, a sex therapist and author. The neck is the perfect place to begin throttling down those stress hormones. Because the nerves and blood vessels are close to the surface of the neck, brushing your lips between her throat and chin will take her mind off the kids or the job. Massage her neck then move to the scalp. It's crucial to keep things non-sexual for her. Thinking you have an ulterior motive will destroy the effect you are going for.

Praise Triggers Passion.

When we asked women to choose the sexiest quality of a man, as we mentioned, most said "his sense of humor," followed by "his kindness," "his brains," and "his powerfulness." "His body" came in fourth place. When we asked the same women to choose the sexiest quality of a woman the vast majority said "her body."

That difference suggests how important a woman's body image is to her feeling attractive and worthy of love. In part because of the evolutionary roots of women's sexual attractiveness— a woman's appearance offered cues to her fertility—a woman's self-esteem is greatly influenced by how she feels about her body, says Cindy M. Meston, PhD, co-author of *Why Women Have Sex: Understanding Sexual Motivations from Adventure to Revenge (and Everything in Between)*. And chances are good that your partner isn't totally thrilled with her looks and is a bit worried about how she looks to you. Not long ago, a survey of 30,000 married and single women in North American found that 55 percent expressed dissatisfaction with their bodies. While her weight, shape, and other physical characteristics play a role in a woman's body image, researchers say that often it's influenced by her perceptions of what her body should look like. (We can thank Photoshopped magazine spreads for some of that.)

All of this can have significant bearing on a woman's desire for sex as well as her ability to achieve an orgasm. A 2010 study of 154 undergraduate women at the University of Texas at Austin explored the association between body esteem and sexual desire, and also assessed the impact of distracting thoughts, including anxiety about their appearance during sex. The researchers found that when a woman worries about how her body looks to her partner during sex, she's more distracted, less aroused, and in the end, less satisfied. So it's up to men to clarify matters. One way to do that is through words and actions—like touching and paying attention to her entire body, instead of making sex all about intercourse.

50

Percentage of women who would lose interest in a man who drinks too much on the first date.

In another study, University of Nevada psychologist Marta Meana, PhD, outfitted 20 heterosexual men and 20 heterosexual women with special goggles to track their eye movements as they looked at erotic and non-erotic images of men and women. The guys spent most of the time looking at images of women. The women's eyes, however, were drawn equally to men and women.

Meana says it's difficult to explain the women's equal-opportunity viewing. Did images of both men and women have arousal value for them, or were they comparing themselves to women? Interestingly, *The Big Book of Sex* survey found that 47 percent of women said they were more likely to check out the bodies of women than the bodies of men, presumably for comparison's sake.

"There's a very self-focused component to female sexuality," says Meana. "Women may need to be convinced that they are desirable in order to believe that anyone else finds them desirable."

So, compliment her often, and not always about her nice ass. Praise her in general terms when she's fully clothed—it will mean more delivered outside of a sexual situation, suggests Suman Ambwani, PhD, a psychologist at Dickinson College who has studied body image and romantic love.

"Women are socialized to think of themselves as bodies; the female form becomes an indicator of a woman's value," says Ambwani. "Praising the individual, paying compliments without focusing on body parts reduces that objectification."

90

Percentage of 700 women surveyed in a *Men's Health* poll who said that a man's primal panting turns them on during sex.

She wants you to be more dominant in bed.

Women desire sexual assertiveness in men because it's masculine and sexy. And surveys show that they want more of it. But men tend to subconsciously check their natural impulses and inhibit their dominance out of concern for her feelings, according to a study in the *Personality and Social Psychology Bulletin*. Surveys show that women want more assertiveness and creativity from men in bed. *The Big Book of Sex* survey, for example, found that 67 percent of women would enjoy a spanking. Well, what do you know? And 56 percent prefer you to be on top most of the time. So, take charge. Ambush her in the shower or when she walks in the door after work. In bed, move her around and be more assertive. Hold her tighter, run your nails up her legs, pin her arms down (if she's comfortable with that). Talk dirty. Tell her what you'd like to do to her. There are lots of things you can do to gain her attention and bring excitement to routine sex. But remember that physical aggressiveness can cross the line, so find out what she'd like before you whip out the leather and duct tape. And that takes—you guessed it—communicating. Always comes back to talking, see? Confess your latest sexual fantasy. Say it's something you dreamt about doing with her. "I might not agree to reenact it, but hearing about it will make me feel like your naughty little confidante, which is really hot," one woman told us.

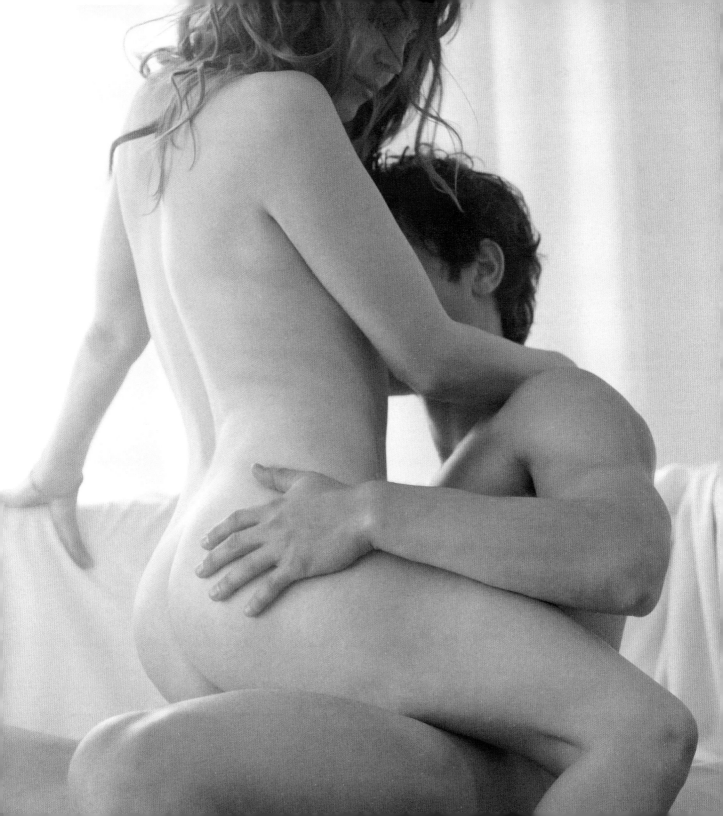

HER TOP 5 REASONS FOR ACCEPTING A BOOTY CALL

1. We're friends

2. He's only calling for sex

3. He's physically attractive

4. Good timing

5. He's interested and available

Your sexual assertiveness may even give her the courage to loosen her own inhibitions. More than a third of the women in one *Men's Health* online survey said that during sex they're thinking of dirty things they're embarrassed to talk about. One in four is imaging a position she's afraid to ask you to try. "Often her hesitancy to speak up is related to other inhibitions, like worrying about how she looks or tastes," says Yvonne K. Fulbright, PhD, the author of *Sultry Sex Talk to Seduce Any Lover: Lust-Inducing Lingo and Titillating Tactics for Maximizing Your Pleasure.* So tell her how sexy she looks and how turned on you are by her scent. Suggest trying a sex toy, new position, or role-playing. The more you open up and show your excitement for her—and the more you take the lead—the more comfortable she'll be.

She needs more than your penis.

The fact of the matter is that intercourse just doesn't do it for the majority of women. That's why women need foreplay, roughly 15 to 20 minutes of sustained play in order to effectively warm up. And why you will need to work your fingers and tongue, and maybe a toy and lube to coax her climax.

"Women require a high level of arousal to reach orgasm, and have difficulty focusing on sexual sensation," says Meston, "The main reason women can have orgasms while masturbating instead of during sex is that they stop worrying about what they think of themselves." So trade your goal-oriented approach to sex for a pleasure-centric one. "Think of sexual activity as a circle rather than a staircase," says Rutgers University sex researcher Beverly Whipple, PhD.

You do that by watching and learning. Masturbation isn't just her release valve; it's your sex school—if she'll let you watch. Encourage her to masturbate for you to share what she likes with you. Take note: When women masturbate they typically rest their forearm on their lower belly and wrist on their mons. Mimic this by having her sit on your lap so you can reach around and place the heel of your hand on her mons, adding pressure as you move it back and forth while stimulating her clit. Ask her to guide your hand to the right spot and rhythm.

Being too rough is the worst mistake men make during oral sex, according to a recent survey of women. Guys think they need to thrust and flick. Often what she wants is a firm, still tongue—a point of pressure—so she can set the rhythm and pace with her own movements, according to Kerner. Ask, watch, and learn what makes her feel best and you'll be the most attentive lover she's ever had. Remember this: A woman's orgasm threshold drops after she has had her first one, so it's often easier to bring her to climax through penetration after she's already had one manually. And that's what Kerner means by the title of his excellent manual of cunnilingus: *She Comes First.*

How's that for incentive to practice these fun, O-producing manual moves?

- Lie next to her, lightly bracing the heel of one hand just above her clitoris. Now run your ring and middle fingers along her outer lips. Do this ever so gently, grazing the skin lightly, then adding pressure as her tension builds. If she is too sensitive for direct clitoral stimulation—most women are—cup the area around her clitoris with your palm to add indirect stimulation, says research scientist and author Debby Herbenick. "As she becomes aroused, brace your hand on her pubic mound, the fleshy area that covers her pubic bone—and tease the clitoris with the middles and tips of your fingers and move your entire hand." For variety, pinch her labia gently. Then insert two fingers, pressing them up against the front wall of her vagina, simultaneously stimulating her clitoris and G-spot. She'll press and grind her clit into your palm. This combo stimulates her entire vulva.

- If your tongue gets tired during oral sex, let her do most of the work, allowing her to press and grind against your firm but resting tongue.

- Use your penis on the outside of her vagina. Press your shaft against her clitoris and thrust gently between the folds of her labia, like a hot dog in a bun.

Don't forget her breasts.

In surveys, women often say that they would enjoy more breast stimulation during sex. So learn to multitask and do it the right way:

- Worship them. Touch them delicately, lick and kiss them in a way that suggests they are the softest, most beautiful parts of her body, says Herbenick. In a *Women's Health* online survey of more than 3,000 women, 20 percent say they most liked to be complimented on their breasts, a score on par with their eyes, and just behind their behinds. Tip: When she is on top during sex, ask her to lean forward and allow them to dangle and sway before your face. Tell her how sexy they look as you lift your head to give them tiny kisses and licks.

- Pay attention to her nipples. Thirty-three percent of surveyed women prefer having their nipples sucked followed in order of preference by licking, nibbling, and rubbing. But explore other regions of the breast, too. The tops and bottoms of the breasts are actually more sensitive than the nipple area.

She thinks slower is better.

Women want rhythm, so relax about the size of your member. In our survey, only 9 percent of respondents said the size of the ship was most important. Twenty-four percent chose "the technique of the tongue," while 67 percent said the motion in the ocean was most crucial for satisfaction. Use deep thrusts at a medium pace. Pistonlike, porn-movie thrusting feels horrible, women say, and can leave a girl dry, sore, and bored. Vary your thrusts, adding side-to-side movement or grinding pelvic pressure against her clitoris when you're all the way inside of her to change up the stimulation. Then, after you've both simultaneously climaxed—no pressure, gents—you can cuddle to release all that good oxytocin you both crave (her, especially).

WHAT SHE WANTS

"The most amazing orgasms I've ever had were when my partner and I were having sex and using a vibrator on my clitoris at the same time."
—Chelsea, 27, Wilmington, DE

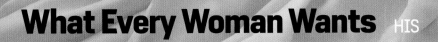

What Every Woman Wants HIS

Her Body/Your Map

INNER THIGHS
Like the inner arms, thin skin here is your opportunity to send shivers down her spine. Kiss her softly starting at the knee and ever so slowly make your way north. Alternate side to side like climbing ladder rungs, kissing and tickling with your tongue. You'll feel her anticipation through her breathing and back arching as your tongue nears her vulva.

GENITALS
Only between 30 and 50 percent of women can achieve orgasm through intercourse alone. Additional manual stimulation ups the odds considerably.

BUTT
"Nice butt." Complimenting her butt should score you points. When *The Big Book of Sex* asked women to name the body part on which they most liked being complimented, the butt won hands down, garnering 33 percent of the vote.

FEET
Packed with so many nerve endings, it's no wonder some women claim that they can reach orgasm just by having their feet rubbed. The key is not to tickle: a real mood buster. It should be a firm touch. Start by holding the ankle then work down the top and bottom of the foot, gently kneading. Tug and massage each toe individually. Linger on the middle toe. Tug on it a bit. Some sexperts believe this toe has a direct nerve connection to the genitals.

BACK
More than 58 percent of women surveyed in *The Big Book of Sex* poll said they preferred having their backs massaged to all other body parts. A lot of guys feel they are so strong, they will hurt her if they massage too hard, when in fact, that's just the kind of deep kneading she needs to work out the tension in her shoulders and help her relax. Go for it. She'll tell you if you're working her too aggressively.

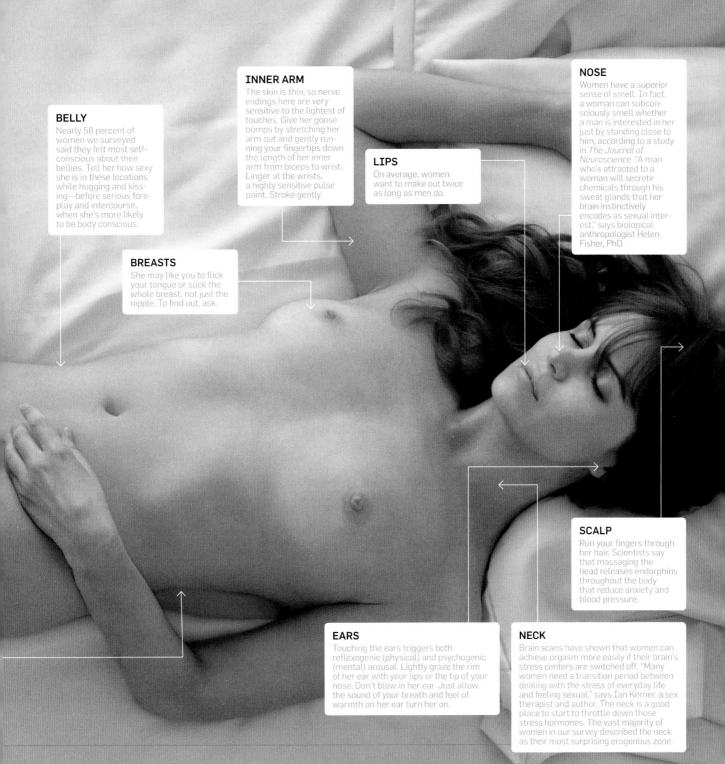

INNER ARM
The skin is thin, so nerve endings here are very sensitive to the lightest of touches. Give her goose bumps by stretching her arm out and gently running your fingertips down the length of her inner arm from biceps to wrist. Linger at the wrists, a highly sensitive pulse point. Stroke gently.

NOSE
Women have a superior sense of smell. In fact, a woman can subconsciously smell whether a man is interested in her just by standing close to him, according to a study in *The Journal of Neuroscience*. "A man who's attracted to a woman will secrete chemicals through his sweat glands that her brain instinctively encodes as sexual interest," says biological anthropologist Helen Fisher, PhD.

BELLY
Nearly 58 percent of women we surveyed said they felt most self-conscious about their bellies. Tell her how sexy she is in these locations while hugging and kissing—before serious foreplay and intercourse, when she's more likely to be body conscious.

LIPS
On average, women want to make out twice as long as men do.

BREASTS
She may like you to flick your tongue or suck the whole breast, not just the nipple. To find out, ask.

SCALP
Run your fingers through her hair. Scientists say that massaging the head releases endorphins throughout the body that reduce anxiety and blood pressure.

EARS
Touching the ears triggers both reflexogenic (physical) and psychogenic (mental) arousal. Lightly graze the rim of her ear with your lips or the tip of your nose. Don't blow in her ear. Just allow the sound of your breath and feel of warmth on her ear turn her on.

NECK
Brain scans have shown that women can achieve orgasm more easily if their brain's stress centers are switched off. "Many women need a transition period between dealing with the stress of everyday life and feeling sexual," says Ian Kerner, a sex therapist and author. The neck is a good place to start to throttle down those stress hormones. The vast majority of women in our survey described the neck as their most surprising erogenous zone.

16 Things She Wishes You Knew About Her

1. She loves when you draw a bath for her without asking. **2.** She longs to receive a handwritten love letter. **3.** She wants your enthusiasm more than your opinion. **4.** She expects you to know that sex involves more areas of her body than just the obvious parts. **5.** She wants more dirty talk, much more. **6.** The top five character traits she's looking for in you, in order of importance: 1. A big package. **Relax, it's a joke.** They are: 1. Faithfulness 2. Dependability 3. Kindness 4. Moral integrity 5. Father-liness. **7.** Don't stick your tongue in her ear. Kiss gently, lick the edges. Hover briefly, then leave it be. It's an ear, not a vagina. **8. She doesn't want you to solve her problems … just listen to them. 9.** It means a great deal to her when you ask her for advice. **10.** She wants you to pay attention to what makes her happy because she knows what makes you happy. **11.** She loves it when you hug her from behind and whisper in her ear. **12.** Sex on the beach, the drink: yummy. Sex on the beach, the act: scratchy. **13.** She'd like you to mow the lawn in tight jeans and no shirt. Then come inside smelling of freshly cut grass and sweat, and make monkey love to her on the dining-room table, just like in *Desperate Housewives*. **Sorry, we're kidding. 14.** She thinks you look really sexy when you fix stuff, shave with a razor, or hold a baby. **No kidding. 15.** Being critical of her in front of others is poor form. Being critical of her in front of others in front of your mother will effectively keep you from having sex for at least a month. **16.** She'd like you to call at 2 or 3 in the afternoon to ask how she's doing.

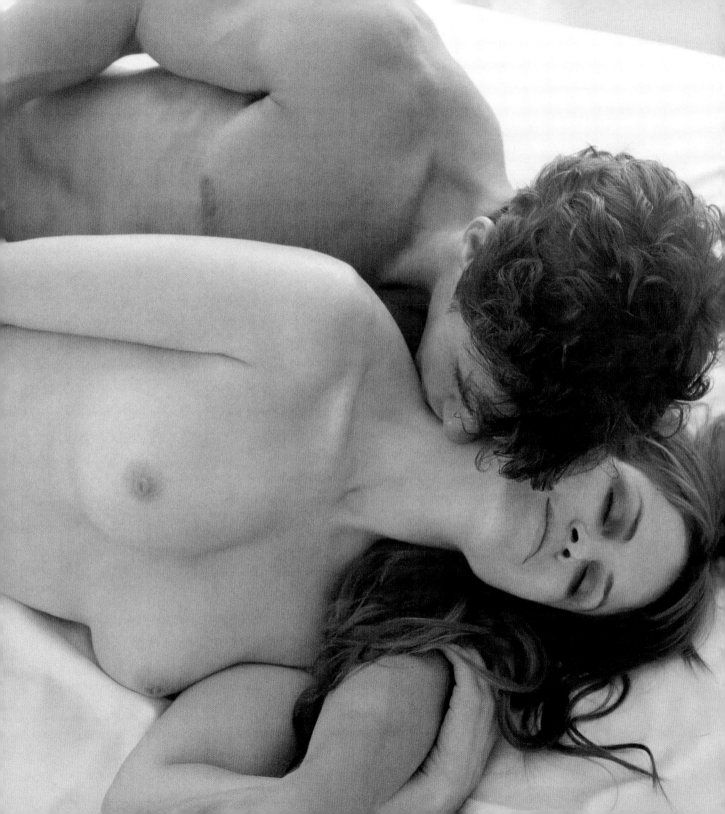

Ask The Girl Next Door

ANSWERS TO FREQUENT QUESTIONS ABOUT WOMEN
BY CAROLYN KYLSTRA AND NICOLE BELAND

Q. She's not that into sex from behind. How can I make it better for her?

A. Easy, cowboy. If you thrust a little too hard, with not quite enough lubrication, this position turns into a real cervix pummeling. Just be generous with the lube, dip shallow, and forget what you've seen on YouPorn (or Animal Planet). Also, maintain the mind-set that you're making love to her, not riding her tush like it's a mechanical bull. To further the intimacy, kiss her neck, gently tug on her hair, whisper dirty words into her ear, and toss in a gentlemanly reach-around. All these tweaks together ought to make doggy style more of a treat for both of you.

Q. The women I'm pursuing often tell me I'm too nice. How can I develop more of an edge?

A. Stop playing the friend. Women have enough of those to lean on, and they (probably) don't sleep with any of them. I'm not saying you should be a jerk, but if you limit your availability—and show a woman you have a life—it certainly won't hurt. Ultimately, sexy is a man who's direct, confident, and independent. Master those qualities and your kindness will be an extra perk, not what defines you.

Q. I read in an article that 51 percent of women say they like to be dominated in bed. What does that mean?

A. For me, being dominated means he's so overcome with passion he can't keep his hands (or mouth) off. It's sexy and exciting to be wanted so intensely. The problem is that in the moment, your girlfriend can't request that you go wild with lust. It has to happen naturally.

Q. The alphabet-with-your-tongue trick: Overrated?

A. Hell, yes. It's a cute tactic, and we admire the effort, but a man who dutifully tries to A-B-C my clitoris won't be seeing my O-face anytime soon. Scrumptious oral sex can certainly include the tip of your tongue dancing across a two-square-inch region, but it also calls for more wide-ranging exploration. Caress her with the smooth underside of your tongue, nuzzle with your lips, and stroke with the pads of your fingers—sometimes all at once!

Q. If a woman is covered in tattoos does it mean she's a freak in the bedroom?

A. No.

Q. After we had sex on the floor last night, my wife said it was nice to "do something different." Am I boring her?

A. Well, not anymore! Her comment was an invitation, not a criticism. Most women want a little craziness; you'd be surprised at how receptive we can be if you take the initiative. And in this case, you already have. Now keep it up.

Q. I can't figure my fiancée out. When she's upset, she wants her space. When I leave her alone, she just stews. Help?

A. If she's asking for space that probably means distance from your analysis, judgment, and solutions—but not from your TLC. Give her some time to calm down. Then circle back with some unrelated, unasked-for tenderness. Don't talk about what's upsetting her unless she brings it up first.

Q. My hook-up friend is visiting for the weekend. What do I plan?

A. If this is just for sex (you're not falling for her, right?), then buy a box of condoms and don't prepare anything else. No romance, no candles, no sex bunker. One reason casual sex can be so hot is that there's no pressure to perform. You're the rare guy she doesn't have to worry about impressing, so the more low-key you are, the more she'll appreciate you. Just be sure to prioritize her pleasure—and by that I mean more than repeated and enthusiastic oral action. Send her flirty and inquisitive e-mails in the week leading up to her arrival. Tell her what you're "so turned on" about doing. And ask, "What about you?" Then do that. With vigor!

Q. Do women ration their freakiness at the start of a relationship so they don't appear slutty?

A. Some do, sure. But it's usually more complicated than that. A woman's transition from demure damsel to sex panther has to do with her level of comfort with both herself and her partner. If you want to speed her intimacy process, never disparage other women as "sluts," kiss her often (before, during, and after sex), and tell her how much it turns you on to give her pleasure.

Q. My fiancée has a complex about her petite breasts. How can I help her overcome it?

A. Give her compliments that you mean, and then back them up with action. Laud her gumdrop nipples, wax poetic about her perk, and then lick her breasts like they're melty double-scoop ice cream cones. Or celebrate her small size, flat-out. One of my

friends told me that the hottest compliment she ever received was, "Wow, you have gorgeous little tits." After the initial shock (did he just call my tits "little"?) it was a huge turn-on to know that he found her A-cups so delicious. Hey, there you go. Tell her you think her tits are delicious. What woman wouldn't love that?

Q. How should I compliment her vajayjay?

A. Well for starters, don't call it a vajayjay. You don't even need to assign a word to it at all—"you" will suffice, as long as the context is obvious. As for specific sweet nothings, most women would feel instantly sexier hearing any or all of the following words: beautiful, hot, tight, intoxicating, and perfect.

Q. Is there a flirting technique that usually works?

A. Shelve the strategy. The most exciting flirt sessions are the ones that zig and zag wildly. The more electric the banter, the stronger the sexual charge. The thing is that type of back-and-forth will never develop if you're too worried about impressing her with your wit or accomplishments. She wants to feel like a co-conspirator, not a target. So here's the secret to sparking a positive reaction: relax. Sidle up to her, smile, and use your surroundings for tangential jump-off points. Then ask her opinion, and respond accordingly. Sounds like conversation, because it is. Oh, and

"Hi, I'm Doug," is a great ice breaker, too, assuming your name is Doug.

Q. On the beach, how do I pick up women?

A. With a six-pack of Corona and a puppy. With a game of bocce or volleyball. Build a serious sand castle. The beach is easy. Next question?

Q. When women offer to split the bill on the first date, is it a test, or sincere?

A. Just assume it's a test. Modern-day etiquette holds that women are fully capable of paying their way and should offer to do so. However, most of us still usually expect the guy to pony up, at least on the first date—and especially if he did the asking. Rest assured that if she truly wants to pay her fair share, she'll insist on going Dutch even after you've waved off her initial wallet dive.

Q. I'm uncircumcised. Is that a turnoff?

A. For some women, maybe. It's about comfort—in what we're used to handling. If a woman hesitates when she sees your penis, she might be feeling like she did back in high school: What do I do with it? That can make her feel awkward, not sex-goddessy. So laugh it off and reassure her: Yes, there are differences (like your sensitivity, so she may need to lighten up on the ol' death grip), and you're happy to explain them. Or better yet, guide her.

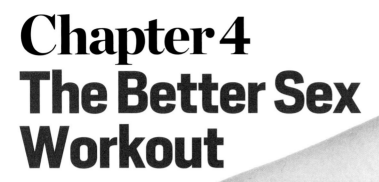

Chapter 4
The Better Sex Workout

BUILD STRENGTH AND STAMINA

FOR PEAK PERFORMANCE

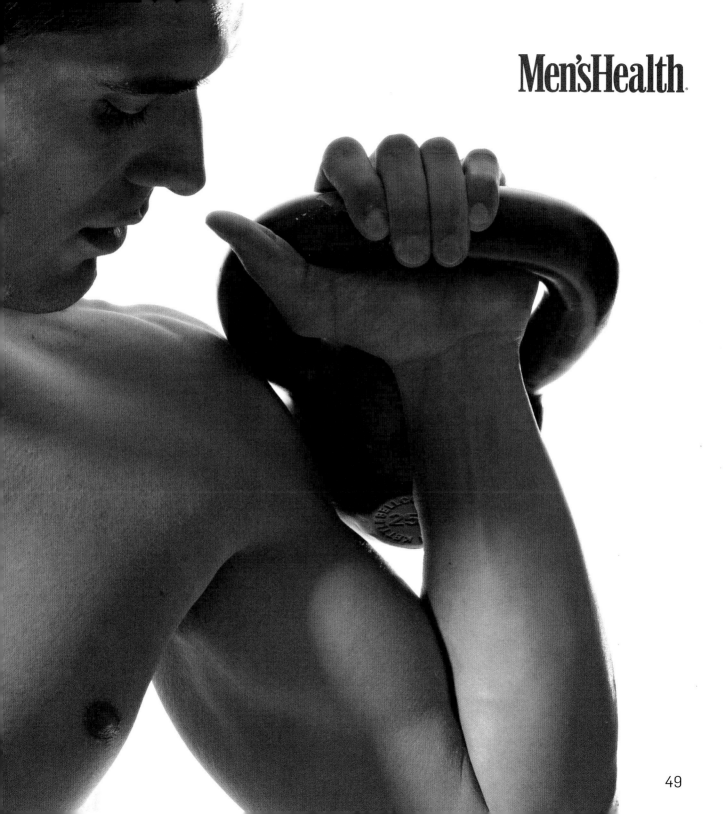

Men'sHealth

49

M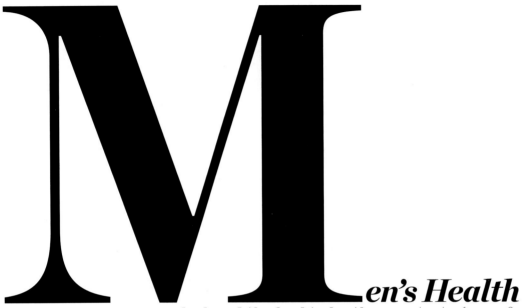en's Health

once declared the bed to be the greatest piece of exercise equipment ever invented. You have to give us props for our enthusiasm, but really there are a lot more efficient ways to burn calories and build muscle.

Walking, for instance.

What we should have said is that sex is the greatest motivation for exercising known to man. Now, that's the truth. Isn't the promise of sex why you go to the gym in the first place and lift heavy objects while listening to "Eye of the Tiger"? Maybe you started lifting weights to make the high school football team. Maybe you joined the health club when your doctor told you to lose weight. All valid reasons to exercise. But, honestly, most guys work out for one thing—to attract women.

Sex is the ultimate carrot before the stubborn donkey. What pries you out of your favorite chair and into the gym when the game's on and there's a six-pack chilling in the cooler? The potential for sex.

What would encourage you to put down that meatball Parmesan sandwich and pick up an apple and a dumbbell instead? The knowledge that women prefer to run their fingers over hard abs rather than a flabby belly.

Sex is one of your most powerful natural urges. So, what more brilliant way to motivate yourself to lose weight, get in shape, build muscle, stamina, and good health? Make some important lifestyle changes and you'll improve not only how you look in a tight T-shirt, but your performance in bed.

Build Here for Sex

Having sex uses a lot of tiny muscles you don't normally use during the course of the day unless you happen to be a gigolo or an alligator wrestler.

"You'll definitely have more enjoyable sex if you don't have to worry about getting fatigued or pulling something," says trainer Jeff Bell, owner of Bell Fitness Company in New York City. Bell is a weight-loss and fitness expert with a specialty in exercise for sexual health benefits. So we asked Bell to put together a workout that's not only a terrific calorie-burning and fitness-boosting routine, but one that preps the body for better performance in bed. It incorporates general fitness, sex-specific training, and moves that can give you more stamina for longer lovemaking sessions. Bell developed this program with men in mind, but women can use it, too.

The Logic Behind the Workout

Upper body strength. Building the muscles of the shoulders, triceps, chest, and back will make it easier to support your body weight for longer periods of time when you are on top or supporting her body weight during moves like standing sex positions.

Flexibility. A cramp in your piriformis at the most inopportune time can do more to cramp your style than her mother walking in on you while you are doing the downward dog to her daughter. By stretching and lengthening your muscles regularly, you'll be more likely to move into more challenging positions.

Core power. The abdominals and low back muscles are used for the thrusting motions of sex. You won't be attempting any of those moves if you are laid up with lower back pain. Finnish researchers say that people with weak core muscles are more than three times more likely to suffer from lower back pain. Strong abs also girdle your belly so it won't flop over and get in the way of business. She wants to wrap her legs around your six-pack, not a keg.

Aerobic stamina. Big, strong muscles may make her swoon, but if you are huffing and puffing you won't have the stamina to maintain your rhythm. Shaping up with endurance workouts like interval training sessions and resistance-training circuits can prevent weaker muscles from quitting too soon.

The Better Sex Workout

A Total-Body Program

This is a four-week program of circuits that become progressively challenging as you build strength, endurance, and flexibility. There are six different circuits. Do them according to the plan below, which schedules workouts 3 days per week, for example on Mondays, Wednesdays, and Fridays, to allow for one day of rest in between for recovery. During off days, do some aerobic exercise such as running, walking, biking, swimming, or playing sports. Select one non-circuit day per week to devote to a high-intensity interval-training workout.

Begin each workout with a brief warm-up to loosen the muscles and send oxygen-rich blood circulating throughout the body. Do the warm-ups for 5 to 10 minutes. Progress from the easier moves to the more challenging ones. We mix up the warm-up exercises for each new circuit to keep workouts fresh and to challenge different muscle groups in various sequences for greater growth and fat burn.

The Four-Week Plan

Week 1	Week 2	Week 3	Week 4
MONDAY	**MONDAY**	**MONDAY**	**MONDAY**
Workout 1	Workout 5, 2 Sets	Workout 4, 2 Sets	Workout 5, 3 Sets
WEDNESDAY	**WEDNESDAY**	**WEDNESDAY**	**WEDNESDAY**
Workout 2	Workout 1, 2 Sets	Workout 2, 3 Sets	Workout 4, 3 Sets
FRIDAY	**FRIDAY**	**FRIDAY**	**FRIDAY**
Workout 3	Workout 3, 3 Sets	Workout 3, 3 Sets	Workout 6, 2 or 3 Sets

The Circuit Program

EXERCISE	SETS	REPS	REST
Workout 1 Warm-Ups			
Jumping Jacks	1	20	0
Low Side-to-Side Lunge	1	10–20 each side	0
Hinge	1	8–10	0
Lower-Back Lie-Down	1	10	0
Workout 1 Circuit			
Stability Ball Decline Pushup	2	10–15	30 sec
Lying Gluteal Bridge	2	10	30 sec
Sandbag Lunge	2	20 alternating legs	30 sec
Kegels	2	10 15-second holds	1–3 min
Workout 2 Warm-Ups			
Squat	1	10–30	0
Jog in Place	1	30 seconds	0
Inchworm	1	6	0
Standing Hip Thrust	1	30 seconds each leg	0
Workout 2 Circuit			
Renegade Row	2	8–12	30 sec
Kettlebell Squat Catch	2	8–12	30 sec
Lower-Back Lie-Down	2	10	30 sec
Kegels	2	10 15-second holds	1–3 min

HOW TO DO A CIRCUIT

Circuits are fast and efficient workouts that combine the heart rate-elevating benefit of aerobics and the muscle building of resistance training. In a circuit, you do one set of each exercise resting only briefly—10 to 30 seconds if at all—between exercises before moving to the next. Only after completing the list of exercises do you go back and repeat the exercises. Rest for 1 to 3 minutes between circuits.

The Better Sex Workout HIS

EXERCISE	SETS	REPS	REST
Workout 3 Warm-Ups			
Jumping Jacks	1	20	0
Squat	1	10–30	0
Hinge	1	8–10	0
Kneeling Leg Crossover	1	10 with each leg	0
Workout 3 Circuit			
Abdominal Tootsie Roll	2	3–4 each direction	30 sec
Spiderman Pushup	2	6–12	30 sec
Gluteal Bridge	2	10–16	30 sec
Kegels	2	15	1–3 min
Workout 4 Warm-Ups			
Low Side-to-Side Lunge	1	10–20 with each leg	0
Jumping Jacks	1	20	0
Squat Thrust (also called Burpees)	1	10	0
Standing Hip Thrust	1	30 seconds each leg	0
Workout 4 Circuit			
Stability Ball Decline Pushup	3	12–16	30 sec
Gluteal Bridge	3	12–20	30 sec
Sandbag Lunge	3	30 seconds alternating legs	30 sec
Sock Slide	3	6–12	30 sec
Kegels	3	10-15 second holds	1–3 min

EXERCISE	SETS	REPS	REST
Workout 5 Warm-Ups			
Cross Back Lunge	1	20	0
Jumping Jacks	1	20	0
Squat	1	20	0
Inchworm	1	6	0
Workout 5 Circuit			
Renegade Row	3	8–12	30 sec
Kettlebell Squat Catch	3	8–12	30 sec
Lower-Back Lie-Down	3	10	30 sec
Hinge	3	8–12	30 sec
Kegels	3	15	1–3 min

ABOUT THE EXPERT

Jeff Bell (ACSM, NASM) is a veteran personal trainer and a frequent fitness advisor to *Men's Health* and *Women's Health* magazines. Bell is the founder of Bell Fitness Company (www.bellfitness company.com) in New York City and has trained thousands of clients and taught more than 18,000 group exercise classes.

The Better Sex Workout

EXERCISE	SETS	REPS	REST
Workout 6 Warm-Ups			
Jog in Place	1	1 minute	0
Low Side-to-Side Lunge	1	20	0
Standing Hip Thrust	1	30 seconds each leg	0
Squat	1	20	0
Kneeling Leg Crossover	1	12–16 each leg	0
Workout 6 Circuit			
Spiderman Pushup	3	10–12	30 sec
Hinge (holding 30 lb. sandbag)	3	6–10	30 sec
Inchworm	3	5–10	30 sec
Sandbag Standup	3	8–10 each leg	30 sec
Single-Leg Hip Bridge	3	8–10 each leg	30 sec
Renegade Row	3	12–16	30 sec
Kegels	3	10 15-second holds	1–3 min

Warm-Up Exercises

This quick warm-up routine will bring blood to your muscles, loosen your joints in preparation for a workout, and stretch and strengthen the stabilizing muscles of the lower body, pelvis and core—used when you get busy. You might be tempted to jump right into the main workout. Don't. Take it slow. Think of this as foreplay for your work-out. On second thought, don't. That would be creepy. Just do the warm-up. It will prepare your muscles so they can work harder and get more from the main workout. And it'll help you avoid injuries that can set you back and keep you out of the sack.

Hinge
Stretches and strengthens core, quadriceps, and hip flexors.

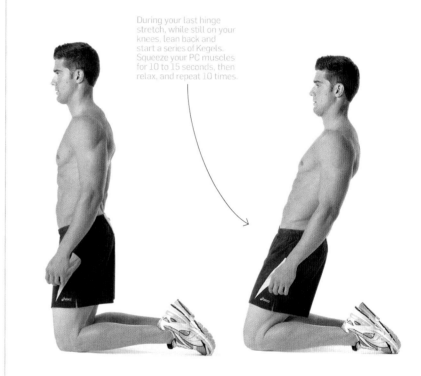

During your last hinge stretch, while still on your knees, lean back and start a series of Kegels. Squeeze your PC muscles for 10 to 15 seconds, then relax, and repeat 10 times.

A
- Kneel on the floor with your hands at your sides. Resist the urge to sit back and rest your weight on your heels. Your back should be straight and your knees bent at a 90-degree angle.

B
- Keeping your head and spine in line with your thighs, slowly lean back a few inches. Hold for 3 seconds then return to the starting position. Do 8 to 10.

Inchworm
Loosens thighs, hips, obliques, back, and shoulders.

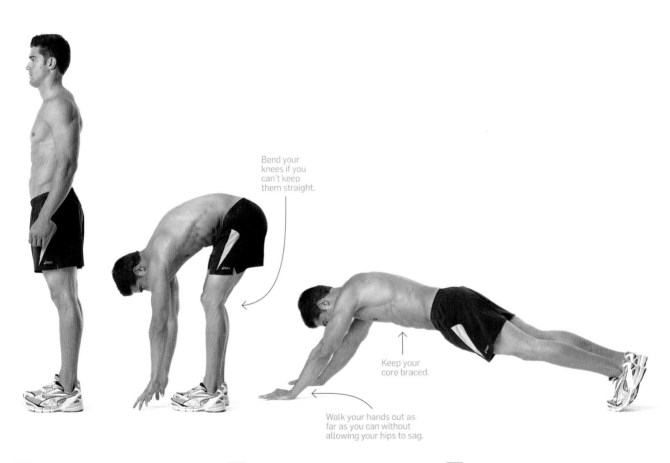

Bend your knees if you can't keep them straight.

Keep your core braced.

Walk your hands out as far as you can without allowing your hips to sag.

A

- Stand with your legs straight, feet hip-width apart.

B

- Bend at the waist and place your hands on the floor.

C

- Keeping your legs straight, walk your hands forward while keeping your abs and lower back braced. Then take tiny steps to walk your feet back to your hands. That's one repetition. Do 6.

Jumping Jacks

Raises the heart rate, lengthens and warms muscles to avoid injury.

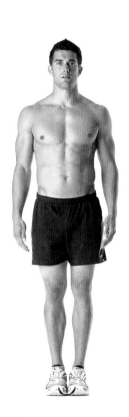

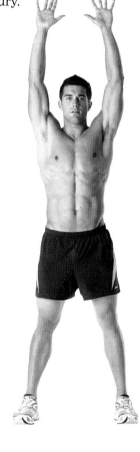

A

- You remember: Stand with your feet together and your hands at your sides.

B

- Simultaneously raise your arms above your head and jump enough to spread your feet out wide. Quickly reverse the movement and repeat. Do 20.

Lower-Back Lie-Down

Stretches the lower back muscles.

A

- Lie flat on your back with your legs bent, feet flat on the floor, and arms at your sides.

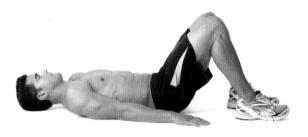

B

- Gently grab your legs just behind the knees. Slowly pull both knees toward your chest as far as you can comfortably go, keeping your back flat on the floor at all times. Hold the stretch for 2 to 3 seconds and then slowly lower your legs. Repeat the stretch for 10 repetitions.

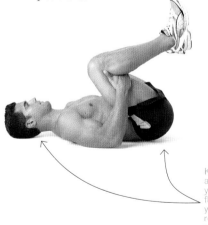

Keep your tailbone and the back of your head on the floor. You'll prevent your back from rounding, which would lessen the effect of the stretch.

The Better Sex Workout | HIS

Low Side-to-Side Lunge

Improves strength and flexibility of lower body, especially hips, glutes, and groin.

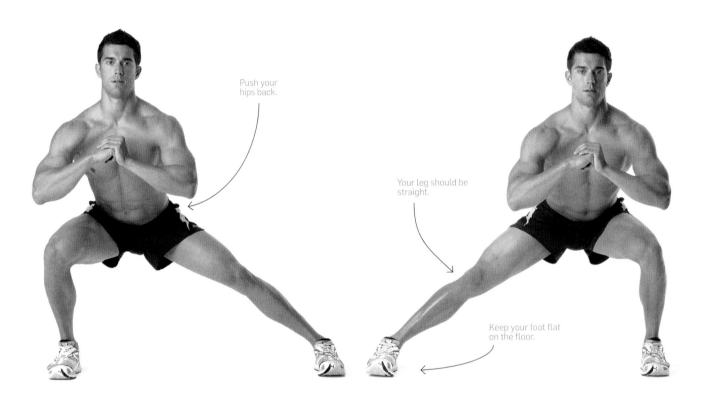

Push your hips back.

Your leg should be straight.

Keep your foot flat on the floor.

 A

- Stand with your feet spread wide, about twice shoulder-width apart, your feet facing straight ahead. Bend slightly at the waist and clasp your hands in front of your chest. Shift your weight over to your right leg as your push your hips backward and lower your body by dropping your hips and bending your right knee. Your lower right leg should remain nearly perpendicular to the floor. Your left foot should remain flat on the floor. Without pausing, reverse the movement and raise yourself back to a standing position.

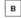 **B**

- Next, repeat to the left side. Alternate back and forth. Do 10 to 20 reps on each side.

Kneeling Leg Crossover

Stretches the adductors and abductors.

A

- Kneel and place your hands on the floor (knees and hands should be shoulder-width apart). Your head should face the floor. Straighten your left leg behind you.

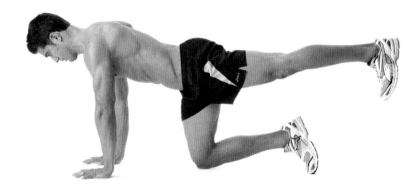

Keep your spine straight throughout the move.

B

- Now, angle your leg to the left, with your toes touching the floor.

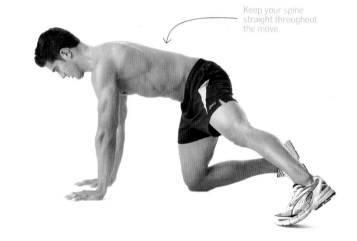

C

- Raise your left leg up and over your right leg, then lower it until your left foot touches the floor just outside your right foot. Reverse the motion to get back to the starting position and repeat 10 times. Then mimic the exercise, this time bringing your right leg over your left.

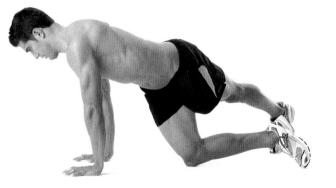

The Better Sex Workout

Squat

Stretches the hamstrings, calves, and quads, and warms the entire body.

- Stand with feet shoulder-width apart. Grasp your hands behind your head.

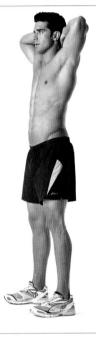

B

- Sit back, bending your knees, until your thighs are at least parallel to the floor (or lower). Stand straight up, pressing through your heels. Do 10 to 30 at a brisk pace.

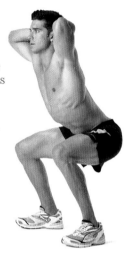

Standing Hip Thrust

Stretches the hip flexors.

- Stand with your feet together, hands on your hips or clasped in front of your chest. Step forward with one foot so that your feet are a couple of feet apart. Keep your toes facing forward and your knees slightly bent.

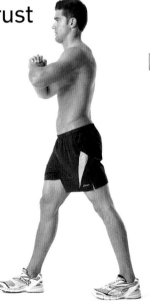

B

- Gently push your pelvis forward until you feel a very mild stretch in your hips. Although this move seems too subtle, don't overdo it: The hip flexors are attached inside the legs in such a way that it takes very little effort to stretch them. Hold the stretch for 30 seconds then reverse leg positions and repeat.

Try to keep the same knee angle throughout the stretch.

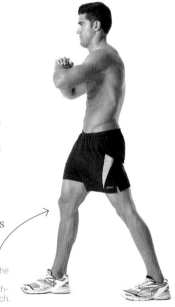

Jog in Place

You know how to do this, but do you know perfect form? You'll burn more calories and warm up faster by doing it right.

- Drive your knees high to get a better stretch and pump. As you drive each knee up, swing your opposite hand upward to get as much vertical lift as possible. If you wish, you can turn this into a high knee skip by adding a hop on the downward step.

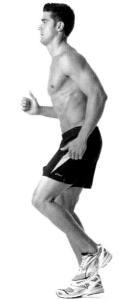

As you run in place, keep your upper body straight. Keeping your head up and looking forward will help your form.

Squat Thrust

Stretches the whole body; also known as Burpees.

- Stand with your feet shoulder-width apart and your arms at your sides.

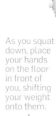

- Push your hips back, bend your knees and lower your body as deep as you can into a squat.

As you squat down, place your hands on the floor in front of you, shifting your weight onto them.

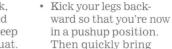

- Kick your legs backward so that you're now in a pushup position. Then quickly bring your legs back to the squat position. Stand up quickly and repeat the entire movement.

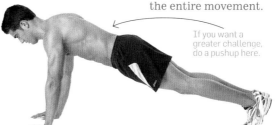

If you want a greater challenge, do a pushup here.

FEED YOUR LOVE MUSCLES

To lose body fat and increase muscle tone:

- **Figure** on eating 10 calories per pound of body weight every day. So, for a 185-pound man that would be 1,850 calories spread over five or six meals.

- **Keep fat** to no more than 20 percent of total calories.

- **Eat** 30 grams of fiber per day. Get a good start by eating at least three pieces of fruit and having protein-rich beans with one main meal.

- **Shoot** for 1 gram of protein and 2 grams of carbohydrates per pound of body weight per day. Canadian scientists recently determined that 130 grams is the bare minimum amount of protein you should eat if you regularly do resistance training.

The Better Sex Workout Circuit

If you want to lose weight, shape up, sculpt an incredible beach body, and fine-tune every muscle required for optimum sexual activity, this selection of exercises is definitely for you. Each has been specifically selected by trainer Jeff Bell, because they do one or more of the following: boost endurance, make muscles and ligaments more flexible, strengthen the lower back and abs, and build upper body power— all the things you need to be a better sexual athlete.

The beauty of this workout is its simplicity and effectiveness. You don't have to go to a gym. Many of the exercises are bodyweight drills that you can do it in the privacy of your home, so it's extremely convenient. However, some key equipment will help you get the most from this workout: a stability ball (also known as a Swiss ball), a pair of dumbbells, a kettlebell, a medicine ball, and a sandbag.

"This is a terrific workout for the busy man who wants to be in top shape for maximum sexual enjoyment," says Bell. "By doing these exercises as a circuit, you can build strength and endurance without spending hours working out. It crams a lot of good work in a short, but challenging workout."

Follow the program schedule and circuit instructions starting on page 52, always beginning your workout with the warm-up corresponding to the circuit number. Commit to this workout for 4 weeks and you'll feel fitter and better prepared to go longer in bed. Later, you can incorporate these exercises into other resistance-training workouts to maintain the sex-specific strength gains you've made. Or you might choose to use it as a once-a-week supplement to the couple's better sex workout found in Chapter 6 in the *Women's Health* section.

Stability Ball Decline Pushup

Works shoulders, chest, triceps, and abs.

A

- Kneel with a stability ball behind you and place your hands flat on the floor, shoulder-width apart. Place your shins or toes on the ball and get into the standard pushup position—arms straight, hands directly under your shoulders. Your back should be flat and your abs drawn in.

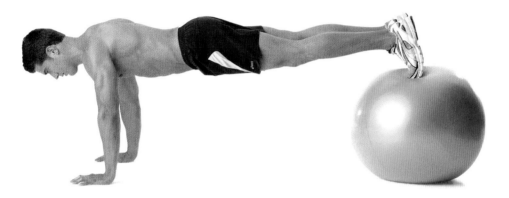

B

- Tuck your chin and, leading with your chest, lower your body to the floor. Push yourself back up. Do 10 to 15 reps.

Keep your head in line with your back and resist looking at the ball. Bending your neck in this position can strain it, and you might lose your balance.

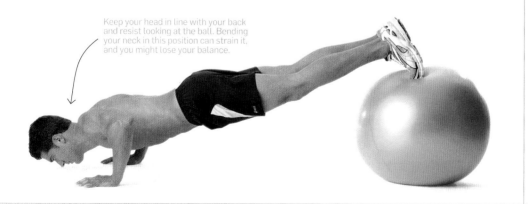

THE HIIT WORKOUT

Fit one high-intensity interval-training (HIIT) workout into your weekly fitness plan. Recent studies show that short bouts of high intensity physical effort interspersed with short bouts of recovery effort burn more fat calories than long aerobic sessions do.

- **Warm up** by running or biking for 3 minutes at an easy pace.

- **Run or bike** for 30 seconds at 90 percent of your best effort.

- **Slow down** to a little less than half speed for one minute to 90 seconds to recover.

- **Repeat** this sprint/recovery sequence six times.

- **Cool down** for 3 minutes.

The Better Sex Workout HIS

Lying Gluteal Bridge

Strengthens gluteals, hamstrings, pelvic muscles, and builds stability in the lower back for lifting and thrusting power through the hips.

A

- Lie on your back with your knees bent and your feet flat on the floor. Place your arms at your sides, palms facing down.

Press with your heels, not toes, when you begin to press up.

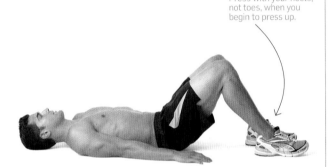

B

- Squeeze your glutes and slowly raise your butt off the floor until your body forms a straight line from your knees to your shoulders. Hold this position for 3 to 5 seconds, then slowly lower yourself to the floor and repeat the move 10 times.

Squeeze your glutes as you lift your hips.

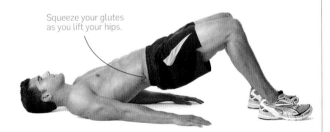

Sandbag Lunge

Targets the quadriceps, glutes, and calves, but also works the arms and back for holding your partner.

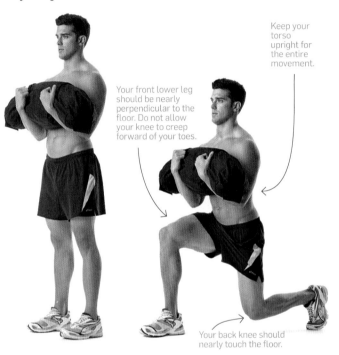

Keep your torso upright for the entire movement.

Your front lower leg should be nearly perpendicular to the floor. Do not allow your knee to creep forward of your toes.

Your back knee should nearly touch the floor.

A

- Hold a 30- to 60-pound sandbag in your arms with an underhand grip. Stand tall with your feet hip-width apart. Brace your core and stick your chest out.

B

- Step forward with your right leg and slowly lower your body under your front knee is bent at least 90 degrees. Pause, then push yourself to the starting position as quickly as you can. Repeat the move, this time with your left leg forward. Continue alternating this way for 20 total reps.

Renegade Row

Works the middle and upper back as well as the chest; ideal for endurance and core strength in the man-on-top position.

- Get into a pushup position with your hands gripping a pair of dumbbells, arms straight and shoulders directly above your hands. Your back should be straight from head to heels. Tighten your core muscles.

B

- Now, keeping your arms straight, bend your right knee and draw it across your torso toward your left elbow. Pause, then straighten that leg, returning your right foot to the floor.

C

- Repeat the move, this time bringing your left knee to your right elbow. Return to the starting position.

D

- Now, balancing on your left hand, row the right dumbbell to your shoulder, pause, then lower it to the floor.

E

- Do the same with the left dumbbell while balancing on your right. That five-part move is one complete repetition. Do 8 to 12.

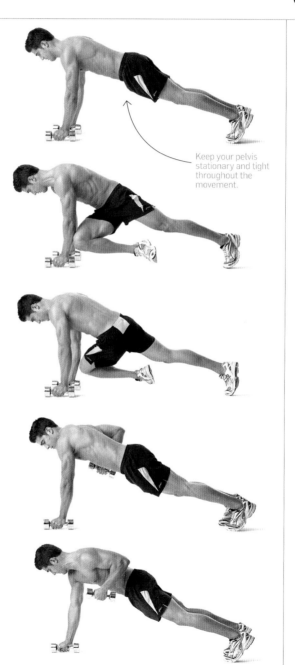

Keep your pelvis stationary and tight throughout the movement.

ERECTION PROTECTION

A study of 31,000 men over age 50 by Harvard researchers proves that daily strolls can keep the lead in your pencil. Men who did aerobic activity equivalent to walking briskly for two miles daily cut their risk of erectile dysfunction by 30 percent.

The Better Sex Workout

Kettlebell Squat Catch

For being able to lift your partner, cardiovascular endurance, leg power, and groin flexibility.

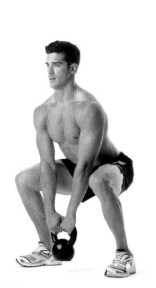 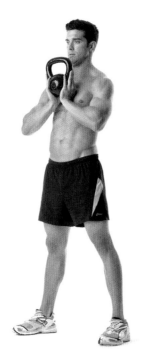 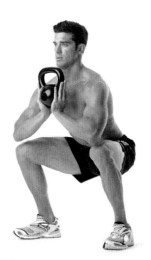 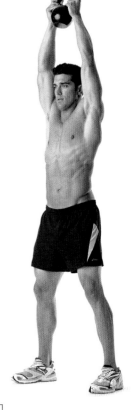

A

- Stand with feet shoulder-width apart and hold a kettlebell by the handle with both hands, allowing the weight to hang between your legs. Bend your knees into a squat position.

B

- Quickly stand up while vigorously pulling the kettlebell up to shoulder height. At this point let go of the kettlebell and scoop your hands underneath to hold it with your palms facing forward, wrists tucked in underneath the weight.

C

- As soon as you "catch" the kettlebell, sit back into a squat position, continuing to hold the kettlebell with hands underneath at the top of your chest.

D

- Now stand explosively and, at the same time, push the kettlebell overhead. Squat again while lowering the kettlebell and grasping the handle with both hands as in the original hang position. That four-move sequence makes one repetition. Do 8 to 12 reps.

Abdominal Tootsie Roll

For a strong, toned waist, and core stability for easily changing sexual positions.

A

- Lie flat on your stomach on the floor with your arms extended out above your head. Lift your chest, arms, and legs off the floor, as if doing a Superman stretch.

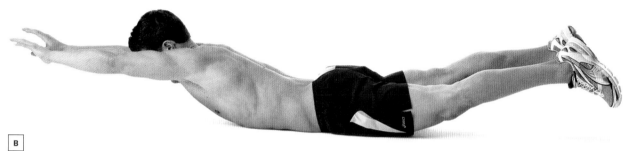

B

- Slowly roll from your stomach to your right side while never losing abdominal control.

The key is not to jerk or use momentum. Stay controlled throughout the entire motion.

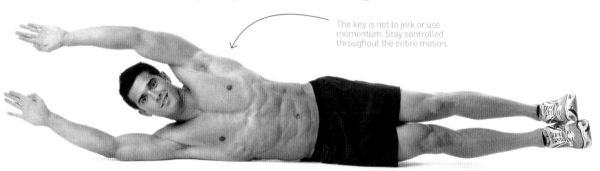

C

- Roll onto your back. Then, slowly reverse the roll first to your side, then your stomach. Relax your arms and legs to the floor. That's one rep. Next, reverse the roll to the left side. Do 3 to 4 reps in each direction.

Spiderman Pushup
Builds core and shoulder/chest endurance and strength.

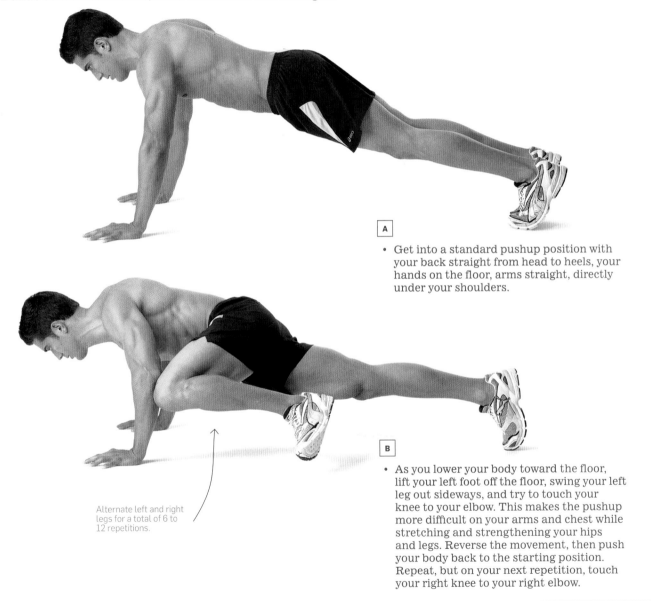

A
- Get into a standard pushup position with your back straight from head to heels, your hands on the floor, arms straight, directly under your shoulders.

Alternate left and right legs for a total of 6 to 12 repetitions.

B
- As you lower your body toward the floor, lift your left foot off the floor, swing your left leg out sideways, and try to touch your knee to your elbow. This makes the pushup more difficult on your arms and chest while stretching and strengthening your hips and legs. Reverse the movement, then push your body back to the starting position. Repeat, but on your next repetition, touch your right knee to your right elbow.

Sock Slide

Strengthens the shoulders, chest, triceps, lower back, and abs.

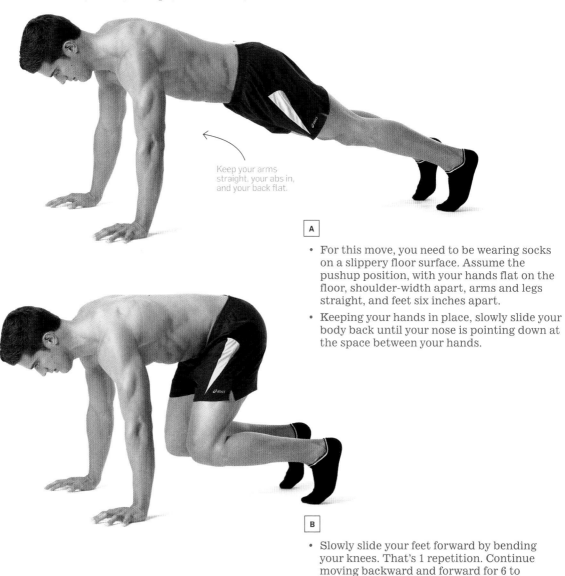

Keep your arms straight, your abs in, and your back flat.

A

- For this move, you need to be wearing socks on a slippery floor surface. Assume the pushup position, with your hands flat on the floor, shoulder-width apart, arms and legs straight, and feet six inches apart.
- Keeping your hands in place, slowly slide your body back until your nose is pointing down at the space between your hands.

B

- Slowly slide your feet forward by bending your knees. That's 1 repetition. Continue moving backward and forward for 6 to 12 repetitions.

Sandbag Standup

Strengthens quadriceps and calves for kneeling, standing, and squatting sex positions—and arms and back for holding your partner.

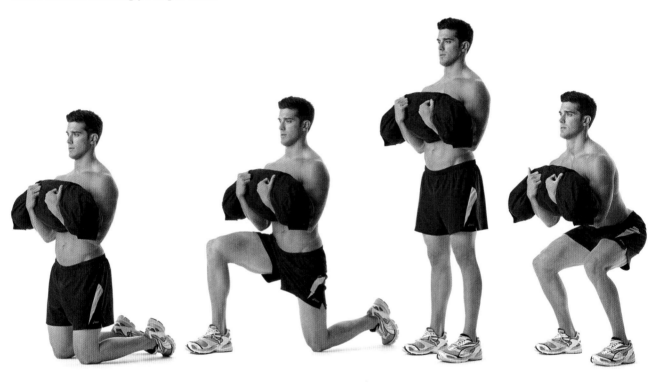

A

- Kneel on the floor and hold a 30- to 60-pound sandbag in both arms. Your arms should be underneath, palms facing up and around the front of the bag. Pull the bag to your chest.

B

- Lift your right leg and place the right foot on the floor to start standing up.

C

- Push through your heel to stand and bring your left foot next to your right to stand completely straight up.

D

- Now bend both knees and move your right knee to the floor, then the left knee until you are kneeling again.
- Repeat, starting with your left foot and pushing through the heel to stand up. Do 6 standups with each leg.

Single-Leg Hip Bridge

A

- Lie face up on the floor with your left knee bent and your right leg straight.
- Raise your right leg until it's in line with your left thigh.
- Keep your back pressed into the floor.

Place your arms out to your sides at a 45-degree angle to your torso, your palms facing down.

You can raise your toes to make sure you're pushing from your heel.

B

- Push your hips upward, keeping your right leg elevated.
- Pause, then slowly lower your body, and leg back to the starting position.
- Complete 6 to 8 repetitions with your right leg elevated.
- Next, repeat the exercise, this time elevating your left leg and working your right glute and hamstring.

Your body should form a straight line from your shoulders to your ankles.

Your right leg stays in line with your left thigh when you raise your hips.

Hard Core

DO YOU HAVE THE BALLS FOR THIS ABS WORKOUT?

You don't need equipment to build impressive abs and a bulletproof core that'll never fail you in bed. But if you're serious about challenging your abs, we recommend you get a pair of balls:

- **A stability ball,** also known as a Swiss ball, also known as a big air-filled ball. When you exercise on it, the lack of stability forces smaller muscles to work hard to keep your body steady. Doubles as a sex toy!

- **A medicine ball**. Buy an 8- or 10-pounder and use it for explosive, rotational exercises that will build a strong, athletic core. Not to be used as a sex toy.

Build a 100-rep abs workout around these abs exercises. Choose five exercises and do 20 reps each (except for the plank, which you'll hold for 30 seconds).

Stability Ball Finger Taps

A

- Lie on the floor, holding the ball between your lower legs. Your lower back should remain on the floor, and your legs should be slightly bent.

B

- Extend your arms straight up as you simultaneously raise your legs and upper body into a contracted position. Keep your upper body in the "up" position for all of your repetitions as your legs move up and down. At the top of the movement, tap the ball to your fingers.

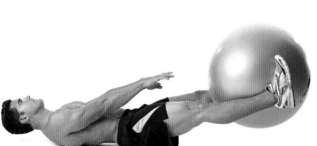

Medicine Ball Situp

 A

- Grab a medicine ball with both hands and lie on your back on the floor. Bend your knees 90 degrees, place your feet flat on the floor, and hold the medicine ball against your chest.

 B

- Now perform a classic situp by raising your torso into a sitting position. Lower it back to the start. That's 1 repetition.

Stability Ball Plank

 A

- Place your forearms on a stability ball and your feet on the floor. Your body should form a straight line from your shoulders to your ankles. Brace your core by contracting your abs as if you were about to be punched in the gut. Hold this plank for 10 to 30 seconds. If you can't hold for 30 seconds at one time repeat as many times as needed to total 30 seconds.

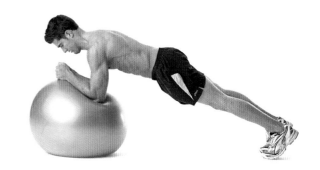

Medicine Ball Standing Russian Twist

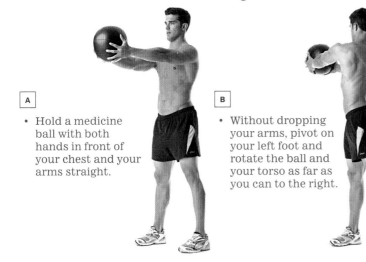

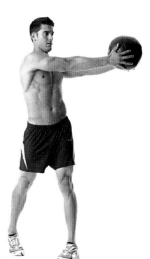

A

- Hold a medicine ball with both hands in front of your chest and your arms straight.

B

- Without dropping your arms, pivot on your left foot and rotate the ball and your torso as far as you can to the right.

C

- Then reverse direction: Pivot on your right foot and rotate all the way to the left. That's 1 repetition.

The Better Sex Workout

Medicine Ball Squat to Press

A

- Stand holding a medicine ball close to your chest with both hands, your feet just beyond shoulder-width apart. Push your hips back, bend your knees, and lower your body until the tops of your thighs are at least parallel to the floor.

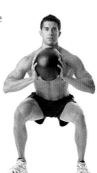

B

- Then drive your heels into the floor and push your body back to the starting position. Simultaneously twist your hips and torso to the right as you pivot on your left foot and press the ball overhead.

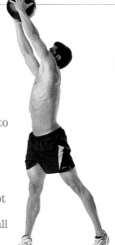

C

- Reverse the motion to squat, then drive your heels into the floor again, this time twisting your upper body to the left, pivoting on your right foot, as you press the ball overhead. That's 1 repetition.

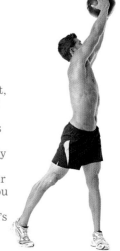

Medicine Ball Suitcase Crunch

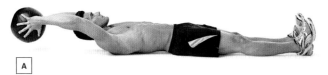

A

- Lie on your back with your legs straight. Use both hands to hold a medicine ball above your head and barely off the floor.

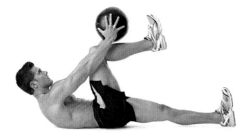

B

- Simultaneously raise your torso and bend your right knee toward your chest as you bring the ball over your knee and toward your foot. Reverse the movement and repeat, this time bending your left knee. That's 1 repetition.

Stability Ball Jackknife

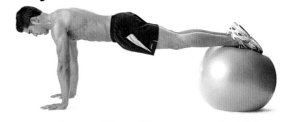

A

- Assume a pushup position with your arms straight. Rest your shins on a stability ball. Your body should form a straight line from your head to your ankles.

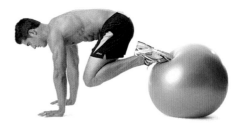

B

- Without changing your lower back posture, roll the ball toward your chest by pulling it forward with your feet. Pause, and then return the ball to the starting position by lowering your hips and rolling it backward.

Medicine Ball Rocky Solo

- Sit on the floor with your legs slightly bent, and hold a medicine ball with both hands just above your lap.

- Twist your torso to the left and place the ball behind you.

C

- Then twist all the way to your right and pick the ball up and bring it back to the starting position. That's 1 repetition. Do 10 repetitions. Immediately do another 10 repetitions, but this time start by twisting with the ball to your right.

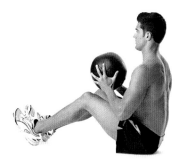
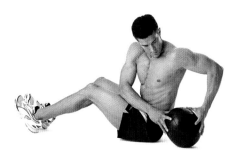
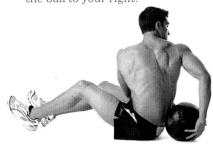

Stability Ball Mountain Climber

A

- Place your hands on a stability ball as if you were doing a pushup.

B

- Your arms should be straight. Your body should form a straight line from your head to your ankles. Brace your core. Now lift your left foot off the floor and raise your knee to as close to your chest as you can. Touch the floor with your left foot. Repeat with your right leg. Alternate raising each knee back and forth for 20 repetitions.

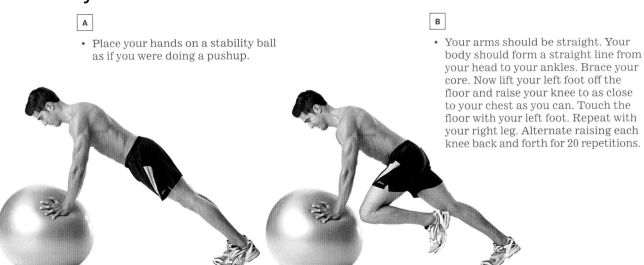

Men'sHealth.

Chapter 5
The Sexual Diagnostic

DOCTOR-APPROVED ANSWERS TO THE MOST COMMON
CONCERNS ABOUT SEXUALITY AND HEALTH

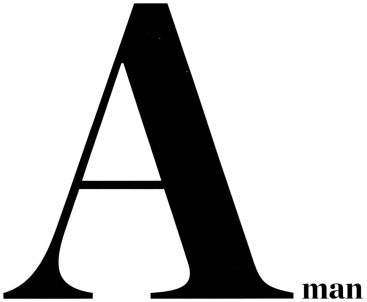

A man
went to his doctor and said, "Doctor, I've got a problem, but if you're going to treat it, first you have to promise not to laugh."

"Of course I won't laugh," the doctor said. "I'm a professional. In over 20 years, I've never laughed at a patient."

"Okay then," the man said and he proceeded to drop his trousers, revealing the tiniest penis the doctor had ever seen. Unable to control himself, the doctor fell laughing to the floor.

When he was able to regain composure, he said, "I'm so very sorry. I don't know what came over me. On my honor as a doctor and a gentleman, I promise it won't happen again. Now what seems to be the problem?"

"It's swollen."

Most sex jokes originate from stuff we're uncomfortable discussing seriously, like displaying our private parts for a doctor's inspection.

Americans are ashamed to talk about penises and vaginas, men more so than women. In a survey of 30,000 men, 33 percent said that they found it impossible to talk face to face with someone about their erections. But even though women visit doctors more regularly than men and tend to be more knowledgeable about their private parts, still one in five admits to feeling uncomfortable discussing their vaginas with their doctors, according to a national survey by the Association of Reproductive Health Professionals.

In this chapter, we hope to create a comfortable and private venue for sexual health information to help you trouble-shoot medical and psychological issues, and make them easier to discuss with your partner and your doctor. On the following pages, we'll cover everything from erectile disfuction (ED) and premature ejaculation (PE) to sexually transmitted infections (STIs) and we'll share frequently asked questions from the readers of *Men's Health*.

But first, one more joke that fell on the barroom floor ...

There was a woman who was interested in getting breast implants, so she went to her physician, Dr. Smith, and questioned him about breast enhancement surgery.

"Before you do anything too serious, you should first try a method that has worked for a lot of my patients," Dr. Smith told her. "Every morning when you wake up, rub your boobs and say 'Scoobie doobie doobie, give me bigger boobies.'"

The woman did this faithfully for weeks and noticed one day that her breasts actually were getting bigger; she was very impressed.

One morning she woke up, late for work and very rushed. By the time she got on the bus she realized that she had forgotten to go through her routine. So, standing on the bus, while rubbing her breasts, she said "Scoobie doobie doobie, give me bigger boobies."

A man standing next to her said, "Oh, you must go to Dr. Smith."

"Yes," she said, "how on earth did you know?"

He replied: "Hickory dickory dock!"

Come on, admit it: you found that one a little funny, didn't you? There's a plethora of penis-size jokes because appendage length holds such universal concern and fascination among men. In fact, every month the Ask *Men's Health* mailbag contains a handful of letters asking the same question: Can I make it bigger? Is penis enlargement possible?

Well, here's the final answer: "All the surgeries, medications, and techniques are ineffective, and some may be unsafe," says Karen Elizabeth Boyle, MD, the director of male fertility at the Shady Grove Reproductive Science Center in Rockville, Maryland.

Oh, you may be able to make it look bigger by losing that belly and trimming your pubes. But, no, despite what you might find being hawked on the internet, medical science has not figured out a safe method for enhancing penis size. To quote an old Texas saying: You have to dance with the one who brung ya. That's because the corpora cavernosa—the two chambers that fill with blood to create an erection—are of fixed length, which no implant, vacuum, herbal tonic, weights or medieval stretch-o-matic device can change. As for phalloplasty, a surgical solution you may have read about, cutting ligaments to make a flaccid penis look slightly longer leads to erections that point down, not up. And there are significant risks, including damage to surrounding nerves and tissues. You may gain up to an inch, but stiffness and strength may be compromised.

Other procedures promise to enhance girth. Typically, fat from another part of your body is pumped below the penile skin, sort of like reverse liposuction. But the body, in time, is likely to reabsorb the fat, leaving you with baggy skin. Doctors are coming up with newer, safer techniques, including skin grafts, but these, too, may result in unevenness, spongy-feeling nodules and deformed units. Buyer beware.

Good thing most men don't need an extension—if your erection measures 4 to 6 inches, you're quite normal.

After penis size, premature ejaculation and erectile dysfunction seem to be guys' biggest private parts concerns. We'll cover those on the next page, but there's another topic that's not talked about as much: prostate cancer. Men are afraid of it, and rightly so because it can be deadly and diagnosis and treatment are risky. What's more, new studies have recently called into question the benefits of the routine screening blood test known as the serial PSA. The test regularly shows false positives, which some experts fear lead to unnecessary painful biopsies. And because the disease typically progresses very slowly, many doctors believe that PSA testing leads to overtreatment.

Our best advice is to discuss the risks and benefits of prostate cancer screening with your doctor. Meanwhile, here are habits to adopt that may reduce your risk of prostate cancer.

1. Have lots of sex. A 2004 study of 29,343 men in the *Journal of the American Medical Association* found that men who had 21 or more orgasm a month were 30 percent less likely to develop prostate cancer than men who had only four to seven orgasms a month.

2. Eat more tomatoes and tomato sauces, which are rich in cancer-preventing nutrient lycopene.

3. Top off your fish oil. Harvard researcher found that men who ate fish rich in omega-3 fatty acids three times a week reduced their risk of aggressive prostate cancer by 25 percent.

4. Move it. Exercise reduces the risk of fatal forms of prostate cancer by 41 percent, according to research at Harvard School of Public Health.

5. Drop the doughnuts. Men with the highest blood levels of trans fats have more than twice the prostate cancer risk of men with the lowest levels.

Staying fit, trim, and healthy is your best option for sexual vitality. Now, let's look at more specific ways to improve sexual satisfaction.

12 Ways to Last Longer

While a longer penis may never be possible, lasting longer during intercourse is certainly achievable for most men. And that's very good news because premature ejaculation, PE, rapid ejaculation, coming too soon, whatever you call it, is the single most common male sexual dysfunction, according to the *Archives of Sexual Behavior*—more common even than impotence. It's estimated that 20 to 30 percent of men suffer from PE—and those figures are based on self-reported studies, so the percentages are likely to be even be higher.

PE is difficult to define. We all kind of know what it's like: she's just getting warmed up and your penis has already hit the showers and is thinking about a snack. But what is too quick from a clinical standpoint? Sex experts say it's any length of time that you and your partner are not satisfied with. In his book *Sexual Behavior in the Human Male*, sex researcher Alfred Kinsey wrote that the average man could maintain penetrative thrusting for about 2 minutes. However, some men's responses are so sensitive that they ejaculate before penetration or within seconds of entry. Other men who say they suffer from PE actually have completely normal levels of sexual stamina, lasting 6 minutes or longer. In 2008, the International Society for Sexual Medicine, hoping to give doctors some frame of reference, published the first diagnostic criteria: A man with lifelong PE cannot last longer than 1 minute, and his time to ejaculation is harming his relationships.

What causes rapid ejaculation is still a matter of debate, too. Some experts chalk it up to performance anxiety, stress, or just having hypersensitivity, like sneezing at the mere hint of pepper or pollen. Others believe rapid-fire ejaculation is a response learned from boyhood masturbation. Most young men, fearing being caught, masturbate quickly, unwittingly training themselves to achieve gratification fast. "Weight lifters talk about muscle memory; I believe that premature ejaculators experience 'penis memory'," says sex therapist Ian Kerner, PhD, a former PE sufferer, who has written extensively on the subject.

Most doctors and sex therapists agree that PE is treatable, with very effective techniques to help men train themselves to last longer, which we will outline below. But it's worth noting here that women are far less likely than men to care or even notice how long intercourse lasts. A study published in the *Archives of Sexual Behavior* found that while 24 percent of men claimed they had a PE problem only 10 percent of their partners agreed. The rest were unbothered. "There's some cultural expectation that the longer you last, the better you are," says Gale Golden, LICSW, a clinical associate professor of psychiatry at the University of Vermont and the author of *In the Grip of Desire*. "[Men] believe that if they last longer, they'll be better able to bring a woman to orgasm." But most women can't reach orgasm through intercourse alone anyway; they need oral or manual stimulation. In fact, women report more orgasms when a vibrator is part of sexual play. So, to be a truly amazing lover, a man needs to understand a woman's need for foreplay and clitoral stimulation. By learning to satisfy a woman in more ways than simply thrusting away, a guy can ease the pressure to perform and focus on relaxing and delaying ejaculation.

Slow-Down Strategies

Most sex experts believe the best course of action for beating PE is to habituate to the sexual stimulation using two similar techniques: start-stop and squeeze. Both work by helping

a guy who ejaculates prematurely to become more aware of his body and the feelings leading up to orgasm so he can learn to back off before the point of no return. Don't be shy about asking your partner to lend a hand. In a *Men's Health* survey, 98 percent of women said they'd be happy to help their partner practice lasting longer.

Start-stop. The idea here is to have her stimulate you until you feel yourself nearing orgasm, and then ask her to stop. Once your sexual tension diminishes (in about 15 seconds), she can continue. It sometimes helps to put a number on the feeling, say, zero for no arousal and 10 representing ejaculation. This way, with practice, you'll be able to tell her you're at a six and can warn her to stop when nearing eight.

Squeeze. This technique is similar: you become more cognizant of your heightening arousal, then just before you reach the point of no return, you or your partner squeezes the head of your penis with a thumb and index finger to thwart ejaculation. Squeeze right below the head, focusing the pressure on the urethra—the tube running along the underside of the penis. This pushes blood out of the penis and momentarily represses the ejaculatory response. You can do this several times during foreplay. It will help you last long enough for her to become really aroused, and you can finish off inside her. In time, as you master the squeeze technique,

HOW TO FIND A GOOD UROLOGIST

The key thing to look for in your specialist is certification by the American Board of Urology (ABU). Certification isn't required to practice, but it indicates that the physician has demonstrated exceptional expertise through both rigorous testing and peer evaluation. For a database of ABU-certified doctors, searchable by zip code or by specialty such as urologic cancer, fertility, or erectile dysfunction, go the American Urological Association's Web site at urologyhealth.org.

you can employ it during intercourse to continue training yourself to last longer.

But don't expect a fast fix from either technique. It can take several months of regular practice to be able to stay at a level seven or eight for minutes at a time. You can get more extracurricular practice by doing these drills alone. Other strategies either used alone or in tandem with the above may help, too.

Have a pre-sex orgasm. Go it alone first and you may last longer in round two, depending on your natural refractory period. But there is a downside: second orgasms are less intense. However, if you have a moderate refractory period, you may find that morning masturbation sets up your nighttime sex for a great start. While masturbating, visualize lasting longer during intercourse. Masturbate with a woman's orgasm in mind, not your own. In other words, take your time: Work up to 15 minutes. Bring yourself close to the point of no return, but don't let yourself ejaculate until 15 minutes is up. It's also a great time to practice the stop-start technique to pinpoint ejaculatory inevitability and control the timing of your ejaculation. The process of sexual response has four phases: excitement, plateau, orgasm, and resolution. The trick is to recognize the spectrum of feelings throughout the process. Rate your sexual excitement on a scale of 1 to 10. Try keeping yourself at 7.

Let her go first. When you help her have an orgasm first, it relieves you of some of the pressure to please and the psychological anxiety that feeds into PE. Many men who suffer from PE become so accomplished in oral sex that they end up giving their lovers better orgasms than they could through intercourse. Use your tongue to bring her to orgasm while your penis is in endurance training. She'll love it.

Try a numbing condom. The lube in Trojan's Extended Pleasure and Durex Performax condoms contains benzocaine, a topical anesthetic that reduces sensation in your penis so you can last longer. The catch: you must keep the condom on. Why? If you take off the condom the residual benzocaine can also numb her vagina.

Another popular home remedy is using an anesthetic gel designed for teething infants or gum inflammation. The gel is applied to the glands to desensitize the penis. But, like the benzocaine in numbing condoms, the medication that isn't absorbed may numb her vagina or her mouth during oral sex.

Have a drink. Some alcohol before sex may depress your central nervous system and delay ejaculation. Don't rely on it, though: You could become sexually dependent on alcohol, and then develop erectile dysfunction while sober.

Breathe from your belly. Fast shallow breathing correlates with ejaculation, so breathe slowly and deeply and you may be able to reduce the anxiety that's contributing to your hair trigger. Try breathing so that your belly rises before your chest does. Try it while practicing start-stop and squeeze. A yoga-style breathing technique may help, too. To learn it, see page 123.

Let her climb on top. When she's on top, your penis is less stimulated. And ask her to go slowly—long and fast thrusting is hazardous to a man's endurance. You might also try entering your partner and not moving at all for a few minutes to acclimate your penis to the feeling of her warm, wet insides.

Practice your short game. Here's another way to habituate to contact with her vagina. After she's sufficiently aroused through oral sex, ride the shaft of your penis through the lips of her vulva, stimulating her clitoris, but never entering her. Do this for a few minutes, then press the end of your penis into her clitoral head. Rub your glans against her clitoris. Linger in her vaginal entrance where the most sensitive nerve endings are. When you do have intercourse, focus on small, shallow movements that penetrate the first 2 to 3 inches of her vagina. When you recognize yourself getting close to coming, pull away and regain your composure. Then enter her again. Switching positions may help also help you prolong sex.

Take a pill. Ask your doctor about trying low doses of Prozac, Zoloft, or other antidepressants called selective serotonin reuptake inhibitors (SSRI). A common side effect of these medicines, delayed orgasm, has proven helpful to some men suffering from PE. Recently, Johnson & Johnson began selling the first prescription drug designed specifically for treating PE in several European countries, including the United Kingdom. In clinical trials, men who took 30 mg of the drug Priligy (Dapoxetine) increased time to ejaculation from 1 minute 45 seconds to more than 2 minutes 45 seconds. Men taking 60 mg lasted more than 3 minutes. Another study of 2,600 patients found the medication increased time a man could last between three to five times their normal. Priligy is an SSRI like Prozac, but with a much shorter half-life; it leaves the body too rapidly to be effective as an antidepressant but may be useful to men who can take the pill only when they expect to have sex. The drug is not currently available in the United States. The FDA rejected Johnson & Johnson's application in 2005, but the company plans to present new studies in new discussions with the agency.

Stop thinking of your orgasm.
The area of the brain responsible for triggering orgasm is engaged whether you're trying to have one or halt one. The more attention you give it, the more likely it is to arrive. Focus on what's happening now—her silky thighs on your hips, say—and you'll diffuse pleasure throughout your whole body.

Erection Protection

Let's move on to a far more critical issue regarding the health and happiness of you and your penis: erectile dysfunction, what used to be called impotence or the inability to maintain an erection strong enough for intercourse. Your overall health plays a huge role in your sexual performance so, there's a lot you can do keep your erections strong.

You see, no penis is an island. If your penis were an island, it would be tempting to think of it as a hot spot in the Caribbean—calm and tranquil during the day, throbbing with activity at night, and the destination of a constant rotation of half-naked coeds. As much as that sounds like paradise, a more precise urological/geographical parallel would be your penis as peninsula—a bodily extension that shares a supply of blood, oxygen, and nutrients with all your other organs. Unfortunately, that means if a natural disaster strikes the mainland, it's likely to affect any protruding landmasses, too.

"ED stands not only for erectile dysfunction but also for 'early diagnosis,' because you can use ED to predict a heart attack, potentially by years—arterial damage from cardiovascular disease affects the small arteries in the penis first," says Christopher Steidle, MD, a clinical associate professor of urology at the Indiana University medical center at Fort Wayne. That's one reason it's a mistake to let Levitra, Viagra, and Cialis lull you into an I'll-fix-it-when-it-breaks mindset. If you like sex, and hope to continue having sex for a long, long time, you'll want to take steps to safeguard your sex life now to avoid ever needing to pop a little blue pill. Or any other shade of erection aid. The peninsula protection steps aren't rocket science—well, in a way they are—but the point is that they aren't any different from what you should be doing to keep the rest of your body strong and healthy.

Swallow anthocyanins. Relax, you find this stuff in dark fruits like blackberries, blueberries, bilberries, and elderberries. Anthocyanins are ultrapowerful antioxidants that attack the free radicals present in our bloodstream. When too many free radicals are present in your bloodstream, nitric oxide goes down—and so does your penis. Remember, nitric oxide is that special blood-vessel-dilating chemical that's crucial to good blood flow to the penis. Indiana University researchers found that arteries treated with anthocyanins retained high levels of nitric oxide even after being flooded with free radicals. "Antioxidants help keep free radicals under control so nitric oxide can do its thing," says David Bell, PhD, the lead study author. And that "thing" is giving your penis the blood it needs to turn excitement into an erection.

Shut down the smokestack. If you still light up, you've probably accepted your increased risk of heart disease, stroke, lung cancer, and bladder cancer. But how about dying young and impotent? A study published in the *Journal of Urology* found that smoking causes arterial damage that doubles a man's risk of total erectile dysfunction. The good news: "If men quit in their 50s or earlier, we can usually reverse the damage," says Andre Guay, MD, director of the Lahey Clinic for Sexual Function, in Massachusetts. When Dr. Guay measured nighttime erections in 10 impotent smokers (average age 49), he noted a 40 percent improvement after just 1 smoke-free day.

Banish stress. Everyone knows stress is a psychological cold shower. But untamed tension also works in a more insidious way—by releasing epinephrine, a type of adrenaline that goes straight to your arteries and slowly wreaks havoc there. "Stress in the long term can contribute to hardening of the arteries," says J. Stephen Jones, MD, FACS, a urologist with the Cleveland Clinic and author of *Overcoming Impotence: A Leading Urologist Tells You Everything You Need to Know*. In a great medical irony, being hard in the arteries can leave you soft in the shorts. The fix: Force yourself to concentrate on

each of your five senses for a few minutes every day—the feel of the steering wheel in your hands, the sound of the engine revving to redline, the sight of the hot brunette in the next car . . . "Obsessing on stressful thoughts will increase your epinephrine," says Jay Winner, MD, author of *Stress Management Made Simple*. "On the other hand, if you focus on current sensations, it decreases the epinephrine and ultimately improves your ability to have an erection."

Check your heart. If you believe that you have ED now, make an appointment with your doctor. Your impotence may be symptomatic of another worry: poor heart health. According to a study from the University of Chicago, about 55 percent of men with atherosclerotic vascular disease have ED. "ED doesn't cause heart disease, but it's an indicator of arterial disease, which may mean your heart arteries are affected as well," says researcher R. Parker Ward, MD, lead author of the study. So pay attention to what may be the best health barometer you have. "Check your erection when you wake up," says John Stripling, MD, a urologist and the cofounder of the Center for Sexual Health and Education. "If it's not totally full, you may have a problem." A urologist can prescribe a device that gauges the state of your nocturnal erections over three nights to determine a physical problem. ED can be reversed without medication.

Lose it so you can use it. One of the best things you can to do to put the lead back

MORNING WOOD

Waking up with a 3-wood in your golf-themed boxers is the sign of a healthy man. Technically, a morning erection is the last in a series of nighttime erections called nocturnal penile tumescence (NPT). Each night a man has between three and seven lasting 20 to 30 minutes during the dream sleep stage known as REM. (Psst: women experience something quite similar nightly, too.) Researchers believe NPTs are nature's way of making sure the machinery is in good working order. If you don't have wood in the morning, how can you be sure if you're having NPTs while you sleep? Go to the post office. Buy a strip of six perforated postage stamps. Bend the perforations back and forth a few times so they will more easily tear. Before going to sleep, wrap the stamps snugly around the shaft of the penis, moisten the last overlapping stamp and glue it to seal the ring. If the perforations are torn in the morning, you know you've had an erection. Do it three nights in a row. If you don't get a tear, a urologist can run more sophisticated tests.

into your pencil is to lower your estrogen by losing weight. Calculate your body-mass index. If your BMI comes in close to or over 25, you may be carrying just enough lard to drag down your erections. "We know that heavier men convert testosterone to estrogen, and that a lower level of testosterone and a higher level of estrogen are not good for erectile function," says Larry Lipshultz, MD, a *Men's Health* advisor and chief of male reproductive medicine and surgery at Baylor College of Medicine. Fortunately, even moderate weight loss can rid you of excess estrogen. A study published in the *Journal of the American Medical Association* found that one-third of clinically obese men—BMI 30 or higher—with erectile dysfunction showed improvement after losing 10 percent of their body weight. Some other strategies to try:

Check your meds. And make a list of all the prescription pills you're popping and discuss them with your doctor. "A lot of prescription drugs may be associated with sexual dysfunction," says R. Taylor Segraves, MD, PhD, coauthor of *Sexual Pharmacology*. One possible culprit is the cholesterol-lowering drug simvastatin, brand name Zocor.

Get pricked. If you think the problem is that you, well, think too much, see an acupuncturist. The results of a study published in the *International Journal of Impotence Research* suggest that acupuncture can help treat psychologically induced erectile dysfunction. (Relax—the prick points are all in your back.) "In psychogenic erectile dysfunction, the patient has trouble with the balance of his sympathetic and parasympathetic nervous systems," says Paul Engelhardt, MD, the study author. "Traditional Chinese medicine tries to restore that balance." Sure, it sounds like using feng shui for your underwear drawer, but it works—64 percent of the men who underwent 6 weeks of acupuncture regained sexual function and needed no further treatment.

Build a stronger floor. Another way to treat erectile dysfunction is to pretend that you suffer from premature ejaculation. British researchers discovered that the traditional treatment for a hair trigger—strengthening the pelvic-floor muscles—is also a remedy for men who can't point their pistols. In the study of 55 impotent men, 40 percent of those who practiced pelvic-floor exercises, a.k.a. Kegels, every day for 6 months regained normal sexual function. Apparently, the same muscle contraction that's used to stop peeing midstream can also prevent blood from escaping during an erection. "Unless they have severe back pain, all men with ED can perform pelvic-floor exercises," says Grace Dorey, PhD, the study author. Here's the workout plan: Contract and relax your pelvic muscles anytime you're sitting, although you can also do them lying down. Work up to doing 50 contractions daily, holding each one for 10 seconds.

Still Not Able to Defy Gravity?

At this point, it makes sense to ask your doctor about a prescription for Viagra, Cialis, or Levitra to stimulate bloodflow to the penis. And who knows what miracles might happen once you prime the pump a few times? "What a lot of men find is that once they start these medications, they may not need them for every episode of sexual activity—they may need them only now and then," says Dr. Steidle. Similarly, if you suffer from performance anxiety, a drug-fueled romp or two may be just what the urologist ordered to restore confidence. And while all three erection medications have the power to prevent you from psyching yourself out in the sack, Cialis's ability to work for up to 36 hours may provide an advantage by giving a man and his partner a lot more time over the weekend to be more spontaneous.

There are solutions even for men with advanced ED who do not respond to medication. For example, a penile implant. It's a very good and very much under-utilized solution, says Ridwan Shabigh, MD, director of the division of urology at Maimonides Medical Center in New York. Most men cringe at the thought of having a bendable rod implanted in their penis but "would you rather stick a needle in your penis every time you want to have sex?" Dr. Shabsigh asks. "When men realize that it's not much different from getting a knee or hip replacement for arthritis or a pacemaker for the heart, it becomes easier to accept." And both partners are usually happy with the results, says Shabsigh "The wife of one implant patient asked me, 'why aren't men born with these?'"

HEALTH RESOURCES FOR MEN

American Academy of Clinical Sexologists:
3203 Lawton Road
Orlando, FL 32803
407-645-1641
esextherapy.com

American Association for Marriage and Family Therapy:
112 South Alfred Street
Alexandria, VA 22314
703-838-9808
aamft.org

American Association of Sexuality Educators, Counselors and Therapists (provides referrals for experts in your area):
P.O. Box 1960
Ashland, VA 23005
804-752-0026
aasect.org

American Foundation for Urologic Disease:
300 W. Pratt Street
Baltimore, MD 21201
410-468-1800

American Psychological Association:
750 First Street, NE
Washington, DC 20002
800-374-2721
apa.org

Centers for Disease Control National AIDS Hotline:
800-342-2437

CDC National STD Hotline:
800-227-8922

HealthyMinds.org
Resource for anyone seeking mental health information from the American Psychiatric Association. Special channels available for men's issues and fatherhood.

National Herpes Resource Center Hotline:
919-361-8488

National Suicide Prevention Lifeline (24-hour hotline for anyone in emotional distress):
800-273-TALK (press 1 for veteran's suicide prevention hotline)
Suicidepreventionlife line.org

UsToo.org
International prostate cancer education and support network for patients, survivors, their spouses/partners and families.

Troubleshooting Your Tallywacker

SOME COMMON, SOME STRANGE THINGS THAT CAN GO WRONG WITH YOUR PENIS AND WHAT TO DO ABOUT THEM

Your penis curves to the right or left when erect.
A healthy penis isn't always straight as an arrow. A minor bend or curve is normal. However, a severe bend right, left, up or down that makes intercourse difficult or impossible requires treatment. **The cause:** Peyronie's disease, a condition first described by a French surgeon named Francouis de la Peyronie. It happens when a plaque or hard lump forms in the erectile tissue causing the shaft to arc significantly during an erection. The lump is benign, but the bend can be painful and cause permanent scarring, which makes intercourse difficult. **The cure:** A doctor injects a medicine called verapamil directly into the plaque to break it down. The most common remedy, however, is surgical. One option is to place two permanent sutures in the lining of the penis opposite the curvature in order to straight it out. The second, patch corporoplasty, is a procedure in which an incision is made through the plaque across the width of the penis to eliminate the pulling that causes the curvature. Then the incision is patched with a skin graft.

There's an agonizing pain in your scrotum.
Possible cause 1: Assuming you weren't just kicked there, one of your testicles is probably twisted around something called the spermatic cord, cutting off the blood supply. "Think of a ball hanging on a rope," says Tony Makhlouf, MD, PhD, a urologic surgeon at the University of Minnesota Medical Center. "As the rope turns, it bunches, and the ball rises." This knotting—testicular torsion, it's called—instantly causes a sharp pain.

The cure: Head to an E.R. "If it isn't treated within four hours, you can lose a testicle," warns urologist Larry I. Lipshultz, MD. "Why take a chance?" The docs at the E.R. will do an ultrasound to assess whether your testicle and cord are indeed twisted. If that's the case, a urologic surgeon will be called to untangle things. Then he'll suture each testicle to the inside of your scrotum to prevent the torsion from happening again.

Possible cause 2: Epididymitis. This is an inflammation of the epididymis, the gland at the top of each testicle that collects sperm and transports it to the vas deferens caused by bacteria. The pain is hard to distinguish from that caused by testicular torsion.

The cure: Head to an E.R. for an ultrasound. If it's not torsion, antibiotics will be prescribed to treat the infection and an anti-inflammatory will ease your pain.

It feels like your scrotum is a bag of worms, and your boys are droopier than normal.

The cause: Sometimes the valves inside the veins of the scrotum don't close properly, so blood pools and they swell. The resulting bundle of enlarged veins, or varicoceles, doesn't always hurt, but the extra blood warms the testes. This jeopardizes sperm production (which requires temps cooler than 98.6°F) and causes the testicles to hang away from the body. About 20 percent of men will experience varicoceles at some point.

The cure: "If you notice you have low-hanging fruit, see a urologist who specializes in infertility," says Harry Fisch, MD, a professor of clinical urology at Weill Cornell Medical College/New York-Presbyterian Hospital and author of *The Male Biological Clock.* Your doctor can stop blood from pooling by tying off the veins or blocking them. It's minor outpatient surgery and you can have sex again in 3 weeks, although you should schedule a follow-up semen analysis in 3 to 4 months. In 60 percent of infertile men, semen quality will improve after surgery, says Fisch. Even if you're not trying to conceive, he adds, the problem should be corrected if it's painful or creates a size discrepancy between testicles.

You think you broke your penis.

The cause: There are no bones in the penis, so what really happens is a tear in the tissue when the erect penis is bent through some trauma during aggressive sexual activity or masturbation. When the spongy tissue that fills with blood during an erection ruptures, blood escapes the membrane causing bruising swelling and pain.

The cure: Immediate medical attention is needed to surgically repair the leak or risk deformity or erectile dysfunction.

There's a bulge in your groin area, and it hurts when you bend over, cough, or try to lift heavy stuff.

The cause: You should have hired movers to lift that fridge. Inguinal hernias occur when part of the intestine protrudes through a congenitally weak abdominal wall. "It's often associated with a major straining episode," says Fisch, but a simple sneeze can set it off.

The cure: If it's small and doesn't bother you, no action may be needed. If it's growing or painful, lying down with your pelvis higher than your head can reduce the discomfort, but ultimately you'll need surgery. This will come in the form of either a herniorrhaphy, in which the edges of healthy tissue are sewn together, or the more modern hernioplasty, a laparoscopic surgery technique in which a piece of synthetic mesh is inserted to cover the entire inguinal area. A surgeon will recommend the option best suited to repair your particular type of abdominal-wall tear. You'll be back to work within a few days.

You have pain in your penis, testicles, lower belly, and down your legs, and it hurts when you urinate or ejaculate.
The cause: Chronic pelvic pain syndrome, usually resulting from an inflamed prostate gland. "It's a collection of symptoms that originates from an injury, often an infection, and the problems come from how the body responds to that infection," says Daniel Shoskes, MD, a Cleveland Clinic urologist.
The cure: Two-thirds of men will get better with antibiotics in the early stages. For those whose inflammation persists beyond initial infection, Shoskes prescribes herbal-based bioflavonoid preparations, such as Prosta-Q and Q-Urol, which reduce inflammation. Flomax and other prescription agents that block an important receptor in the region also reduce pain and can improve urinary flow. Still other men suffer from nerve and muscle spasms, requiring muscle relaxants and physical therapy. See a urologist in any case, but you can help your own cause by taking hot baths; by avoiding alcohol, spicy foods, and caffeine; and by using a doughnut-shaped cushion when sitting for long periods of time.

You took your ED medication and your erection won't go down even after your second orgasm.
The cause: An erection that lasts more than 4 hours and isn't relieved by orgasm is a medical disorder called priapism, named for the Greek fertility god Priapus, who was endowed with an exceptionally huge, always-erect penis, which he wielded against intruders.

Priapism happens when blood that flowed into the penis to inflate an erection doesn't properly drain out. There can be many causes beyond a reaction to an ED drug or other medication, including injury or drug and alcohol abuse. It's very rare, but dangerous. For most men who experience it, the pain prods them to the E.R.
The cure: Medications are used to decrease blood flow to the penis and a needle may be used to drain the blood because a prolonged erection can cause scar tissue to develop.

Your semen has a reddish tint, and it drips out rather than shoots when you ejaculate.
The cause: When infections begin to heal, scar tissue can form and create a blockage in the ejaculatory duct. "It's like a five-lane highway becoming a two-lane highway," says Fisch. The red tint is blood from the initial infection. Your ejaculate volume may drop below the average of half a tablespoon and continue to dribble like an NBA point guard after you achieve orgasm.
The cure: You can function with a dribbly ejaculate, but it's kind of a buzz kill. Fortunately, there's a surgical solution. The formal term is "transurethral resection of the ejaculatory ducts," but it's simpler than it sounds. "We just scrape out the scar tissue, and that opens it all up," says Fisch. You can resume sexual activity in 7 to 10 days.

You are under age 30 and in great shape, but have trouble maintaining an erection.
The cause: According to the American Urological Association, about 25 percent of erectile-dysfunction cases are psychological, and the cause could be anything from relationship issues to performance anxiety. For example, a man may have a sexual experience after drinking and fail to get it up. "In subsequent sexual attempts without alcohol, he'll remember that episode, think something's wrong with him, and be unable to perform," says Karen Boyle, MD, director of reproductive medicine and surgery at the Johns Hopkins Brady Urological Institute.
The cure: Try having sex after breakfast. Your testosterone levels peak around 7 a.m., so your hormones, and your penis, should be at full attention then. If that doesn't work, see a urologist to rule out physical factors and then try counseling to address any underlying issues. Even if a psychological cause is suspected, a pharmaceutical option can offer a helping hand. "A little added self confidence—such as receiving some extra lift from Viagra—goes a long way in this arena," says Andrew McCullough, MD, director of the male sexual health program and male fertility and microsurgery at New York University Medical Center.

When you use the rest room, the urine sometimes dribbles out. You are over age 50 and you have to pee more frequently than ever before.
The cause: A weak urine stream, dribbling after urinating, and feeling that the bladder is not completely empty are some classic symptoms of something called BPH, benign prostatic hyperplasia, a common problem among men your age and older. It's caused by an enlarged prostate, which presses down on the urethra (urine tube) and disrupts the flow of urine. BPH is not prostate cancer, but it does need to be diagnosed and treated by a urologist.
The cure: Doctors usually take a step-by-step approach, starting with behavioral changes such as diet and exercise in combination with medications like Flomax to help ease symptoms. If symptoms

persist or the prostate is large, urologists can use minimally invasive techniques, such as microwave and laser therapies, and transurethral needle ablation. Another effective technique is TURP, for transurethral resection of the prostate, which involves removal of the core of the prostate using an instrument passed through the urethra. It typically requires a two-day hospital stay.

You're 35, and your orgasms seem less intense than they once were.

The cause: As a man ages, he gradually begins to lose smooth-muscle sensitivity in his penis, a process that can affect ejaculation. And while this can certainly hinder orgasm intensity, it's more of a problem for men 50 or older. "A 35-year-old man should have strong orgasms—so if there's a problem, head to your physician," says Steven Lamm, MD, a professor of medicine at New York University and the author of *The Hardness Factor*. There could be a number of causes, including a new medication (such as the hair-loss treatment Propecia), too much booze, or too little testosterone.

The cure: If your doctor rules out the above and other possible causes, start employing this variation on the stop-start technique: Before you reach the point of no return, stop thrusting, pull out, and ask your partner to gently squeeze the head of your penis. Wait a minute or two until you've cooled down, and then rev your engine again. Have her hit pause once more. When you finally ejaculate, the feeling should be significantly more intense from all the anticipation.

You're depressed and your sex drive seems non-existent.

The cause: Lethargy and no interest in sex are among the classic symptoms of clinical depression, but they are also common in men with hypogonadism. Doctors use this term to describe below normal blood levels of testosterone when the testicles have stopped producing enough of the male hormone. Depression, belly fat, and erectile issues are other symptoms of hypogonadism. Testosterone levels in men normally decrease with age starting around year 30. Testosterone supplementation isn't recommended unless there is a significant drop off in T levels, which your doctor can detect through a blood test.

The cure: Testosterone replacement therapy, where the hormone is added through a patch placed on the body or a gel applied to the shoulders, chest, arms and abdomen. But testosterone supplementation should be considered carefully. Pumping added testosterone into your body can cause your system to cut its own production, meaning your testicles will shrink over time. There are health concerns, too. For example, testosterone therapy may contribute to baldness, sleep apnea, lowering of HDL (good)cholesterol, breast enlargement, risk of heart disease, and possibly stimulate the noncancerous growth of the prostate or possibly fuel the growth of existing prostate cancer.

PREVENTING PREGNANCY

For *The Big Book of Sex* Birth Control Guide, see page 76, in Chapter 5: The Sexual Diagnostic/Hers.

Better Safe Than STI

WHAT TO KNOW ABOUT SEXUALLY TRANSMITTED INFECTIONS

There are 19 million new cases of sexually transmitted infections (STIs) each year, according to the Centers for Disease and Control. In 2007, chlamydia and gonorrheal infections saw their highest increase in cases in history, most likely due to better screening. But STIs across the board are on the rise in the United States.

Due to anatomical differences—women have a greater chance of being infected with an STI. Roughly 25 million women in the US are currently infected with human papilloma virus, which causes cervical cancer, and another 6.2 million are diagnosed every year. Women now account for more than a quarter of all new HIV/AIDS diagnoses.

But preventing STIs is everyone's responsibility. It starts with knowledge of the risks, which leads to making smarter safe-sex decisions. The following chart provides an at-a-glance overview of basic STI information for both men and women. If you are sexually active with multiple partners, we recommend you get tested for STIs every 3 to 6 months and ask your partner if he or she has been tested, too.

	Symptoms	How it spreads	Prevention	Treatment
Chlamydia	May be asymptomatic; a burning sensation when urinating; abnormal discharge from penis or vagina; untreated cases can lead to complications that can cause pain, fever, pelvic inflammatory disease, and (more rarely and mostly in women) sterility.	Oral, anal, and vaginal sex through bodily secretions; mother to child.	Mutually monogamous relationship with an uninfected partner; use a condom; screen annually if you have new or multiple sex partners.	Antibiotics **Extras** Fastest spreading infection disease in the United States. Many infected people don't know they have it. Women should be screened annually during pelvic exams.
Gonorrhea	Usually develops within 10 days. Often there are no symptoms early on; discharge from the penis and vagina; frequent urination and discomfort during urination; may lead to pelvic inflammatory disease in women and epididymitis in men, which can cause infertility.	Transmitted through semen and vaginal secretions during intercourse. Gonorrhea—also known as "the clap"—is actually easily cured. Like chlamydia, it's caused by bacteria, so a simple course of antibiotics will zap the clap right out of your system. According to the CDC, it's the second most reported infectious disease, with nearly 356,000 infections in 2007, but it's estimated that about twice as many new cases actually occur but are undiagnosed and unreported.	Use a condom; mutually monogamous relationship with an uninfected partner; testing if you have new or multiple partners.	Antibiotics **Extras** Gonorrhea has shown resistance to certain drugs so as of 2007 treatments are limited to one type of antibiotic, the CDC reports. Women should be screened annually during pelvic exams.

The Sexual Diagnostic

	Symptoms	How it spreads	Prevention	Treatment
Herpes	Genital: Itching, burning, soreness, and small blisters in the genital area and possibly headache, and fever usually within 2 weeks after contact; small sores when blisters break; enlarged or painful lymph nodes (swollen glands) in the groin area.	Oral, anal, and vaginal sex; contact with infected skin.	Mutually monogamous relationship with an uninfected partner; use a condom.	No cure, but symptoms can be controlled to reduce recurrence. **Extras** There are two strains of the virus: herpes simplex virus type 1 (HSV-1), which causes cold sores, and herpes simplex virus type 2 (HSV-2), which is responsible for genital herpes. At least 50 million people in the country have genital herpes.
Hepatitis B	Flu-like symptoms, fatigue, abdominal pain, jaundice, joint pain, although there may be no early symptoms in up to one third of cases.	Through the passing of bodily fluids such as semen, blood and vaginal fluid, during all types of intercourse; IV drug use with shared needles; mother to child.	Hepatitis B vaccine; mutually monogamous relationship with an uninfected partner; condoms but they don't fully protect against the infection; do not share needles.	Symptoms usually clear up in a few months with rest and fluids. Drugs are prescribed for chronic infection but there is no cure. Left untreated, Hepatitis B can cause cirrhosis, liver cancer, and liver failure. **Extras** The virus can be transmitted through contact with contaminated medical instruments and tattoo and piercing needles. Hepatitis C virus is similar to Hepatitis B.It can be sexually transmitted, but is most often passed through IV drug use.
HIV/AIDS	Flu-like symptoms, or no early symptoms; fever, swollen glands, weight loss, fatigue, rash, weakened immune system.	The Human Immunodeficiency Virus is transmitted primarily via bodily fluids through sex, blood transfusions, or contaminated syringes. Semen to blood contact through anal intercourse is the greatest risk.	Mutually monogamous relationship with an uninfected partner; condoms reduce, but don't eliminate risk; do not share needles; wear latex gloves when treating open wounds of others.	No cure, although antiretroviral drugs are effective at suppressing the virus, increasing CD4 cell count, and strengthening the immune system. **Extras** If you think you've been exposed to HIV, contact your doctor immediately. The risk of getting HIV/AIDS can be decreased with post-exposure treatment with highly active antiretroviral treatment. Always inform your past partners if you've been diagnosed with HIV. Note that nonoxynol-9 spermicide irritates vaginal tissues, increasing risk of HIV infection in women.

	Symptoms	How it spreads	Prevention	Treatment
Human Papillomavirus (HPV)	Often no symptoms occur, but some people can get genital warts, small raised bumps on the genitals, which may be itchy.	Skin-to-skin contact with the vagina, penis, vulva, anus, scrotum, and other genital areas; mother to child.	Mutually monogamous relationship with an uninfected partner; HPV vaccine available for some strains of HPV; condom use reduces but does not eliminate risk.	No cure, but genital warts can be removed by laser, with chemicals or by freezing with liquid nitrogen. Women should be tested and treated to avoid cervical cancer. **Extras** According to the CDC, 50 percent of women are infected with HPV within two years of becoming sexually active. HPV can increase the risk of cervical cancer in women. Regular pap tests can catch cancer early when treatment is most effective.
Syphilis	**Primary:** An ulcer or sore at the infection site. **Secondary:** A rash, which may look like "copper penny" spots or fine red dots on palms or soles of feet; a skin rash on arms, legs, and trunk, sore throat, sores in throat, fever. **Latent stage:** Typically syphilis then goes undercover for years, and can eventually cause severe and fatal complications.	The microorganism passes from sores through tiny breaks in the uninfected partner's skin during vaginal, oral, or anal intercourse.	Mutually monogamous relationship with an uninfected partner; use condoms, but they don't fully protect against the disease since it can be spread through unprotected areas of skin.	Antibiotics, but permanent damage may have occurred prior to treatment. **Extras** Syphilis peaked in the nineteenth century, but there was a re-emergence of the disease in the past decade. This disease is highly infectious and can be deadly; it's crucial to receive treatment in its early stages.
Trichomoniasis	Men typically have no symptoms or a minor irritation of the urethra. Women may experience vaginal discharge, itching, and pain during urination or intercourse.	The one-celled parasite passes between partners through vaginal intercourse. The protozoan can also be passed from one person to another via wet towels and washcloths, sex toys, and other moist objects.	Mutually monogamous relationship with an uninfected partner; use condoms but they don't fully protect against infection since the parasite can be spread through unprotected areas of skin.	Antibiotics **Extras** It can take weeks or months before symptoms show up.

For more information, contact the National Center for HIV/AIDS, Viral Hepatitits, STD, and TB Prevention at www.cdc.gov/nchhstp/ or call the National STI Resource Center Hotline at 1-919-361-8488.

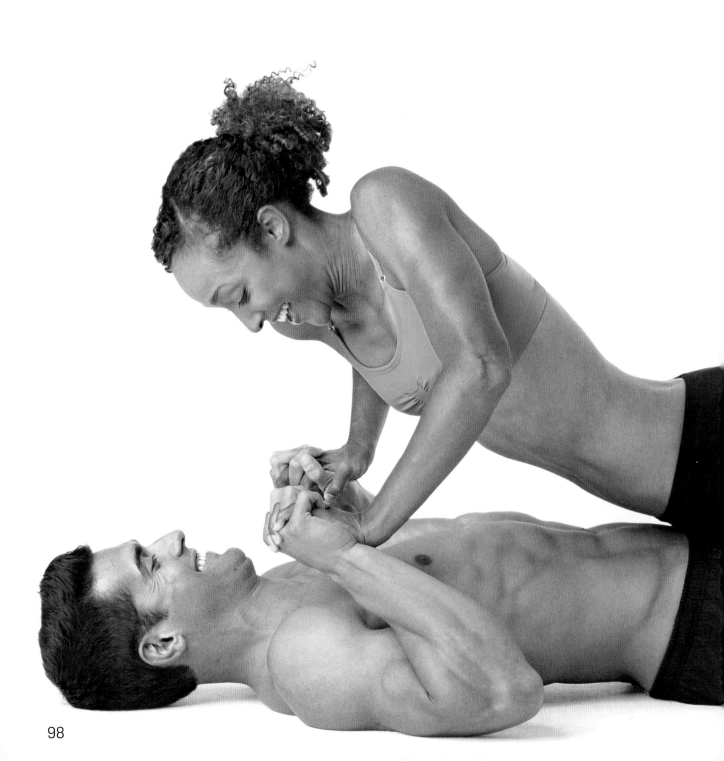

Chapter 6
The Couple's Workout

STRENGTHEN YOUR LOVE LIFE WHILE TONING YOUR BODY

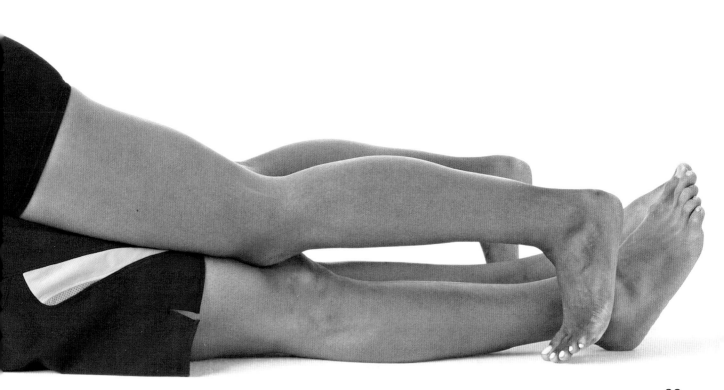

You see all types

at the gym. Chicks in cut-off Metalica T-shirts pumping dumbbells. Guys contemplating their abs in the mirrors. Runners with longing looks on their faces waiting for the next available treadmill.

What you rarely see in health clubs are happy couples. Couples, period, working out together. Strange, isn't it? Exercise is something that most people do solo, even in a crowded health club. When you look around what do you see? Dozens and dozens of people communing with iron bars and robotic-looking machinery. The closest they get to touching another human being is accidentally bumping rumps in the locker room.

People! You are missing a terrific opportunity to spend honest-to-goodness quality time with your best friend, your spouse, the significant other person in your life. How? By working out together. What a concept!

Engage, interact. Grab hold of her sweaty glutes. Whisper sweet encouragements into his ear: Push … harder … yes! That's it! Feel the burn!

It's completely G-rated.

The marriage counselors and sex therapists agree that what's missing in many long-term relationships is a non-sexual connection—engaging with one another on physical and emotional levels that don't necessarily lead to sex (although that wouldn't be a bad thing). And surveys show that couples who share common passions—and have more fun—outside of the bedroom tend to enjoy hotter passion inside the bedroom. In fact, laboratory studies of brain scans of married people show that having new experiences together as a couple triggers the release of dopamine, the neurochemical associated with the brain's reward system and those obsessive feelings so prevalent at the beginnings of lusty courtship.

Listening to John Coltrane's jazz together? That works. Downhill skiing? Even better. But how about doing something challenging and physically interactive like a strength and cardio workout, relying on each other's body-weight for resistance and connecting intimately through touch, sight, sound, and smell? That's hands-on. That's good for the muscles, heart, brain, and—who knows—it just might recreate those urges you had on your third date.

Working out in tandem at home works on a practical level, too. It's efficient and inexpensive: you don't need equipment and you don't have to drive across town to the health club. It can help you both lose weight, strengthen your relationship, and motivate yourselves to keep on keeping on. A study by researchers in Australia suggests that couples who embark on a weight-loss program together are significantly more successful than those who attempt it on their own. The research at Royal Perth Hospital found that married couples who participated in a nutrition and fitness program that included 50 minutes of brisk walking together weekly lost more weight than the individual dieters did and maintained their weights and overall fitness for an entire year after the 16-week study ended. What's more, while 43 percent of the singles dropped out of the fitness program, only 6 percent of the couples did, suggesting that husband and wife motivated each other through the physical and mental challenges.

Another study at Brigham Young University analyzed the lifestyles of more than 4,000 middle-aged married couples and found that husbands and wives typically mirror each other's physical health. A man who's in great shape was highly unlikely to have an out-of-shape, overweight wife and vice versa. Similar research at the University of Pittsburgh School of Health and Rehabilitation Services determined that physically active men were three times more likely to have active wives than inactive men were. Use the power of your partnership to get into the best shape of your life.

You can lift weights with your spouse

STICK TOGETHER

To stay true to your fitness goals, "your training partner needs to be someone who will hold you accountable," says Jack Raglin, PhD, professor of kinesiology at Indiana University. A study by Raglin found that 92 percent of couples who went to the gym together continued to do so after a year. By contrast, the couples who exercised separately had a 50 percent dropout rate.

The Couple's Workout | OURS

or toss a medicine ball back and forth, but the natural differences in size and strength between men and women can make working out this way difficult and slow things down. Plus, using equipment separates you from one another, which defeats a big part of the purpose of couples exercise. "Holding your partner's bodyweight, looking into his or her eyes like you do with a dance partner creates a natural connection that strengthens relationships … while building muscle," says Dean Graham, a yoga and martial arts instructor in New York City.

And there's always the hot shower to look forward to after the workout!

Taking inspiration from ballroom dance, yoga, jujitsu, and Kung fu, Graham developed a series of bodyweight exercises for couples. They build muscular strength, balance, core stability, and cardiovascular endurance if you do them in circuit fashion as prescribed below.

How to do the workout

- Design your own couple's circuit from the following 13 exercises. Choose seven.

- Do as many repetitions as you can until your form starts to suffer, then stop. Each one of you can complete the full circuit before the other starts exercising, or you can take turns and use the non-working set as active rest.

- For the first 2 weeks, do just one circuit three days a week. During weeks 3 and 4 complete a second circuit after resting for at least 90 seconds. On week 5, do three complete circuits with rest periods in between. Moving forward, trim down the length of the rest periods.

The Couple's Circuit

Create a seven-exercise circuit by choosing one exercise from Groups 1 through 6 and ending with the resisted side plank. Do the exercises in the order shown, as many reps as you can, before moving to the next group. You can make copies of this chart to keep track of "his" and "hers" reps.

ABOUT THE EXPERT

Dean Graham is a co-creator (with Lori Lim) of the WeFitFor2 Couple's Workout from which our BBOS Couple's Workout is adapted. A 3-disc DVD set of the full WeFitFor2 Couple's Workout is available for $39.95 at www.wffor2.com.

Build Your Workout

EXERCISE	HER REPETITIONS			HIS REPETITIONS		
	Weeks 1&2	Weeks 3&4	Week 5	Weeks 1&2	Weeks 3&4	Week 5
Group 1						
Single-Leg Lunge						
Lying Hamstring Curl						
Group 2						
Lying Leg Adduction						
Lying Leg Abduction						
Group 3						
Decline Pushup						
Mirror Pushup						
Group 4						
Horizontal Pullup						
Single-Arm Row						
Group 5						
Back Extension						
Throw-Down						
Group 6						
Decline Situp						
Weighted Situp						
Include in Every Circuit						
Resisted Side Plank						

FARTLEK FOR TWO

Running with a slower partner can be frustrating for both runners. Here's one way to make it work with an interval concept originated in Sweden called the fartlek or speed play. Run together at a warm-up pace for about a mile. Then select a landmark (a telephone pole, mail box, the end of a block) and pick up your pace until you are running at your typical race pace. The faster runner will reach the landmark first and start walking in a circle to wait for his or her partner. Walk or jog together for about 2 minutes, then look for your next landmark and take off again. Repeat this sequence (you can vary the length between landmarks to adjust speed-play segments) for six to 10 rounds. Then resume easy running together for 10 minutes to cool down.

The Couple's Workout

Single-Leg Lunge

Works the quadriceps and calves as well as backs of the thighs, butt, and the muscles supporting the knee.

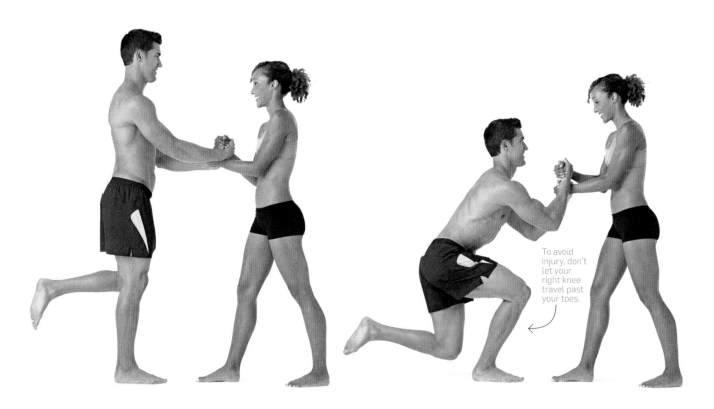

To avoid injury, don't let your right knee travel past your toes.

A

- Stand facing your partner and grasp hands, your right to his or her right. Your partner bends slightly at the waist, knees, and arms to offer support as you lunge. Bend your left leg to 90 degrees, putting all your weight on your right leg.

B

- Starting the movement at your hips, begin descending and bending your right leg until your back knee nearly touches the ground.
- Pushing through your right heel, stand straight up on your right leg. Repeat. After you've done as many as you can with good form, stand on your left leg and repeat the lunge with your right leg bent.

Lying Hamstring Curl

Exercises the large muscles in back of the thighs.

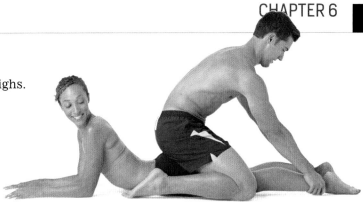

- Lie face down on the floor and have your partner sit on your hips, facing your feet, and hold your ankles.

Squeeze your glutes as you curl your legs up.

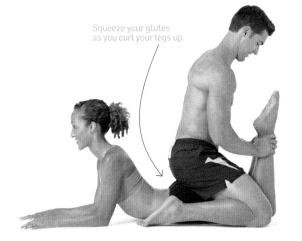

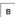

- Slowly bend your knees to raise your lower legs against your partner's downward press.

If you feel a strain in your back, you may rest your chest on the floor during this exercise.

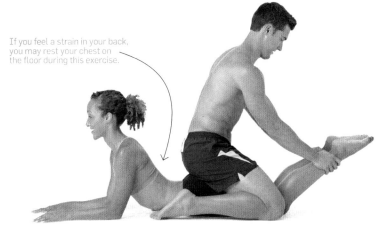

- Lower your feet to the floor against your partner's upward resistance.

Lying Leg Adduction

Strengthens the inner thigh muscles, the adductors.

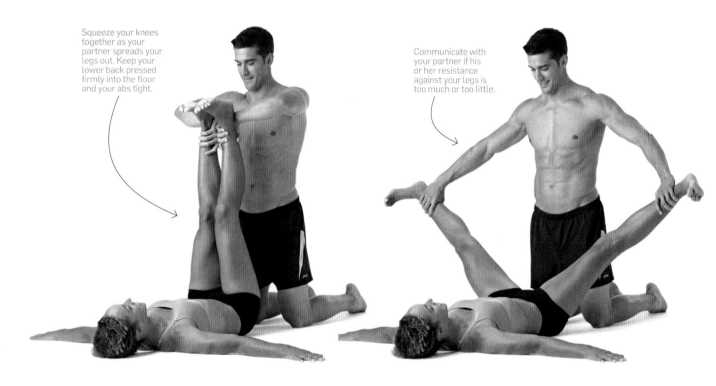

Squeeze your knees together as your partner spreads your legs out. Keep your lower back pressed firmly into the floor and your abs tight.

Communicate with your partner if his or her resistance against your legs is too much or too little.

A

- Lie on the floor on your back with your arms out to your sides and your legs held together straight up in the air.
- Your partner will kneel, with hands on the inside of your lower legs.

B

- Resist the pressure of your partner spreading your legs outward to the limit of your comfort.
- Close your legs against even more partner resistance until they are once again together. That's one repetition.

Lying Leg Abduction

Works the muscles of the outer thigh, the abductors.

- Lie on your right side, supporting your upper body by leaning on your right elbow and forearm and keeping your left leg stacked on top of your right.
- Your partner should kneel behind you, placing one hand below and one hand above your left knee.

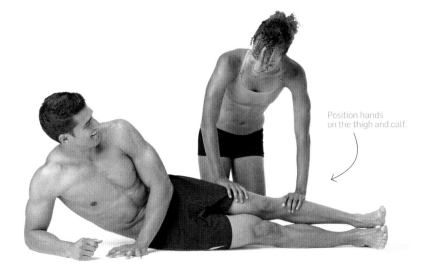

Position hands on the thigh and calf.

B

- Slowly raise your straight left leg against your partner's downward pressure to an elevation of about 45 degrees.
- Keep your abs tight while you slowly lower your leg against your partner's downward pressure. Repeat until you are fatigued. Then turn over to lie on your left side and repeat the exercise with the other leg.

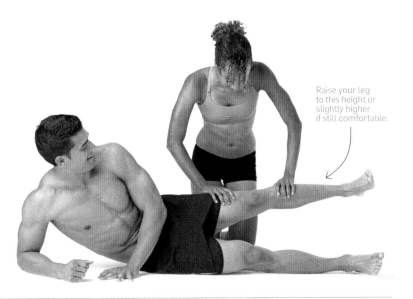

Raise your leg to this height or slightly higher if still comfortable.

Decline Pushup

Raising your feet makes your chest and arms work harder during a pushup.

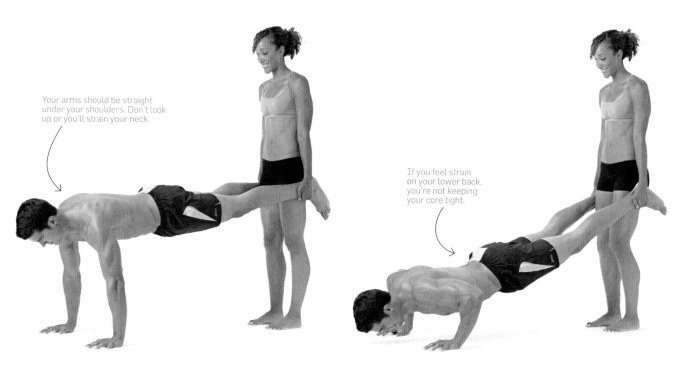

Your arms should be straight under your shoulders. Don't look up or you'll strain your neck.

If you feel strain on your lower back, you're not keeping your core tight.

- Lie on the floor, placing your hands directly under your shoulders as in a classic pushup position.
- Have your partner grab your ankles and lift your legs until your straight back creates a 30- to 45-degree angle from heels-to-head.
- Do not arch your back in either direction, but keep your torso straight from head to feet and your core tight.

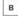

- Lower your body as far as you can without allowing your hips to sag.
- Press up forcefully. That's one repetition.

Optional

- You can also do a weighted standard pushup. While in the up position, hands and feet on the floor, have your partner press down on your back to add resistance going down and pushing up.

Mirror Pushup

Targets the chest muscles, but also works your shoulders, triceps, back, and core.

- Have your partner lie back on the floor. Straddle his legs and grab his hands, interlocking your fingers. Assume a pushup position, supporting yourself on the balls of your feet and with arms straight and hands on his directly underneath your shoulders.
- The backs of his upper arms rest on the floor, elbows bent at 90 degrees, to support your weight. This is the starting position.

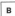

- Lower your body until your chest nearly touches his.
- The instability of this move calls more tiny muscle fibers into play as you naturally balance yourself on his hands.

C

- Pause at the bottom, then push yourself back to the starting position.
- Don't drop your hips. Keep your core stiff.

Optional

- While you are in the up position, he can do a chest press, pushing you up until his arms are straight, and then lowering you at which point you can do a full pushup.
- You can keep alternating this way for as long as you can without sacrificing form or safety.

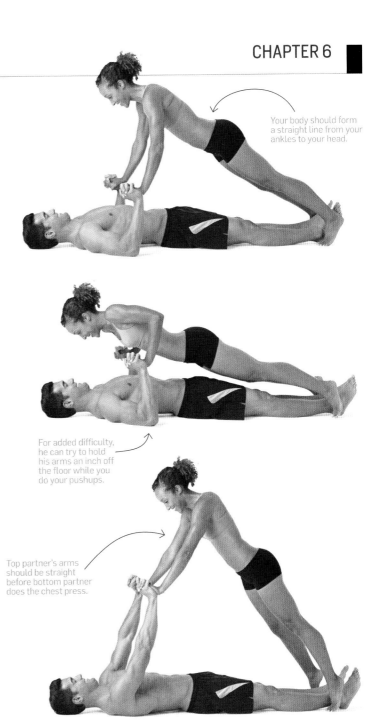

Your body should form a straight line from your ankles to your head.

For added difficulty, he can try to hold his arms an inch off the floor while you do your pushups.

Top partner's arms should be straight before bottom partner does the chest press.

Single-Arm Row

Works the upper back, rear deltoids, and arms.

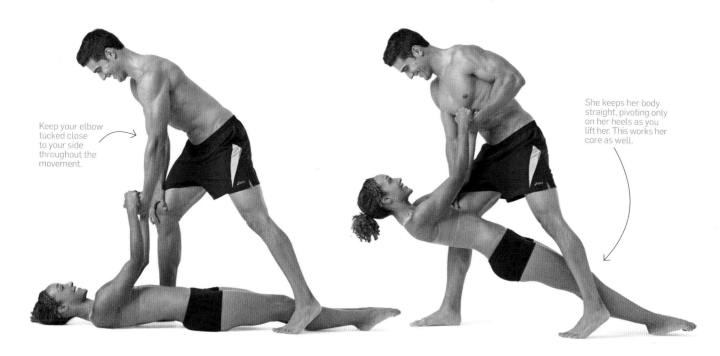

Keep your elbow tucked close to your side throughout the movement.

She keeps her body straight, pivoting only on her heels as you lift her. This works her core as well.

A

- Have your partner lie flat on her back. Straddle her body in a split stance, right foot forward, and left foot back, both knees bent slightly.
- Bend at the waist so your torso forms a 45-degree angle and grasp her left hand with your left. Have her wrap her right hand over top of yours for a secure grip. Brace yourself with your right hand on your right knee.

B

- Keeping your back flat, pull your left hand to the side of your torso, lifting her arrow-straight body off the floor. When your forearm meets your biceps, slowly lower her until your arm is straight, and repeat. After doing all your reps, switch foot and arm positions and work the other side of your back by rowing her with your right arm.
- Don't lift your torso or rotate it as you row your partner's weight.

Horizontal Pullup

A good move to build back and arm strength in preparation for regular bar pullups.

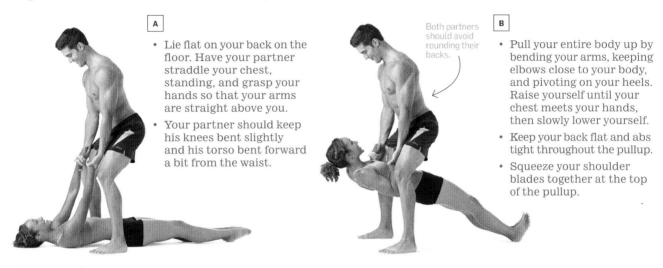

A

- Lie flat on your back on the floor. Have your partner straddle your chest, standing, and grasp your hands so that your arms are straight above you.

- Your partner should keep his knees bent slightly and his torso bent forward a bit from the waist.

Both partners should avoid rounding their backs.

B

- Pull your entire body up by bending your arms, keeping elbows close to your chest body, and pivoting on your heels. Raise yourself until your chest meets your hands, then slowly lower yourself.

- Keep your back flat and abs tight throughout the pullup.

- Squeeze your shoulder blades together at the top of the pullup.

Back Extension

Works the lower back and core.

A

- Lie facedown on the floor and have your partner sit on the backs of your lower legs. Extend your arms out to your sides, palms down so your body forms a T.

B

- Slowly raise your torso as high as you can.

- Pause for a second, then slowly lower your body to the floor. That's one rep.

Don't hyperextend your back, but rise to a comfortable height.

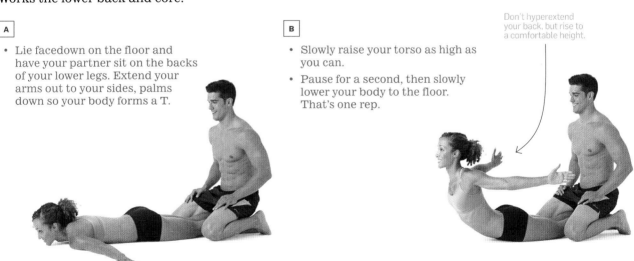

Throw Down

Works the abs and lower back muscles.

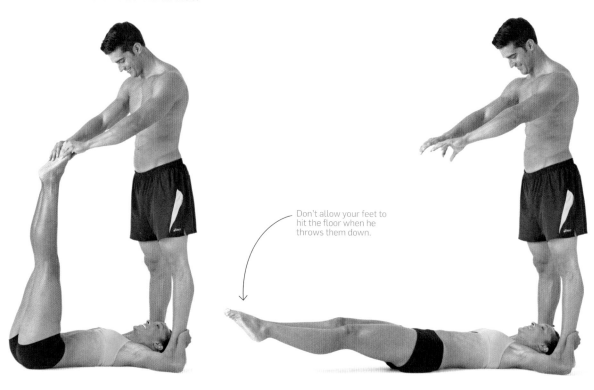

Don't allow your feet to hit the floor when he throws them down.

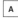

- Lie on your back with your head between your standing partner's feet. Reach back and grab his ankles.
- Press your lower back firmly into the floor (don't arch your back) and raise your legs straight up together toward him so he can grab your feet.

- Your partner will push your feet down toward the floor. Allow your legs to come close to the floor but not touch. Lift them up again, using your abs.

Optional

- You can also work your obliques by adding a move.
- To hit those love handles, have your partner push your feet down toward the left. Raise them again, so he can push them down to the right. Alternate straight, left, and right until your abs fatigue.
- All the while, keep your abs engaged.

Decline Situp

Works the upper and lower abdominals (and the obliques, if done with a twist). The angle allows for a greater range of motion.

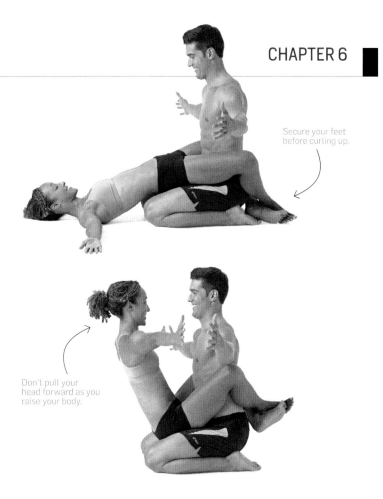

Secure your feet before curling up.

A

- Have your partner kneel on the floor, and rest his butt on his ankles. Sit high on his thighs and wrap your legs around his back to hold yourself there. This will also exercise your inner thighs.

- Engage your thighs and lower yourself back until your head is on the floor. This is the starting position.

Don't pull your head forward as you raise your body.

B

- Keep your arms out to your sides forming a T. Slowly sit up all the way using the full range of motion. Pause, then lower yourself.

C Optional

- To work your obliques, alternate twisting to the right or left after every other straight situp. Keep a slow and even tempo.

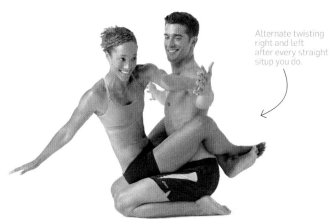

Alternate twisting right and left after every straight situp you do.

Weighted Situp

Exercises the lower back and front abdominals.

A

- Sit on the floor with your knees bent and feet flat. Have your partner stand on the tops of your feet and grasp your hands, fingers interlocking. Her arms should be locked straight. Bend yours to right angles and keep them at your sides as you lie back flat and her torso leans over you.

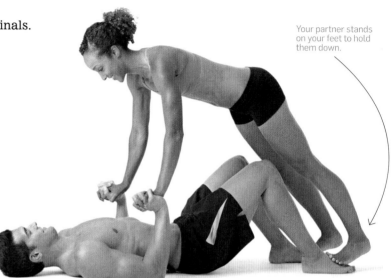

Your partner stands on your feet to hold them down.

B

- Pressing your lower back into the floor, sit up to at least a 45-degree angle against her weight. Keep your arms to your sides so your arms, shoulders, and torso rise as one unit.
- Do not allow your elbows to stay on the floor.
- Use a slow and controlled movement as your rise up, pause, and lower yourself back to the floor.

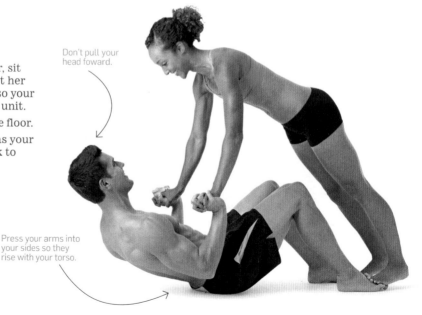

Don't pull your head foward.

Press your arms into your sides so they rise with your torso.

Resisted Side Plank

Works the obliques.

A

- Lie on your right side with your left leg stacked on your right. Bend your right elbow and place it on the floor directly under your right shoulder.
- Have your partner kneel behind you and place her hands on your hip and thigh to add resistance as you lift into a side plank.

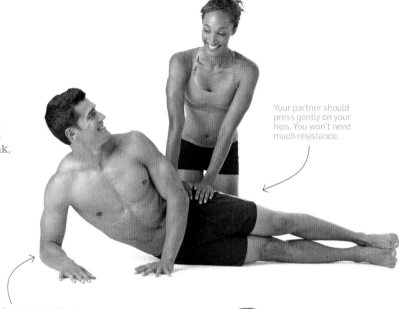

Your partner should press gently on your hips. You won't need much resistance.

Position your elbow under your shoulder.

B

- Keeping your belly drawn in tight, raise your hip against her downward pressure. Try to lift your left hip to the height of your supporting arm's shoulder. Pause for three seconds, then lower yourself slowly against constant pressure.
- After completing as many repetitions as you can with good form on one side, repeat the side plank by lying on your left side with your partner behind you.

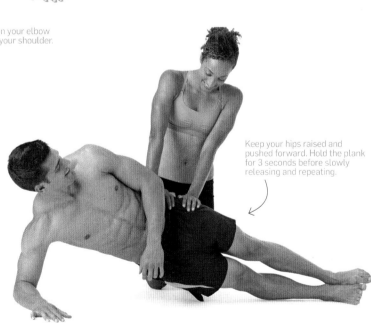

Keep your hips raised and pushed forward. Hold the plank for 3 seconds before slowly releasing and repeating.

Yoga for Both of You

REPOSITION YOURSELVES FOR GREATER PLEASURE

Here's something to meditate on: Research suggests that women and men who can perform a proper Bhujangasan (serpent-like) posture enjoy more satisfying sex. That may not come as a surprise to practioners of yoga. The ancient Indian healing and flexibility exercise has long been shown to offer a host of physical and mental health benefits including easing joint pain, lowering blood pressure, and relieving anxiety and symptoms of depression. And now it appears that yoga practice is really great mind-body training for the sexual health of both women and men.

"Yoga truly is *sexercise*," says Vikas Dhikav, MD, senior research officer at All India Institute of Medical Sciences in New Delhi. "It improves strength and tone of the abdominal-perineal muscles (abs and pelvic muscles), it reduces anxiety, and affects the endocrinal glands, all of which play an important role in good sexual functioning."

Two studies in the *Journal of Sexual Medicine* recently demonstrated the beneficial effects of yoga on common sexual dysfunctions. One study conducted at medical universities in Mumbai and Delhi, India, involved 68 men suffering from premature ejaculation. Thirty-eight of the men were told to practice 12 yoga poses and a relaxation breathing technique called anulomvilom, in which you alternatively close one nostril at a time and breath deeply (see A Nose for Sex later in this chapter). The rest of the men were given fluoxetine, an antidepressant medication often used to treat PE. After eight weeks, 25 of the 30 men on Prozac had clinical improvement in staying power while all 38 men practicing yoga were able to last significantly longer (according to evaluations by their wives). And the men who did asanas and yogic breathing reported no adverse side effects, unlike the drug-taking group.

The women's study, also conducted at those medical universities in India, involved 40 women, ages 22 to 55, who were enrolled in a 12-week yoga program. At the end of the experiment, nearly 75 percent of the women reported greater satisfaction with their sexual life after learning yoga. Researchers found significant improvements in sexual function scores assessing desire, arousal, lubrication, orgasm, pain, and overall satisfaction. Worth noting: women over 45 showed the greatest improvements in arousal, lubrication, and pain reduction.

Flexy is Sexy

Yoga enhances blood flow, and many poses direct it right toward the pelvic region, heightening sensitivity and desire. Yoga improves flexibility by toning and strengthening the core, including your pelvic floor muscles. Greater range of motion in your legs, hips, and back helps reduce pain in women who find some sex positions uncomfortable. And fitter pelvic floor muscles (the muscles you use to stop the flow of urine) can elevate pleasure. Exercising these muscles "gives you stronger contractions and releases, which can help you experience a more intense orgasm," says Becky Jeffers, fitness director at the Berman Center in Chicago, which specializes in female sexual health and menopause management.

"Men tend to be really tight in their hips, hamstrings, and lower back and they carry a lot of tension in their shoulders, too," says Tara Stiles, founder of Strala Yoga in New York City and yoga expert for *Women's Health*. "All that can put limits on performance, but it can be remedied with some simple yoga poses."

Stiles, also the author of *Slim, Calm, Sexy Yoga*, suggests five must-do poses that'll benefit anyone in the bedroom, man or woman. Do this 15-minute beginner's sequence in order once a day. After completing the sequence once through, repeat it, this time doing the first two positions using opposite legs. Remember to keep your breathing easy—inhaling and exhaling with each shifting movement.

Asana	Hold For
Fire Log	10 breaths
Pigeon	10 breaths
Upward-Facing Dog	5 breaths
Bow	5 breaths
Bridge	5 breaths

Fire Log

Opens the hips, stretches the thighs and groin, and strengthen the abs.

A

- Sit on the floor and bend your right knee, bringing your shin in front of you, parallel to the front of your yoga mat. Bend your left knee to place your left ankle directly on top of your right knee so that your left shin is parallel with your right. Inhale deeply and gently, and allow your knees to relax down toward the floor to open the hips. Sit up straight, keeping your back flat and chest open. Flex your feet. Exhale and move your torso forward. If you can, walk your torso forward over your shins. Hold this position for 10 long, deep breaths. After completing all 5 poses, repeat the Fire Log pose with your right ankle on top of your left knee.

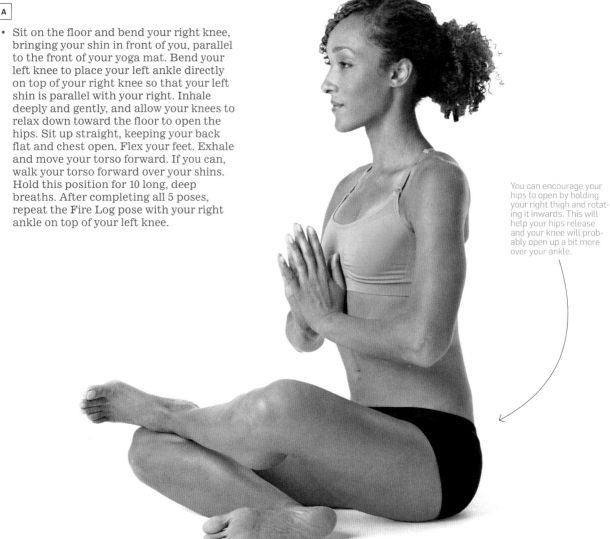

You can encourage your hips to open by holding your right thigh and rotating it inwards. This will help your hips release and your knee will probably open up a bit more over your ankle.

Pigeon

Stretches the hip rotators (gluteal area), the hip flexors (the long muscles that run along the front of your thighs and pelvis), and the piriformis muscle deep in the butt that can press on the sciatic nerve.

- Start on all fours with your hands below your shoulders and your knees below your hips. Bring your right knee forward and slowly turn your right foot out and to the left side of your yoga mat. Position your right foot below your left hip; for a more intense stretch, move your right shin toward the front of your mat. Now straighten your left leg behind you. Walk your hands back toward your hips and lower your pelvis to the floor. Press your hands into the floor to lift your torso away from the thigh and lengthen your spine.

Be sure your hips don't lean to the right.

B

- Now, inhale deeply. Exhale as you walk your hands forward, bending your torso toward the floor. Try to rest your forehead on the floor if you can. Hold for 10 deep breaths. After completing the full sequence, repeat the sequence again, this time doing pigeon with your left leg bent and right leg extended behind you.

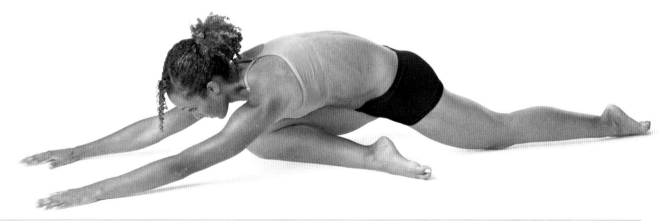

Upward-Facing Dog

Strengthens arms, relieves stress, opens chest; releases tension in the neck, shoulders, and upper back.

- Lie on the floor with your toes pointed back, tops of your feet on the floor. Bend your elbows and place your palms on the floor near your waist. Your upper arms should be parallel with the floor. Inhale and press into the floor with your hands to straighten your arms and push your torso up. Your hips and legs should rise a few inches off the floor. Roll your shoulders down and back and press your chest forward. Look straight ahead. Hold this pose for 5 deep breaths.

At the top of the position, bend your elbows slightly and sway your torso from side to side to release tension.

Bow

Opens the chest and shoulders and flexes the hips, quadriceps, and spine.

- Lie on your belly on the floor. Bend your knees and reach back with your hands to grab your ankles (not the tops of your feet). Keep your knees hip-width apart. Inhale deeply and gently press your ankles into your hands. This will pull your upper torso, head, and thighs away from the floor simultaneously. Look straight ahead and drop your shoulders away from your ears. Hold for 5 long, deep breaths.

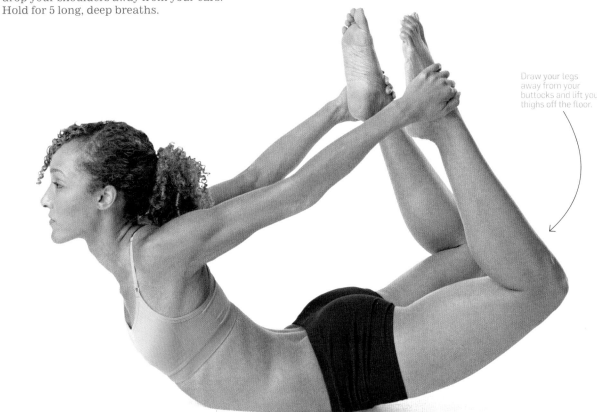

Draw your legs away from your buttocks and lift your thighs off the floor.

Bridge

Opens the chest and rib cage, improving lung capacity, and flexes shoulders, spine, and hips.

- Lie on your back with your knees bent and feet flat on the floor. Place your hands on the floor next to your hips and gently lift your hips, pressing your arms into the floor. Grab your ankles with your hands. Keeping your feet flat on the floor, try reaching your hips up farther. Hold for 5 deep breaths.

For a better shoulder stretch, let go of your ankles and lace your fingers together between your feet. Wiggle your shoulder blades together and press your chest toward your chin.

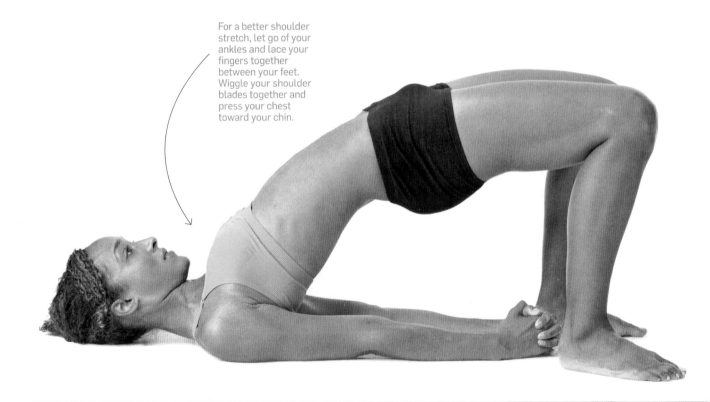

A Nose for Sex

TRY THIS ANCIENT YOGIC BREATHING EXERCISE TO EASE ANXIETY

Practicing alternate nostril breathing, an ancient meditation technique used in yoga, can reduce anxiety and improve sexual performance in men and satisfaction in women. A study in the journal *Applied Psychophysiology and Biofeedback* offers a possible reason why: lower blood pressure. Researchers say nerves in each nostril reach different parts of the hypothalamus that regulate blood pressure. Stimulating the nerves separately by breathing through one nostril at a time activates the hypothalamus and triggers the parasympathetic nervous system calming effect. It also forces you to breathe deeply, filling your lungs and bringing more oxygen to the bloodstream.

"Performance anxiety is an important precipitating factor for premature ejaculation," says Vikas Dhikay, MD, who has researched this at All India Institute of Medical Sciences in New Delhi. "Deep yoga breathing teaches men to control anxiety in body and mind. If someone is relaxed they can hold on for more time."

Try it yourself: Sit in a comfortable position. Place your right hand over your nose so that your thumb rests near your right nostril and your ring finger is positioned next to your left. Close your right nostril with your thumb and inhale through your left nostril for a count of four. Close your left nostril with your ring finger and hold your breath for a count of four. Now release your thumb and exhale through your right nostril for a four-count. Breathe in through the right, pause, close that nostril and release the left and breathe out through the left nostril. That's one round. Continue this pattern for about 5 minutes. Practice a couple of times a week.

Chapter 7
Make Lust Last

MONOGAMY IS THE MOST
CHALLENGING COMMITMENT
YOU'LL EVER MAKE.
KEEP THE FAITH WITHOUT
LOSING THE EXCITEMENT.

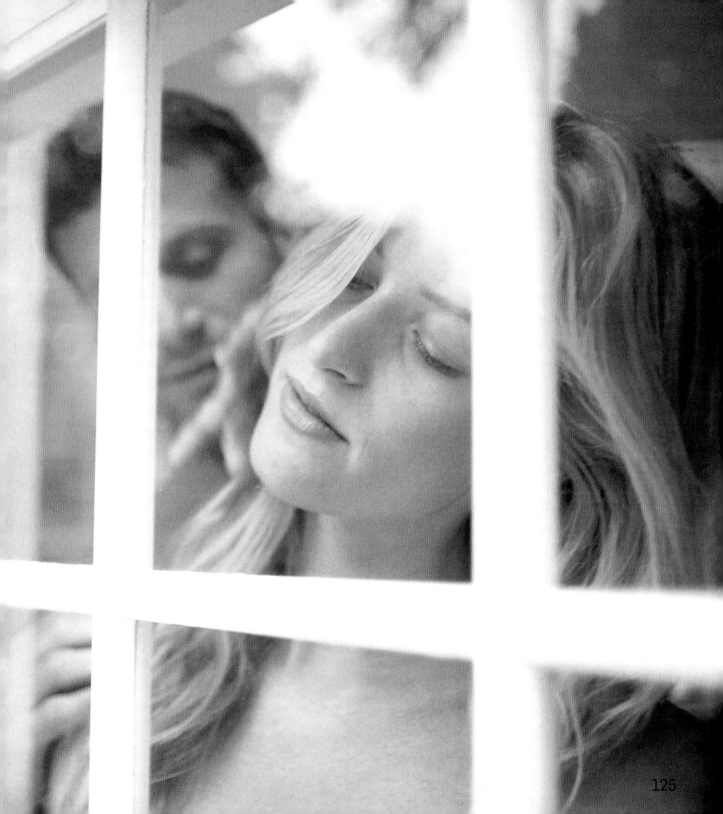

My friend

Frank was living with a woman who had the whole checklist—looks, brains, goodness, sass, a tolerance for sports, even family dough. Clearly, marriage should have been next. But our boy couldn't pull the nuptial trigger.

"Why no wedding?" I asked him over a beer one night.

"48th and Madison," he said, as though a busy intersection explained it all. "Every day . . . that corner . . . all those women . . . shining in the morning."

I said nothing.

"I've been monogamous for 3 years," he said, staring at me with haunted eyes. "But I don't think I can do it forever."

He was a lost boy, skewered on the horns of the monogamy . . . monogamy . . . monogamy.

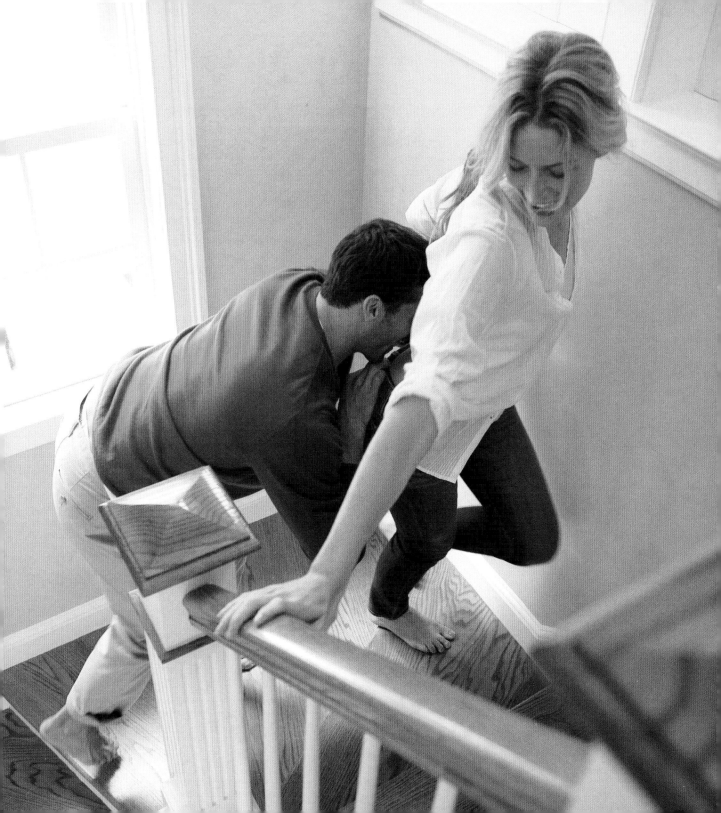

Make Lust Last HIS

20

Percentage of couples who are too tired to have sex, according to the National Sleep Foundation.

Sounds an awful lot like monotony, doesn't it? Or Monopoly? Do we hear mahogany? Not exactly a sizzling trifecta: tedium, an endless board game, and your great-aunt's dining table. Monogamy just doesn't sound like much fun, certainly not in comparison to its alternative.

Still, a hunch lingers that true happiness—the deep, sustaining contentment we seek—lies somewhere down Monogamy Road. If only we could find our way past all the soft, warm, scented bodies of this tempting world.

Well, here's a little help from a friend. If you have no interest in forgoing the carnal cornucopia of this blessed land, skip this chapter and head over to the A to Z Guide to Sex Tips. But if you'd like to be captain of your ship, master of your longing, faithful to a person with whom you just might build an enriching life, read on. In the beginning of this chapter, we suggest six essential things you ought to know if you've got wild oats you'd rather not sow. Later you'll find a practical (and fun) homework assignment for stoking your sex life to red hot status in just 16 days. The road to sizzling monogamy, for the most part, is simply a matter of mind over monotony. It begins with a pledge to resist the cliché that familiarity breeds lower temperatures, a decision that you will not be doomed to a bleak future of ho-hum, twice a month sex, and the determination to bring the same appetite for excellence to exalting your partner's body that you bring to every other arena of your life.

Throw Down the Gauntlet

First, it's important to understand that you're not in this alone. All men wrestle with the call of the wild. Some will argue this proves all men are pigs. Wrong. It proves all men are brothers. Those thoughts about Myrna at the FedEx place don't make you a bad guy. They just make you a guy. Are we clear on that? Lust is not a virtue. Lust is not a vice. It's just a fact.

Why is monogamy so tough for men? Some women favor polemical explanations featuring reptile analogies and the phrase "incapable of commitment." But the truth bears no grudge. Fact: Men get hammered by two powerful, antimonogamy forces—our Darwinian hardware and our cultural software. Plain and simple: The monogamous man must battle both his genes and his mythology.

Blame it on biology. According to Darwin, life is just DNA working like mad to reproduce itself. Our sex drive is the vehicle for spreading our genes. We're in thrall to a biological imperative, hard-wired to want anybody who might carry our double helix down the line.

Aha! cry the women. We have DNA, too. How come we don't mount anything with a blood pressure?

Darwin has an answer women hate: Women are more finicky because they've only got a few hundred eggs in a lifetime. Can't afford to waste one on a loser. Since we have a billion sperm in a nanosecond and remain fertile till

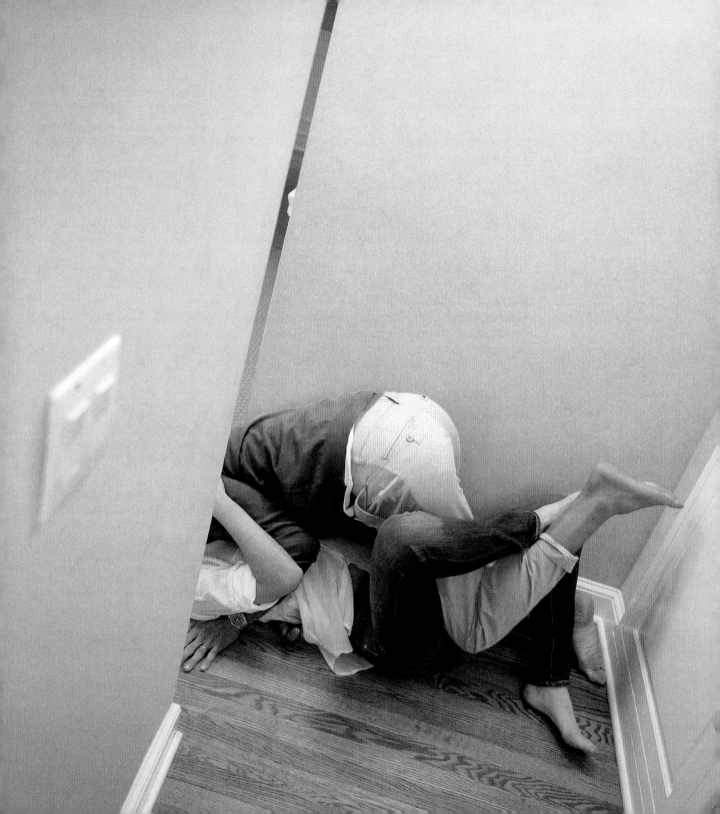

we die, there's no need to hold our fire. We've got tons of ammo. Again: Not a virtue. Not a vice. Just a fact.

Blame it on Rio Bravo. However strong the innate male drive to dance with many partners, it's nothing compared to the potent cultural messages that hurl us into the arms of other women. Our nature is polygamous; our nurture doubly so.

What's that you say? But we're a Puritanical culture, built on the nuclear family? Hah! We admire the monogamous man? Hah! again. Oh, sure, for the record, our official position is that we respect the steadfast guy. But be serious. We're cowboys. Nobody wants to be Ward Cleaver.

Quick quarterback quiz: Would you rather be Roger Staubach or Joe Namath? The answer you just gave is revealing.

We claim to look up to Staubach— the God-fearing, steadfast naval officer and family man. Roger even has more championships than the bad boy from Beaver Falls. But we'll take Joe's little black book over the Book of Ezekiel any day. The one-woman man is seen as something less than a man. He's a cowboy turned sodbuster, a wimp who has surrendered his freedom, tied his horse to the hitching post. He's henpecked, emasculated, a rooster without his comb, a stallion without his—well, his stallion stuff.

With our bodies crying out for communion and our culture pulsating with conquistador signals, it's no surprise that for men, monogamy's a long shot.

But, hey, that's the good news. That's what makes monogamy worth chasing. After all, there's no glory in the easy stuff. Lindbergh didn't become famous for Boston-to-Philly. Ripken didn't play most of those games for 13 years.

Monogamy is tough? Bring it on, baby. Hard is good. Hard is a chance to show what we've got. You know what else is hard: winning a Medal of Honor, amassing wealth, having washboard abs at 45. We hate easy. Hey, we're the gender that brought you Magellan and Martin Luther King, the gender that scaled Everest, discovered the New World and invented the Ironman Triathlon. Why monogamy? Simple. Because it's there.

Don't Fight the Feeling

When early Christian theologans made lust one of the seven deadly sins, they were talking about bad lust. You know, the kind that hoots at and objectives women, that stupid, grunting, hubba-hubba kind of lust. I'm talking about good lust, the kind that might even be described as zest or vitality, maybe reverence, perhaps an appreciation of all God's children. A man without good lust is an insensate mass, a lump. I ask you: Is a proper man unmoved by the sight of the Teton Range? The sound of Beethoven's best? The smell of freshly mown grass? Surely, Debbi at the pizza place—she of those green eyes and that sweaty nape—should stir our blood as well.

Remember: The feelings are not a problem; acting on them is. It's perfectly okay to covet thy neighbor's wife. What's not okay is sneaking into thy neighbor's shed for a quickie with his missus.

The point is: You can't stifle the feelings that emerge while relaxing on a beach crowded with women wearing tiny strips of colorful fabric. Grass grows through concrete, and male vim will find a way. When you're feeling lusty, it won't help to think of your old coach, Mr. Jantz. In fact, it may actually make monogamy even tougher. A steam engine needs a release valve. Bottle things up and it's surely gonna blow.

True monogamy—full-blooded, masculine monogamy—requires lusty thoughts. Just as St. George needed his dragon, Connors needed McEnroe and Wyatt Earp needed the Clantons, he who would be monogamous needs temptations over which to triumph. You don't pretend your rival doesn't exist. You tip your hat to him, then kick his ass.

So enjoy your lust, up to a point. You're a connoisseur of fine females. Be not ashamed. You have biceps and quads and pecs. You also have sharp eyes and an inquiring mind. Praise the Lord.

Stoke Up the Home Fires

Lots of guys who step out plead sexual deprivation or boredom at home. And, often enough, a good case can be made. But here's an important monogamy pointer. If your sex life isn't everything you dreamed, make sure you've given it everything you've got. Ask yourself how much ingenuity, improvisation, energy, joy, and lust you bring to the sheets. The danger is that because the cliché of the not-tonight-I've-got-a-headache wife is so deeply embedded in our heads, when a couple's sex life withers, men assume it's because chicks are under-sexed, that they just don't dig it as much as we do. Maybe. But maybe not.

You must remember this: A kiss is not just a kiss. A woman's interest in sex can have quite a lot to do with the practitioner. Doing the carioca with a klutz is one thing; a fandango with Fred Astaire is something else entirely.

Technique matters. And you should work on yours. Try the Peruvian wiggle, the Sicilian spider. Read all the books, especially the centuries-old Asian classics. Experiment. Stay out of rutting ruts. Remember: Sex is like golf insofar as little things can mean a lot. Just a little bit slower may be a lot warmer. Sometimes counterclockwise stops time. A slight sideways shift can turn ho-hum into hallelujah. But . . .

Technique is just part of the game. Even more important is to be in the moment while in the act. Feel her skin. Inhale her scent. Inhabit the moment with all of your attention. Be intimate. Murmur. Remember, she's going for monogamy, too. You're her only access to Eros.

80

Percentage of divorced men and women who say their marriages broke up because they gradually grew apart. Only about 20 percent of couples say an extramarital affair was even partially to blame.

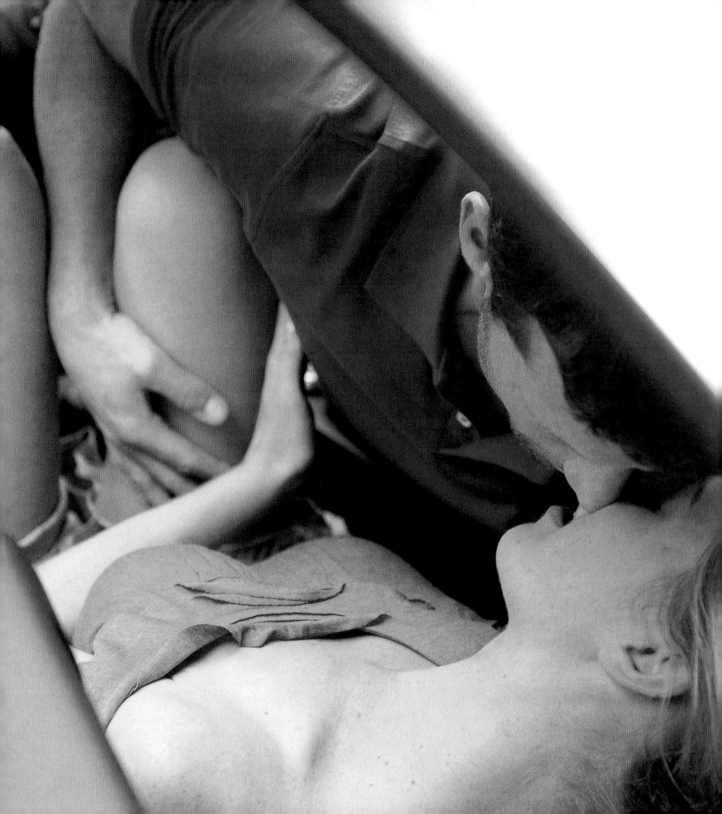

It's simple: If you're a badda-bing, badda-boom kind of guy, if you've got one move and one speed, it's no wonder she'd rather watch Bucks-Nets garbage time than go one-on-one with you. If, on the other hand, you're a virtuoso, if you make waves crash upon her shores, if she finds herself slipping in and out of consciousness under your touch, you'll be too busy pulling command-performance nooners to scan the horizon for other partners.

Stay lusty out of bed, too. Talk to her, for God's sake. Express yourself. Confide in her. Listen to her. Don't let this venture flounder because you didn't give it enough gas. Trust is a turn-on. It'll fire up the old slap-and-tickle. (See page 136 for a 16-day fire-up plan for red-hot monogamy, then saunter on over to page 154 for even more bed-rocking practical tips.)

Don't Do the Crime if You Can't Do the Time

You'll tell yourself that nobody will know. But that's not true. Don't argue with me. Trust me. Your partner will find out.

Infidelity staying a secret? It's 20 to 1, against. You may be so guilty that you actually drop the dime on yourself. (Remember Raskolnikov in *Crime and Punishment*?) Or your partner in crime may be a wild card. Even if she doesn't boil the family bunny like Glenn Close in *Fatal Attraction* she could get careless with her smile when she runs into your wife at Costco. Is it worth it?

The Cost-Benefit Analysis.

The benefit most often cited is sexual—the chance that Judy from accounting will be a human dynamo, a dominating dervish of delights, that sex with La Judithe will elicit tantric visions of burning wheels, lots of yelping, perhaps regression to past lives.

Well, maybe.

People can do invigorating things to each other. But the plain fact is that most sex is not apocalyptic. Most sex does not include fireworks and parades. Most men who fall off the monogamy wagon find themselves thinking of singer Peggy Lee's classic "Is That All There Is?" Right after, disappointment is common. Sometimes it becomes a lifelong thing.

Though the bodily bennies of cheating are uncertain, its costs are crystal clear. Some couples survive it. But, boy, it's a grenade in the garden. Do it and an efficiency apartment is in your future. Do it and tucking in the kids will mean taking a 10-mile drive on the expressway instead of a 10-step walk to their room. Do it and lawyers and words like "chattels" and "adultery" will become a part of your life. But more important, somebody's feelings will be hurt—big-time.

At the close of the day, the equation is exquisitely simple: Less monogamy equals more pain.

Just use this simple test. Imagine you just learned your wife did the hokey pokey with the house painter. Ouch! Ruins the day, doesn't it? It doesn't matter if the 'Canes and 'Noles are tied with a few ticks left; the news that your

Priscilla partied in a panel van can take the edge off even the Orange Bowl.

Repeat after me: I'd rather forgo erotic pleasure than cause [fill in name of loved one] pain. Just do as I say. Repeat after me: I'd rather forgo erotic pleasure than cause [loved one] pain. Plenty of pain out there already, pal. The hump just ain't worth the heartache.

Invest in Accident Insurance

How many bad television movies have you seen where some feckless cheating husband claims that "it just happened?" It is, of course, salt on a wound to hear sexual betrayal described as if it were no more serious than a fender bender.

But you know what?

It's true. Lots of guys veer off Monogamy Road accidentally—or rather, unintentionally. Make no mistake, it's not an excuse. At some point, there was a deliberate act of cuddle or thrust. But it is an explanation. Cheating happens when people are careless. Human beings have an appetite for each other. Putting them together in certain situations is asking for trouble, like storing oily rags in an overheated attic. For example, consider that most virulent of monogamy manglers, the business trip. Let's say you and Martha have one of those flirty office friendships. You're both happily married and monogamous, but you've also both thought about what it would

be like. Cut to the regional sales conference: the presentation you give together is a smash and you stop by her room to celebrate. Or your presentation implodes and she stops by your room to work on resumes. Either way, euphoric or depressed, next thing you know, you and your good bud, Martha, are doing the horizontal hora.

Safety rule number one: Don't ever be alone in a hotel room with a woman who is not your mom, your sister, or your wife. No exceptions. Don't stop by just to pick up the new sales data or drop off the old sales data. Forget the data, all right? Just don't go there. Period. Hotel rooms cry out for sex. It's against some law of nature for a man and a woman to be in one together and not have sex. If you don't want to dive, why walk out on the board? You could fall in. In fact, don't limit this rule to hotel rooms. Never be alone with a woman anywhere. This is the single best monogamy tip there is. If your son goes to Camp Iroquois with Joey from next door, for God's sake, don't drive up to get the boys with Joey's mom. You know you've watched her bend over her tomatoes. Why tempt fate? Would you run an extension cord across the steps? Why make yourself resist the urge to pull into a scenic overlook and overlook her scenery? The point is, defense wins championships—see the '69 Knicks, the '85 Bears, the Devils of '95. He who would be king of constancy has to

72

Percentage of women who say it turns them on when a man helps out around the house.

protect his goal. Make sure that sexual duplicity requires at least several purposeful, underhanded steps. A lot of us are weak, but far fewer of us are capable of cold-blooded mendacity. Avoiding what the Sisters of Mercy used to call the "occasions of sin" will minimize inadvertent adultery.

Safety rule number two: If, by some remote chance, you've broken rule number one and find yourself still faithful, do not—under any circumstances—have a drink. I know six guys who've cheated on their mates. Four of them said the last thing they remember was twisting open one of those tiny vodka bottles from a hotel minibar. The other two were bourbon guys. Alcohol hates monogamy.

Remember: Home Is Where The Sex Is

It's really none of their business, but statisticians have determined that monogamous, married men actually get laid more often than any other group of men. Of course, in any particular week, month, year, or even decade, single guys and tomcats can get more nookie than stalwarts. But over the course of a lifetime, Ozzie Nelson does okay for himself, thank you very much. Sometimes slow and steady—three times a month till you die—really does win the race.

Now, granted, this says nothing about the quality of said sexual events. Just that when the final score is tallied,

Staubach bests Joe Willie. Home can be hot. The key is to make your mind monogamous. See it clearly. Monogamy is not a lack of other women, it's expertise in one. It's an opportunity to specialize—like the neurosurgeon who studies the cerebral cortex or the fiddler who masters Haydn. The monogamous man hones his craft, refines technique, learns subtleties of terrain, and comes to understand a lot about both his partner's pelvis and her point of view.

When you've promised to drink only from one spring, its water will be sweet. Surely, when a woman knows that she is it for you—that she is the alpha and omega of your erotic world—she'll be emboldened by that responsibility. Surely, she'll answer the call and offer all of life's juice. When two people are entwined, for better or worse, lips get liquid with loyalty, hips bring wholesome heat, skin comes alive in partnership. Lust is intensified by trust, made fierce by faith and impassioned by a promise kept.

Six hours after Frank and I started talking about the "m" word, we walked up Broadway through a bright Manhattan dawn. He stopped at a pay phone, woke up his sweetheart, and proposed.

Six weeks later, I was his best man. He was buoyant at the reception. Happiness seemed within his grasp. He did, however, ask me if I'd gotten an eyeful of the girl singer in the band.

20

Percentage of women who have higher libidos than the average guy.

Heat the Sheets

16 DAYS AND DOZENS OF WAYS TO REIGNITE ROMANTIC LOVE—
START ANYWHERE, PICK A DAY, HAVE FUN

Every couple reaches a point when the wild lust of exploration becomes a distant, exotic memory. Some of us, when the friskiness fizzles, turn elsewhere for passion. Others stay faithful and figure that contentment (or boredom) is the price paid for commitment. The smart ones know that great sex after those first wild months can still be had—and even made better—but it takes a bit more effort. It's less about touching her in the right physical spot (although that always helps) and much more about touching her in the right mental spot by honoring her feelings, validating your love for her, and showing your unwavering support.

Day 1. Appreciate How Good You've Got It

The grass, as they say, is always greener on the other side of the fence. So is the ass. And you may be tempted, especially when your relationship is in the doldrums, to think how much better sex and everything would be with someone else, someone younger, funnier, smarter, richer, more attentive, and hotter looking.

If you find yourself doing that, realize this: finding someone new, having an affair, and getting a divorce is a lot easier to think about than to do, actually. And just dwell for a moment on the misery of the standard broken marriage:

anxiety, animosity, depression, psychological damage to the kids, and the tens of thousands of dollars that go away from you and toward your attorney's new Mercedes. But, hey, look at the bright side; only one in five second marriages fail!

The two leading causes of divorce are lack of communication and lack of patience to work on the marriage; people want a quick fix. Why not just take the affair and divorce cards completely off the table? They are not an option. Then you are left with only looking for ways to make things better. The rest of the suggestions in this chapter should help, but start here:

71

Percentage of women responding to a *Women's Health* sexual satisfaction survey who said they value the emotional aspect of sex over the physical pleasure.

136

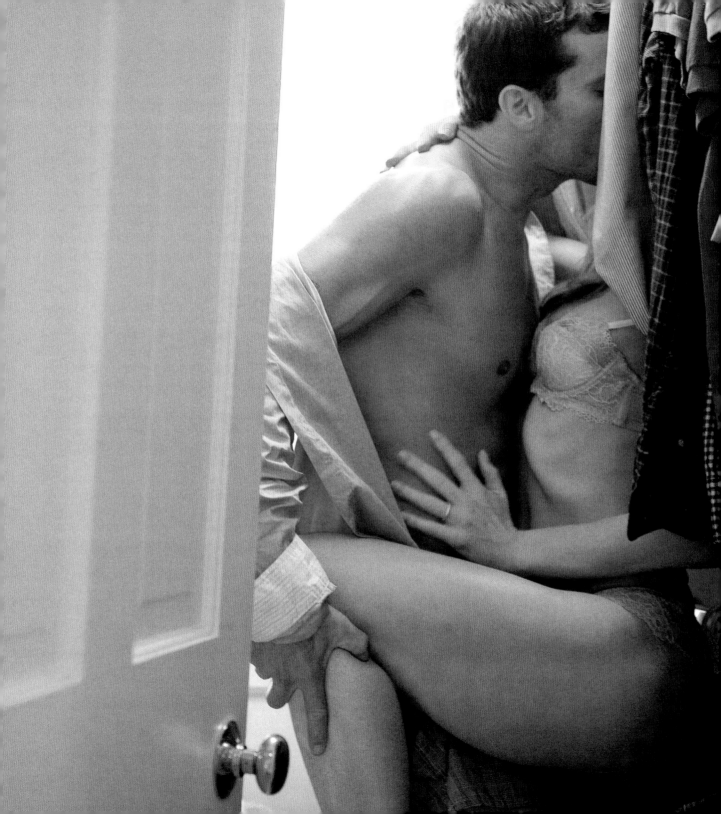

Make Lust Last | HIS

Grab a pad of lined paper and jot down all of the things you love or loved about your partner, the sound of her laugh, how good she is at her job, her ability to pick out just the right gift. Take your time—a couple of days. Avoid writing down anything negative, only the positives, the things you appreciate about her. Don't leave out the little things. Write it all down.

Write down memorable things you've done together: vacations, parties, trips, dinners, etc., on a second sheet of paper. Include situations and brief moments of sadness, tenderness, laughter, love, challenge, and great sex. Think about ways to recreate those times. What can you do to initiate those situations again? Write down your ideas.

Reflect on all the ways you are better off in your relationship than people who are single or divorced. Remember that committed couples generally are happier, healthier, less overwhelmed by stress, have stronger immune and cardiovascular systems, sleep better, and enjoy more frequent sex.

Review your lists every day over the next 2 weeks. In all likelihood, you'll develop a much greater appreciation for your partner and your good fortune. One more tip: Be optimistic about your partnership. Did you know that 70 percent of men and 68 percent of women describe their marriages as "very happy," and 96 percent of men (and 91 percent of women) would marry their current spouse if they had it to do over again? An online survey we recently posted on MensHealth.com and WomensHealthMag.com showed that 77 percent of married women and 78 percent of married men claim to be more in love with their spouses than on the day they were married. Well, what do you know?

Day 2. Tell Her a Secret

Peggy Vaughan knows a lot about secrets. Many years ago, she discovered one about her husband James: He had been having affairs for years. Since then, they have overcome his infidelities, are happily married, and are highly sought-after experts on affairs, having written five books, and the popular and informative website DearPeggy.com. Peggy believes what ultimately saved their marriage—and the critical ingredient to sustaining a loving relationship—is "responsible honesty." What she means by that is having regular, honest communication that goes beyond being truthful in what you say. It means volunteering all your thoughts and feelings that are relevant to the relationship.

"A lot of people think being honest is not telling lies; that's not honesty," says Vaughan. "Real honesty is not withholding information relevant to the relationship. Responsible honesty is sharing your deepest hopes, fears, and dreams on an ongoing basis, and it can be sexier than all of the sex manuals combined."

Even little white lies or withholding

information out of fear of hurting your partner is poisonous to relationships because it creates emotional distance, says Vaughan. Both men and women do it all the time. It's a way of rationalizing one's unwillingness to devote the time and energy to deal with the complexity of honest communication.

"When you are strong enough to expose yourself and make yourself vulnerable, you show your partner the real you." The benefits of such honesty can be life-altering, according to Vaughan:

- It fosters a deeper level of intimacy that leads to a more lasting trust. Vaughan calls trust the most important element for love and good sex.

- It allows your relationship to keep pace with the changes occurring in each of you.

- It keeps channels of communication open and provides constant challenges that can be used for growth.

- It allows each of you to know your-selves at ever-deeper levels and use all of your resources to build the best relationship possible.

No lie.

Day 3. Learn Her Language

The things that make you feel loved (like sex with handcuffs) can be very different from what makes your partner feel loved (a diamond bracelet). Marriage counselor and best-selling author Gary Chapman says couples often speak different emotional love lan-guages . . . as different as Chinese is from English. "No matter how hard you try to express love in English, if your spouse understands only Chinese, you will never understand how to love each other."

Chapman went through 12 years of notes from his counseling sessions and identified five types of emotional lan-guages: Quality Time, Words of Affirma-tion, Receiving Gifts, Acts of Service, and Physical Touch. They formed the basis for his book *The Five Love Languages*, which has sold more than six million copies. "One reason couples argue so much is that they don't feel loved," says Chapman. "And that makes their differ-ences seem so much bigger."

If you feel most loved by having sex (physical touch), and your partner feels most loved when you clean the house (acts of service), then scrubbing the toilet may be your sacrifice for a better sex life.

"Love is intentional; it takes work," says Chapman. Start by doing some investigative reporting. Ask your spouse or partner what you do that makes her feel most loved. Or identify your personal love languages by taking Chapman's quiz together. Number the following boxes in order of importance with "1" being what matters most. Numbers 1 and 2 are your primary and secondary love languages, respectively.

__ I feel especially loved when someone expresses how grateful they are for me, and the simple things I do.

__ I feel especially loved when a person gives me undivided attention and spends time alone with me.

RED-HOT MONOGAMY TIP

"Facial skin is incredibly sensitive, so a sensual, sexy exploration of your partner's face can be very erotic," says Stephanie Buehler, PsyD, a sex therapist and the director of the Buehler Institute in Irvin, California. "Use your finger-tips, lips, or tongue to get intimate with each other's faces and create sexual arousal."

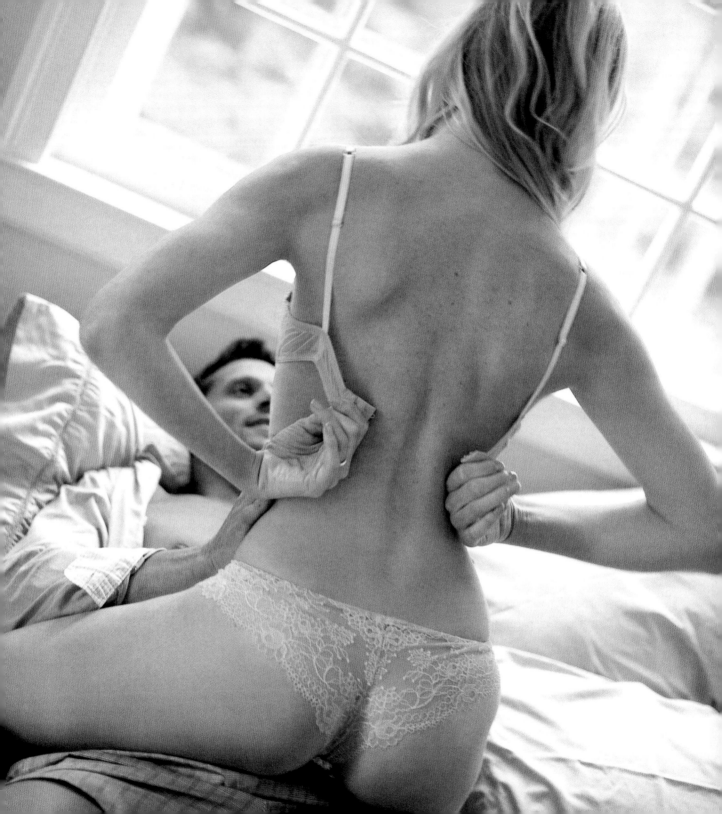

— I feel especially loved by someone who brings me gifts and other tangible expressions of love.

— I feel especially loved when someone pitches in to help me, perhaps by running errands or taking on my household chores.

— I feel especially loved when a person expresses feelings for me through physical contact.

Got it? Spend the rest of the week focusing on meeting your partner's top two love needs.

The results, Chapman promises, will be dramatic. "I had a guy say to me, 'My wife's language is Acts of Service. If I had known that taking out the garbage before she asked me to was sexy to her, I'd have communicated that love to her long ago,'" says Chapman.

And think of how much he might have saved on jewelry.

Day 4. Put Sex on the Calendar

Busy couples must be intentional about sex or they will never get around to it. That means scheduling it. Sure, no one wants to schedule sex. After all, it's supposed to be spontaneous, motivated by pure lust? Right. In the movies. In college. In your dreams. But not in the reality of today's world with two working partners and a houseful of kids and a Pinewood Derby car to whittle by Friday. That's reality. And if you don't have a game plan, you'll end up sitting on the bench. Couples who try carving out time for sex often find that they end up looking forward to it. And even if they are too busy to look forward to it, if they keep that special meeting on the calendar, they are so glad they did afterward. Be creative. Build sexual traditions into your year beyond Valentine's Day, your wedding anniversary, and Father's and Mother's Day. Use annual sporting events as occasions to celebrate naked. Have your own post parade on Kentucky Derby afternoon, with mint juleps by the bedside in case anyone gets thirsty in the backstretch. Game 1 of the World Series deserves a sexual salute. How about the Final Four? Better yet, make it a Sweet 16. On Election Day, for that matter, celebrate democracy and America by shedding your grace on each other.

Day 5. Start Foreplay at 6:30 a.m.

Building on yesterday's concept of planning sex, be intentional about foreplay, too. "To a man foreplay is just the three minutes before insertion," says psychologist Louanne Brizendine, MD, author of *The Male Brain: A Breakthrough Understanding of How Men and Boys Think* and *The Female Brain*. "But for a woman foreplay is everything that happens 24 hours before sex."

In other words, getting in the right frame of mind for great sex takes all day long communication, sending frequent signals that say, "I'm thinking about you," "I want to get close to you."

RED-HOT MONOGAMY TIP

Use double digits. Insert two fngers into her vagina and open them up in a V-shape. "Making a 'come here' motion, like [you] would for the G-spot, will stimulate the roots of the clitoris inside the vagina and bring on different orgasmic sensations," says Jaiya Hanauer, co-author of *Red Hot Touch*.

Dozens of little things you can do to and for your partner will encourage her to think of you in a positive, romantic way that can trigger desire on a hormonal level. Besides, anticipating sex is sometimes even hotter than the act itself. Try a few of these:

Start the day with a long embrace.
A 20-second hug releases the hormone oxytocin, which produces feelings of trust and attachment, according to researchers at the University of Virginia. Holding hands triggers it, too.

Send a dirty text message. Slip a note underneath the windshield wiper of her car saying, "I can't wait to get my hands all over you tonight." A Nielsen survey a few years back found that more than 67 percent of unmarried texters use text messaging to flirt, so why don't you involved folk give sexting a try. Send a daring "Hard4U" or in the subject line or "You've got me wanting to . . ." says Yvonne K. Fulbright, author of *Sultry Sexy Talk to Seduce Any Lover: Lust-Inducing Lingo and Titillating Tactics for Maximizing Your Pleasure.* "Use the first line of your text to complete your sexy subject line."

SEX RULES!
Old Rule: Say "I Love You" Every Day
New Rule: Verbalizing Feelings Should be More Than Just a Habit

Mumbling those three little words through mouthfuls of cornflakes every morning or tossing them at the end of every phone call dilutes their importance and impact. To keep them meaningful: Say "I love you" only when you are really feeling it. Better yet, say it in new and interesting ways. For example, try a compliment ("You are seriously the greatest wife on Earth"), a term of endearment ("Honey" or "Babe"), or a statement of appreciation ("It was so thoughtful of you to let me watch the Giants get clobbered last night"). They all send the same message of affection without becoming rote.

Day 6. Use the Whole Field
Your home probably has five or more rooms—a dining room, kitchen, bathroom, living room, heck some even have a home theater room, a rec room, a mudroom. But no dedicated sex room. Not even a sex nook. So why do we feel compelled to have sex in just one place—the bedroom? Why not utilize all 3,000 square feet of that two-story suburban colonial, and the cabana by the pool?

Living room: Have sex on the living room coffee table the night before a party at your house and see if that doesn't bring a naughty smile to your wife's face during hors d'oeuvres.

Laundry: On the Maytag, during the spin cycle. Have her sit on the edge of the machine with her legs bent and feet on your shoulders. As the machine agitates, bend over and stimulate her orally.

Bathroom: Make use of the mirror and steam things up. Ask her to hold onto the sink and watch the reflection of you entering her from behind. The unusual eye-contract during the G-spot-targeting doggy-style creates instant intimacy.

The stairs: Sit on the stairs facing the railing with one leg braced two steps down and the other leg slightly bent. Lower her onto you while she's facing the rail and holding it for support.

On the sofa: She straddles the arm of the couch facedown grinding her mound on the arm as you enter her from behind. Place a silk scarf on the arm of the couch ahead of time and her breasts and clitoris will rub against the fabric, creating multiple stimulation points.

Outdoors: Eighty percent of surveyed *Men's Health* and *Women's Health* readers said they would love to try outdoor sex. "There's something incredibly raw and primal about having sex outside. It awakens the senses," says sex therapist Sandor Gardos, PhD, founder of MyPleasure. com. You'll feel the cool breeze on your naked skin, smell the sweet peonies and Aphrodite hostas, hear the crickets, the screech owls, the neighbors stopping by for a visit. "The fear of getting caught can add to the thrill," says Gardos.

Day 7. Be Assertive, Not Insertive

Men feel intimate as a result of being sexual; women feel sexual as a result of being intimate. Man or woman, if you can understand the profound truth in that statement, you will be well on your way to building a more romantic and engaging intimacy.

"A lot of women come into the clinic complaining of low libido," says sexual health expert Laura Berman, PhD, founder of the Berman Center in Chicago. "They say they've lost the intimacy in their relationship. The want to cuddle with their guy but the second they do, he thinks it's an invitation for sex. Then the woman has to reject him because she's not in the mood and the whole process begins again." To break this cycle explore VENIS: "very erotic non-insertive sex." This is sexual contact without penetration, where you focus on romantic, playful eroticism through verbal and physical communication. "It removes the pressure of goal-oriented sex, and as a result sex becomes less predictable and more pleasurable," says Berman.

What kind of activity qualifies as VENIS? It could be as tame as brushing each other's hair or as erotic as covering yourselves in oil and wrestling playfully. Try bathing together by candlelight, massage, licking whipped cream off of each other, cuddling in bed, or masturbating together. "The point is to have one night when intercourse isn't the focus," says Berman.

RED-HOT MONOGAMY TIP

Don't call your spouse "Mom." You don't want to have sex with mom, so use your wife's name both in and out of bed.

143

Day 8. Have Morning Sex

There's no sweeter wakeup call.

"Having sex in the morning releases the feel-good chemical oxytocin, which makes couples feel loving and bonded all day long," says Debby Herbenick, PhD, author of *Because It Feels Good*. Put a smile on both of your sleepy faces by starting the day off very right.

Get fresh: Sneaking off to the bathroom to brush your teeth will do more than ward off dragon breath. "Not only will your kisses be minty, but the menthol in your toothpaste can give her a tingly thrill during oral sex," Herbenick says.

Try a cozy move: Since you'll both be groggy, try a position that requires little to no effort: spooning. If she's facing away from you, snuggle up to her back, help her part her legs, and allow her to guide you inside of her. Your hands will be free to caress her breasts and stimulate her clitoris. And you can whisper sweet somethings in her ear.

Day 9. Control Anger

Despite what they say about makeup sex, screaming matches are a poor foreplay choice. Learning how to control major outbursts of anger can go a long way to improving the health of your relationship—and making it hotter.

What gets us so angry? It almost always has to do with feeling disrespected by your partner. Disrespect is just a type of attack, and when we feel threatened and defensive our bodies react as if we are being mugged by a knife-wielding hoodlum, not the person

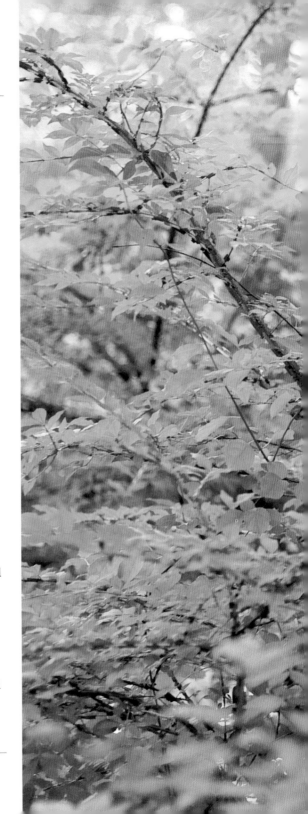

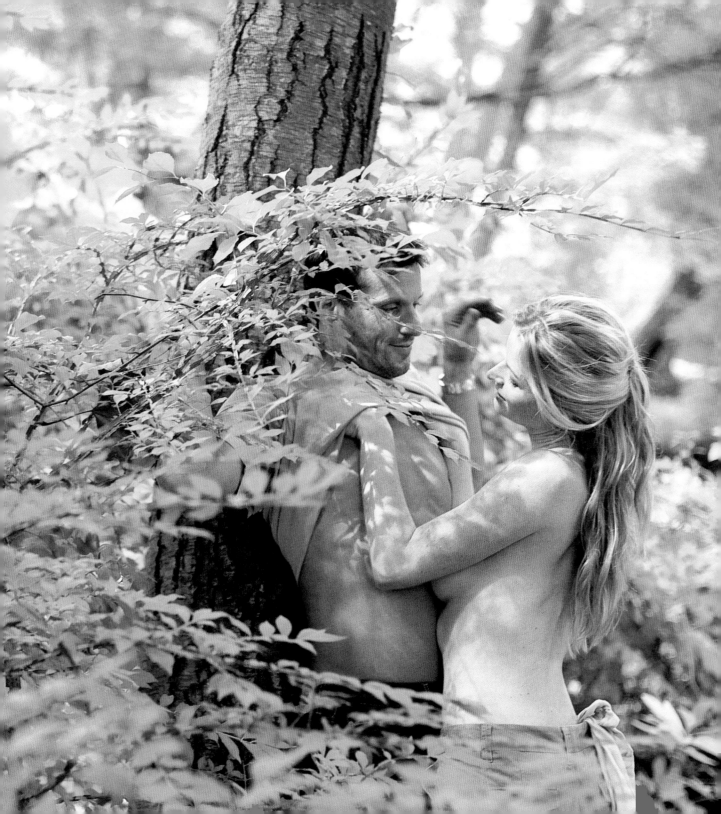

whose bed we share. Your body releases the fight or flight hormones adrenaline and cortisol into your bloodstream and you become so pumped up with righteous indignation that you may explode and say or do foolish things that can be very hurtful to relationships and may take days, weeks, even years to mend.

"A perceived injustice is a tasty looking bait on the fish hook of anger," says Robert Allan, PhD, a clinical psychologist and author of *Getting Control of Your Anger*. "It can be helpful to recognize reasons for anger as baited fishhooks and realize that when we bite, we lose our freedom."

What to do when you feel anger welling up inside you? Don't take the bait and let loose. "The emotionally intelligent fish swims on by the hooks," says Allan. "As the sixteenth century philosopher Montaigne said, 'there is no passion that so shakes the clarity of our judgment as anger.' Things truly seem different once we have quieted and cooled down."

Thomas Jefferson advised pausing 10 seconds before responding if you are angry, 100 if you are very angry. Not only can that strategy improve your love life; it may save your life. A large clinical trial for treating type-A behavior called the Recurrent Coronary Prevention Project, which reduced second heart attack rates by 44 percent, rated recognizing the hook of anger as the single most effective tool for controlling damaging outbursts.

"Anger management is like toilet training," says Allan, "something we should begin early in life before we get involved with someone."

While controlling outbursts of anger is a useful relationship skill, learning how to argue right is even more constructive. "It's not the arguing that kills marriages; it's the arguing style," says John Gottman, PhD, the author of *Why Marriages Succeed or Fail: And How You Can Make Yours Last*. Make sure you have five positive interactions for every fight. Smart arguing can even make the heart grow fonder.

Studies have shown that partners can draw closer together during significant arguments when the volley is constructive and demonstrates how much each partner values the other's opinion. That result comes from choosing words carefully and understanding the art of negotiation. Consider a long-term investigation of 154 married couples reported in the journal *Psychology and Aging* that examined their conversation styles by monitoring physiological responses with heart rate monitors and video cameras. During arguments, the research found, couples who more often used the pronouns "we," "our," and "us" tended to be calmer and more emotionally positive than couples who used more individual pronouns such as "I," "me," and "you."

"This is our problem," is one of the most effective things you can say to your spouse in a conflict, according to Kenneth Silvestri, PhD, a psychotherapist in New Jersey. "It puts you on common ground."

PLAY THINGS

Ten percent of Americans routinely incorporate toys into their lovemaking. (Tip: If you mention this to your partner, don't use the word "incorporate.")

Silvestri is all about achieving harmony, having practiced aikido for 20 years. He believes the martial art's principal of redirecting the energy of an attack through graceful blending movements that bring your opponent into your range of influence is the ideal strategy for marital sparring.

"If you push hard against someone, they will push back just as hard. Aikido teaches that you must yield to win. In a marriage, backing down offers signs of appreciation for your partner's feelings. It creates a positive volley that leads to win-win," says Silvestri.

Day 10. Enjoy a Quickie

Women don't always need 10 or 20 minutes of foreplay to enjoy great sex. Studies published in the *Journal of Sexual Medicine* found that if women ignore outside distractions (kids, TVs blaring, Blackberries humming) they can start to become aroused in just 30 seconds. The heart-pounding adrenaline of spontaneous sex can be a huge erotic rush for her as well as you. Quickie sex can resurrect the feelings of the early days of your courtship when you did it everywhere you had the opportunity.

Rediscover the joys of dry humping, ideal for when you are lying on the couch watching TV. During a commercial break, roll on top of her and target her neck with your mouth while slowly grinding your crotch against hers until she is reaching for your zipper. Or while you're both making dinner, lean in for a long, wet, romantic kiss. Continue making out and press her back up against the kitchen cabinets. When she melts into your arms, push up her skirt and lift her onto the counter. Remember, you're not being rough. You're being direct in a gentlemanly way. Think James Bond in Goldfinger.

Day 11. Scare Your Pants Off

Take a kayaking course. Go rock climbing together. Ride a roller coaster for better sex? Get risky then get frisky. "Trying something new or exciting before sex delivers a burst of dopamine, a chemical that activates the pleasure centers of your brain," says Gail Saltz, MD, author of *The Ripple Effect: How Better Sex Can Lead to a Better Life.* The brain chemical also influences attraction, as one study at the University of Texas at Austin demonstrated. Researchers from the Meston Sexual Psychophysiology Laboratory at the University of Texas in Austin visited a theme park and asked women there to rate the attractiveness of an average looking guy. They showed the women a photograph of the man and asked them to gauge how much they would like to kiss him or date him. Some women were questioned while standing in line for a roller coaster ride; others were questioned right after they got off the ride. It turned out that those who'd just come off the coaster, jacked on adrenaline, rated him as much more dateable and kissable than did the women who were still waiting in line.

Day 12. Knead Each Other

Stand up. Look down. You will see a body part of amazing erotic ability just below waist level—your hands. Use them to massage your mate; a massage is romance you can both appreciate even if it doesn't lead to sex. Start with a good massage oil such as Neal's Yard Remedies Ginger and Juniper Warming Oil ($15 for 1.7 fluid ounces, nealsyardremedies.com) or Naturopathica Arnica Muscle and Joint Massage and Body Oil ($28 for 4 fluid ounces, naturopathica.com). Avoid mineral or baby oils because they are absorbed too quickly into the skin. Don't forget to rub your hands together to warm them before applying the massage oil and performing the following techniques:

1. **Stroke toward the heart.** That means when you're working on her legs, stroke upward. On the arms, stroke downward.

2. **Ease with effleurage.** The French are experts at more than retreating. They know their massage. Effleurage is a simple loosen-up stroke. Light, long, and rhythmic, it generally runs with the grain of the muscle. On the legs, for example, use your cupped palms and gently glide upward. On the back, flatten your hands and broaden your strokes.

3. **Play with petrissage.** This circular stroke is designed to squeeze the muscles and wring out tension from the shoulders, upper arms, legs, and buttocks. Use both hands to work the muscles in opposite directions: When stroking thighs, for example, move one palm away from you as you slide it forward, and move the other toward you.

4. **Roll your thumbs.** This is best for working on tension knots. Use your thumbs, one after the other, to press into the flesh, sometimes moving circularly and other times just holding pressure on one point. Lean your weight into it.

5. **Be generous.** Don't forget the body parts that rarely get touched, such as the backs of the arms and knees, feet, fingers, and scalp.

Day 13. Watch an Erotic Film Together

Watching other people have sex—even viewing a hot scene in an R-rated flick—can trigger lusty thoughts about your partner and spice up your sex life, especially when you view it together, say many sex therapists. And while more men watch porn than women do, many women do find that sexually explicit material is a way to satisfy their natural human curiosity about sex, how bodies look aroused, and what others do in bed.

A study by the University of Denver Center for Marital and Family Studies analyzed the association between viewing sexually explicit films and relationship quality in a random sample of 1,291 unmarried people in romantic relationships. While men tend to watch porn alone (77 percent), the study found that more women watch porn with their partners than by themselves (46 percent versus 32 percent). The researchers also looked at measures of communication, relationship strength, commitment, and sexual satisfaction. "We found that couples who view sexy movies together are more dedicated to each other and more sexually satisfied than those who watch them alone," says study author Amanda Maddox. The only difference between people who reported never watching erotica and those who view it only with their partners was that the porn teetotalers had lower rates of infidelity.

From a purely physiologic standpoint, women and men appear to be equally stimulated by porn. A 2006 study at McGill University found that both men and women started displaying arousal within 30 seconds of turning on the video player. But that doesn't mean cuing up *Edward Penishands* will be everyone's cup of tea. Tastes in erotica differ. And there are psychological downsides to weigh. Many men and women find porn terribly degrading to women and a huge turnoff. A woman may feel threatened if her partner turns on a porn video (Am I not pretty enough? Am I not doing it right?). Watching porn can make both women and men feel inadequate if they don't stack up to the lean, muscular bodies, and large breasts and penises. Remember, body image has an enormous impact on a woman's comfort level. Will you/your partner get too caught up in body comparisons to enjoy the visuals? And, of course, a lot of porn is just plain hokey.

So, before you hunt for porn websites or head to the adult video store, have a talk. Reassure her that you are happy with your relationship and sex life, but want to try something new for inspiration that you both can enjoy together. Talk about what kind of film you'd both like to see. After all, you wouldn't go to the multiplex without talking about it first. Women tend to be more aroused by films that have a good romantic plot that takes its sweet time to ease into the sex scenes, and includes a lot of foreplay. Fifty-six percent of women say seeing more regular or realistic-looking female bodies in films would make watching porn more enjoyable for them. So, look for films that use wide angles rather than genital close-ups, because full bodies (and faces in particular) help women identify with and feel like the turned-on women in the video. Those kinds of films tend to be made by women directors. Check out Pornmoviesforwomen.com for movies by Candida Royalle, Anna Span, and Annie Sprinkle. Or try Comstock Films, which features sex between actual couples. Also consider films like *The Elegant Spanking* or *Silken Sleeves* by Maria Beatty, which feature lesbian sex and look like 1920s noir films with slow, teasing sex scenes that women may find arousing.

Day 14. Become a Stranger

Do you realize how different you became after you got married? Write down a list of 10 things you used to love to do before you got hitched. How many of those activities that made up your core being are you still doing? If you are like many people in long-term relationships, you've cut a big part of what made you feel vital—what attracted your partner to you in the first place—right out of your life. Why not fill up the tires on your old road bike? If you don't have the time to get back into golf or the sense of adventure to start river running again, figure out something new to reinvent yourself. You'll immediately boost your attractiveness to your mate because the newness will tickle those areas of his or her brain that get off on novelty.

Men are typically better at this reinvention game than women are. That's why it's crucial for husbands to do everything in their power to help their wives grow their interests and explore their passions.

SEX RULES!

Old Rule: The Sex Gets Better Over Time

New Rule: The Sex Gets Better Over Time—If You Help it Get Better

"Women voluntarily make more sacrifices and accommodations in a marriage, especially if there are children," says Vaughan. "Eventually that can fester into resentment toward her husband, who she sees as being self-centered."

Encouraging her to get a sitter so she can go out with friends doesn't fly with women. That's not a solution. "That just builds more resentment," says Vaughan. "You are equal people, equal parents. Establishing equitable duties

and taking over to give her freedom to reinvent herself, that's what makes women feel loved."

"As couples get to know each other's bodies, there's a reliability in sexual response," says Yvonne K. Fulbright, PhD, *Women's Health* columnist and author. Familiarity also can breed a deeper intimacy and greater willingness to explore new territory together—two things that are sure to keep you both extremely satisfied for years to come.

Day 15. Employ Some Toys

Using a vibrator, dildo, cock ring, anal toy, clitoral pump, or other toys during sex can enhance the entire experience—if you feel comfortable using them. Many Americans do. Studies by researchers at the Center for Sexual Health Promotion at University of Indiana not only found that 53 percent of women and 45 percent of men have used vibrators during sex, but that those who used them reported more positive sexual function.

Here are some of the most popular sex toys for women and tips you can glean by getting in on the action:

The classic dildo.

Unlike porn actresses, most women first focus these male stand-ins on their clitoris, penetrating only as climax nears, says Lisa Lawless, PhD, cofounder of the National Association for Sexual Awareness and Empowerment.
The lesson: The penis isn't just for penetration. Use it to stroke the outer labia and clitoris during foreplay, says

Vivienne Cass, PhD, author of *The Elusive Orgasm*. Gyrating along these pleasure points while steadily increasing pressure will push her desire to the tipping point, so once you penetrate, you'll deliver orgasm-inducing thrusts.

The G-spot stimulator.

These instruments of pleasure target the spongy, sensitive area in her upper vaginal wall, 2 inches from the opening. **The lesson:** G-spot (as opposed to clitoral) orgasms come from strategic pressure, not size. "Those huge, man-made members aren't what she's hiding under the mattress," says Lawless. To put pressure on this sensitive area with each thrust, a man should enter a woman when she's on her back, with her knees resting on her chest.

The Rabbit vibrator.

With two vibrating petals shaped like a set of hare's ears, this Bugs-inspired toy rubs both sides of her clitoris. **The lesson:** Gently stimulate the clitoris from all sides. First, use your index and ring fingers to rub the sides. Then simultaneously stroke the top of her clitoris with a middle finger, completing the chorus that will send her over the edge.

The classic vibrator.

This multispeed massager lets her focus on her most nerve-rich erogenous spot, the clitoris, as intensity increases. **The lesson:** A little change is good; too much can capsize an orgasm. Always start slow, with gentle, broad strokes of your finger or tongue. Build toward a climax, instead of rapidly changing techniques and intensity.

Day 16. Turn Her on in the Kitchen

No, not that way, but by making dinner and doing the dishes afterward. Recognizing all she does and giving her a well-deserved break is one of the most loving things a guy can do. And it will work in your favor, too, by eliminating the stresses that stifle her sexual thoughts and motivation. "Women need a certain context in place before they can focus on feeling sexual and recognize desire," says sexual behaviorist Brooke Seal, PhD, an assistant professor of clinical psychology at the University of The Fraser Valley.

Remember that, unlike you, a woman is not going to be interested in sex if she's exhausted, stressed, and has a lot on her mind. She needs to feel relaxed, admired, and loved. "Being responsive to your partner's non-sexual needs is so important because it signals that you are really concerned with her welfare," says sex and relationships researcher Gurt Birnbaum, PhD, of the Interdisciplinary Center Herzliya in Israel. Use touch without a sexual motive to endorse her, a caress, a kiss, a tender tap. Touch connects emotionally much deeper when it is set free from the link to sex. But the validation it offers is just the kind of thing that turns kittens into tigers, once the kids go outside to play.

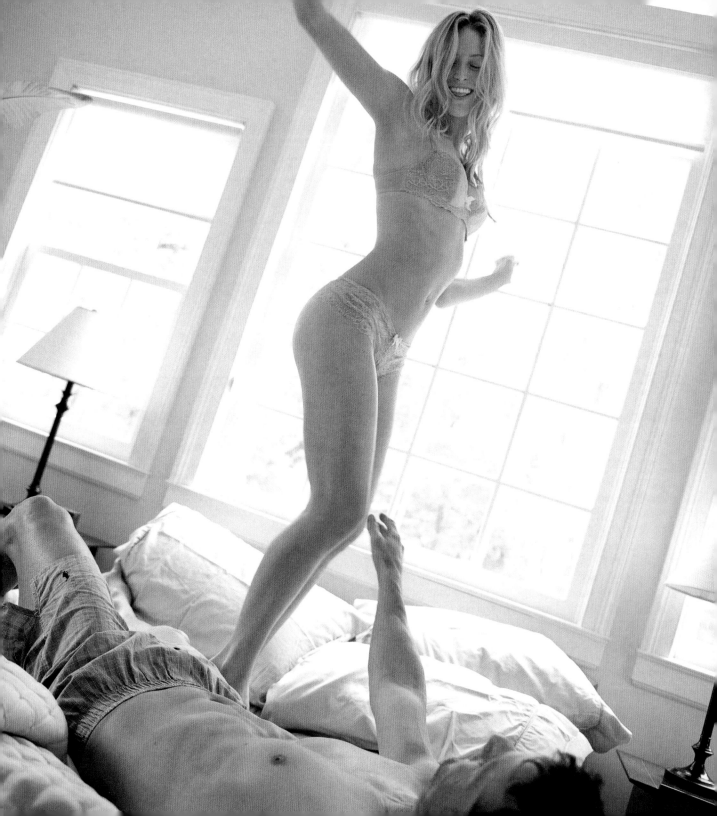

Love Lifts

FIVE EXERCISES FOR A STRONGER RELATIONSHIP

You can build a better relationship just as you can build strength with a couple of dumbbells. Here's a weekly training plan that'll pump up your love life. Designed by John Gottman, PhD, it's based on his research at the Love Lab at the Gottman Institute. It takes less than 5 hours a week and you can expect to start seeing results within 2 weeks.

Exercise 1

Before saying goodbye to your partner in the morning, learn one important thing that's happening in her life that day. This is designed to break the "habit of inattention" that can turn couples into strangers.

Sets:
1 per
working day
Repetitions:
2 minutes
Time:
10 minutes
per week

Exercise 2

When you get home from work, decompress by discussing the most stressful parts of your day. This will prevent job frustration from spilling over into your home life all evening. When it's your partner's turn to vent, resist the urge to give advice. Instead, just listen, be supportive, and say you understand.

Sets:
1 per
working day
Repetitions:
20 minutes
Time:
1 hour, 40 minutes
per week

Exercise 3

Spontaneously tell your partner that you appreciate something she has done or some quality you admire in her.

Sets:
1 per day,
7 days a week
Repetitions:
1 to 5 minutes
Time:
up to 35 minutes
per week

Exercise 4

Show affection out-side the bedroom by occasionally kissing or touching.

Sets:
7 days a week
Repetitions:
5 to 50 times
a day, the more
the better
Time:
a couple of seconds
each is all it takes

Exercise 5

Plan a date once a week, just like when you were single. Get out of the house, even for just a walk, but preferably someplace a bit special, just the two of you, and get reacquainted with each other.

Sets:
1 per week
Time:
30 minutes to
2 hours

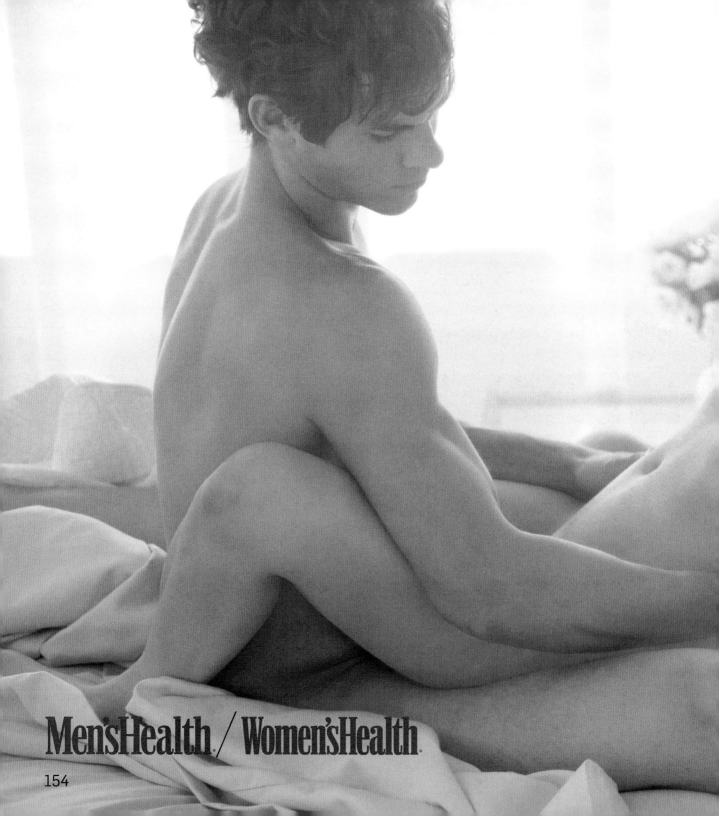

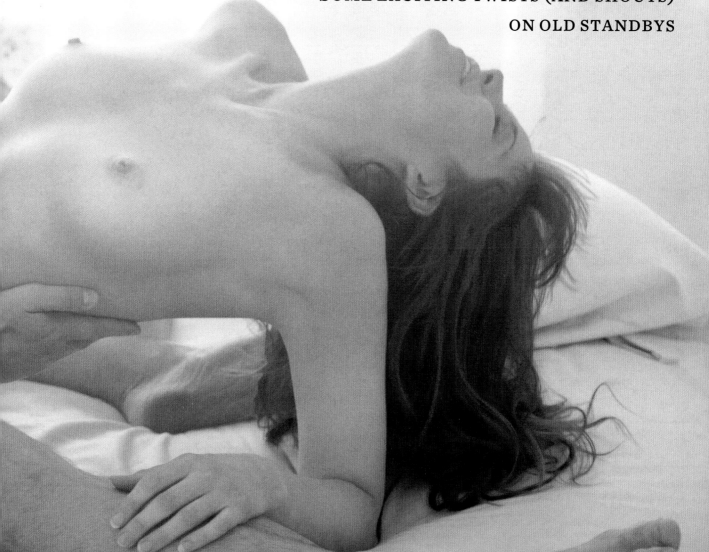

Chapter 8
The Big Book of Sex Positions Sampler
SOME EXCITING TWISTS (AND SHOUTS)
ON OLD STANDBYS

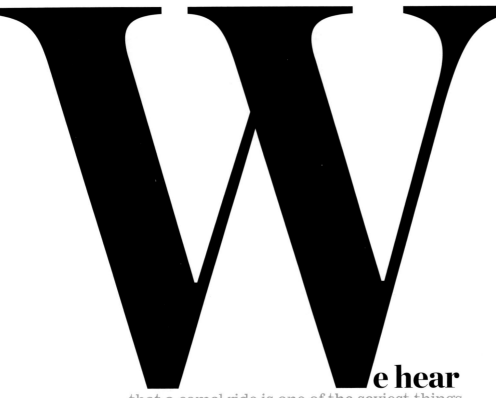

We hear

that a camel ride is one of the sexiest things a couple can do together.

Not into traveling the desert on the backs of sweaty beasts? That's fine. Because the camel ride is a sex position. You might call the move something completely different in your bedroom, but it gave one *Women's Health* reader her first official body-quivering, no-batteries-required orgasm.

"It . . . was . . . a . . . mazing," she says. "My boyfriend Charlie was on top and then he switched positions. He did this thing with his you-know-what and it was like waves of little ripples that kept coming faster and

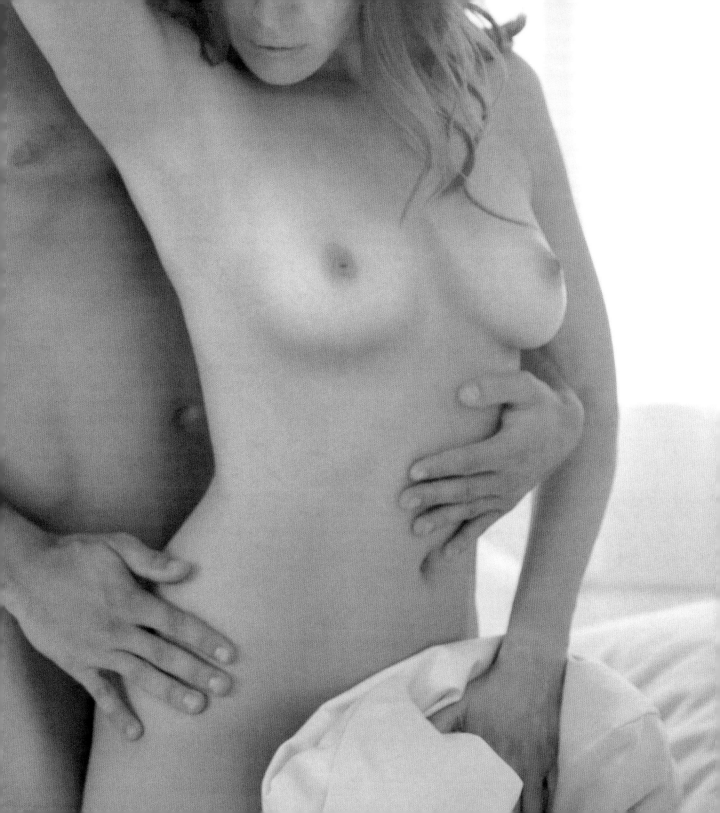

faster. I was tingling everywhere from little explosions and then—oh my God—it was like a warm water balloon burst inside me."

Whew! Like we said, hot. (See The Camel Ride, a.k.a. The Pretzel Dip, page 167.)

When you have sex the same way, in the same place and position, same mmmms and grunts, going through the same foreplay sequence time after time, sex can become, well, not so hot. Warm milk. About as exciting as watching Adam Lambert's hair move.

"Trying something new, such as giving oral sex after eating extra-strength Altoid mints—a craze we were asked about in 2008—creates new sensations, catches your attention, and spices things up," writes Cindy M. Meston, PhD, and David M. Buss, PhD, in their book *Why Women Have Sex*. Maybe adding curiously strong mints isn't your idea of romantic night, but the point is that great sex sometimes takes effort and creativity. Just trying something a little different can fix bedroom boredom and spark greater intimacy in your whole relationship. And, who knows, your partner might look even cuter from that new angle!

But here's the important thing to know about trying sex positions: it's really about the journey, not necessarily reaching a particular destination. "People can twist themselves into the most creative sexual positions, but if they're not feeling relaxed, open to pleasure or present in the moment, they are unlikely to find that sex feels good,"

says Debbie Herbenick, PhD, a research scientist at Indiana University's Center for Sexual Health Promotion, and sex columnist for *Men's Health*.

In other words, go ahead and try the Tilt-a-Whirl or the Reverse Flying Lariet for fun and variety but remember that sex shouldn't resemble a Cirque du Soleil audition. Too much contorting can backfire. "Unlike men, women can lose an orgasm almost in the midst of having one," says sex therapist Ian Kerner.

Instead, play Marco Polo in bed. Be Christopher Columbus to her Vasco da Gama. Become comfortable with touring each other's skin beyond the peaks and crevasses. Did you know that your largest sex organ is your skin? Explore the landscape. Make total-body massage part of a long prelude to lovemaking. Ask your partner, "How does this feel?" "Tell me if this is too much or too little pressure." And answer honestly. This is a team effort.

One of the smartest things a man can do to learn what she likes best is ask her to touch herself. Watch as she brings herself to the brink of orgasm. Notice the rhythm of her finger strokes.

Visit various types of penetration to see what feels best, and don't hesitate to go back to an old standby. The most common positions—man on top, woman on top, spooning, and rear entry—are popular for a reason. Every couple may have their own preferences, based on the size, shape, and angle of a man's penis and a woman's vagina, but couples always seem to return to one of these four because they feel so good.

80

Percentage of women who want to stimulate themselves while you watch (and learn). "The fact that she's turning you on while bringing herself to orgasm makes her feel incredibly sexy and compounds her pleasure," says sex therapist Sandor Gardos, PhD.

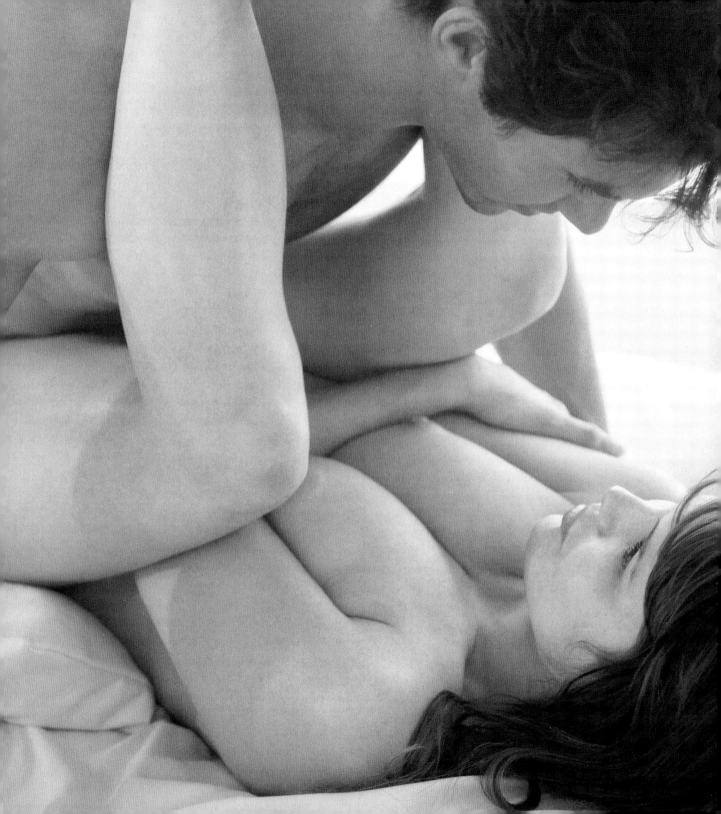

Man on Top

Missionary

a.k.a. The Matrimonial, Male Dominant
Heat Index: ★★
Benefits: Lots of eye and body contact.

The most commonly used position in the world, the missionary is an especially intimate position allowing for face-to-face contact. You like it because you can control penetration depth and speed of thrusting. She enjoys feeling your weight on her body, and the maximum skin-to-skin contact. Note that this position can make it more difficult to hold off ejaculation because of the intense friction and deep thrusting. To lengthen love-making, start there then switch to a position that maintains clitoral pressure without so much pelvic back and forth. **Now try this:** Push up to create space in between you to sneak a small vibrator down for buzzing the top of her mound.

YOUR NEXT MOVE

Quicker Picker Upper

Place a pillow under the small of her back or her buttocks to tilt her pelvis and change the angle of your penetration for different sensations. Bracing yourself with your hands on the bed as in a pushup position, you take your weight off of her body.

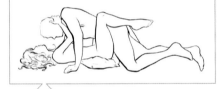

Hot Tip —**His**

Raise her left leg so her knee is level with your right shoulder. Keep her other leg flat on the bed. Thrust toward the inner thigh of her raised leg. This adjustment forces tighter penetration and more clitoral pressure.

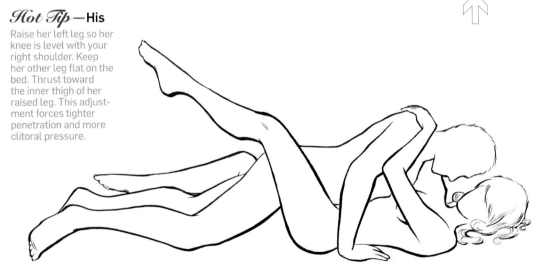

Hot Tip —**Hers**

Raise both legs in the air and spread them wider to shorten the vagina and feel tighter around his penis. If you want him deeper, bend your knees and lift them to your chest.

The CAT

a.k.a. Coital Alignment Technique
Heat Index: ★★★
Benefits: Strong clitoral stimulation. In one study in the *Journal of Sex and Marital Therapy*, women who were unable to have an orgasm in the missionary position reported a 56 percent increase in orgasm frequency using the coital alignment technique.

The CAT is just like the missionary except that your body is farther up and to one side. Instead of being chest to chest, your chest is near her shoulders. Have her bend her legs about 45 degrees to tilt her hips up. This causes the base of your shaft to maintain constant contact with her clitoris.
Now try this: Ask her to straighten her legs. Push your pelvis down a few inches while she pushes up.

Hot Tip —His

Instead of thrusting up and down, rock forward and back to, hopefully, provide enough stimulation for her to orgasm. Also try grinding your pelvis in a circular motion. Other studies suggest even greater success, with up to 73 percent of women achieving orgasm with CAT.

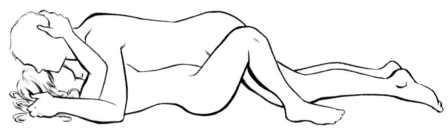

Mountain Climber

a.k.a. The Pushup
Heat Index: ★★★
Benefits: Creates great eye-to-eye contact. Keeps your weight off her body.

There's a reason women swoon when they see a six pack. They know a man with strong abs is going to be great in the sack. The mountain climber position shows off your strength and hard abs (if you have 'em). While between her legs, assume the standard "up" position.
Now try this: Lower yourself to kiss her teasingly while thrusting with your shoulders as well as your pelvis.

Hot Tip —Hers

Ask him to tease you with a series of moves: by entering you with just the tip; thrusting just halfway in; then removing himself and stroking you outside with his member. You can reach down and grab his shaft and rub your clitoris with it.

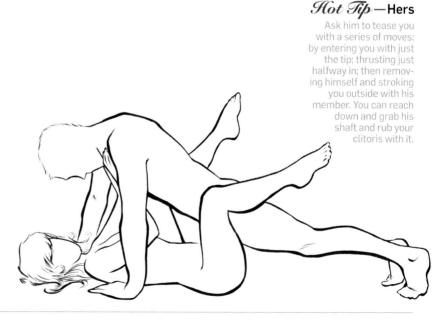

Standing, Rear Entry

Quickie Fix

a.k.a. The Bends, Drop the Soap
Heat Index: ★★★★
Benefits: Greater thrusting power, and good for quickie sex in your kitchen, or a bathroom at a party, especially if she is wearing a skirt.

Ask her to bend at the waist and rest her hands on a piece of furniture, her knees or the floor for support. You enter her from behind and hold her hips for support as you thrust. **Now try this:** Reach below to caress her clitoris for extra stimulation.

Hot Tip — **His**
Massage her shoulders or stimulate her breasts by bending over her.

Hot Tip — **Hers**
Cross your ankles. This will squeeze your vaginal and gluteal muscles tightly around his penis.

Take It Out of the Bedroom

VARIATION #1

Couch Surfer
Ask her to bend her body over the arm of a couch as you enter her from behind. She can grind on the firm but cushy arm for multiple stimulation with minimal effort.

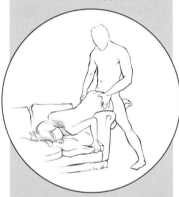

VARIATION #2

Restroom Attendant
Slip into a bathroom and ask her to look into the mirror while you enter her from behind. It lets you have eye contact during the G-spot–targeting rear-entry position.

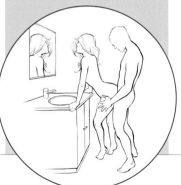

Standing Tiger, Crouching Dragon

a.k.a. Crouching Tiger, Hidden Serpent
Heat Index: ★★★★
Benefits: An ideal position for G-spot stimulation. Seeing the round curves of her rear tends to be highly erotic for you.

Stand and enter her from behind as she poses on all fours on the edge of the bed and arches her back to lift her buttocks.
Now try this: With your legs outside of hers, use your thighs to squeeze her knees together, which tightens her vagina around your penis.

Hot Tip—His
Make some noise. Explore the deeper sexual response and energy by letting lose with powerful sounds, a roar, perhaps?

Wheel Barrow, Standing

a.k.a. The Hoover Maneuver
Heat Index: ★★★
Benefits: Calorie burner because it's so athletic. You can stroll around the house in this position, but draw the shades first.

You enter her as you would in standing, rear entry, but lift her up by the pelvis and have her grip your waist with her legs. Summer camp wheelbarrow races were never this much fun!
Now try this: Ask her to rythmically squeeze her PC muscles to help her climax.

Seated Style
Try the wheel barrow while sitting on the edge of a bed or chair. Movement is limited, but penetration is deep.

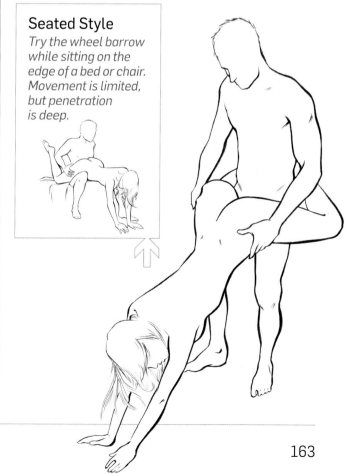

Standing, Front Entry

The Ballet Dancer

a.k.a. Get a Leg Up
Heat Index: ★★★★★
Benefits: Erotic move for quickies in tight quarters. Good option for outdoor sex. Allows for easier penetration. She has control of thrusting, depth, and angle.

You stand facing one another. She raises one of her legs up and wraps it around your buttocks or thigh and pulls you into her with her leg.
Now try this: If her wrapped leg gets tired, cradle it with your arm. If she's very flexible, lift her leg over your shoulder.

Hot Tip—**Ours**
Try this standing position in a hot shower. During the steamy foreplay, rub each other's entire body with a coarse salt scrub to stimulate nerve endings and blood flow.

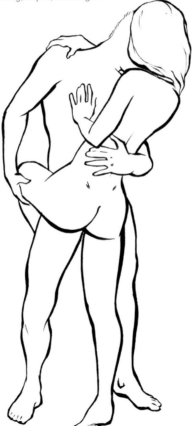

Take It Out Of The Bedroom

VARIATION #1

H2Ohh Yeah
Her buoyancy in the water makes this position easier to hold. And all you need to do is shift some bathing suit material out of the way of certain body parts; the lifeguards will be none the wiser.

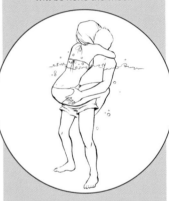

VARIATION #2

Iron Chef
Your kitchen counter is the perfect height for this standing-to-seated appetizer.

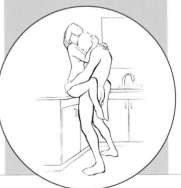

164

Stand and Deliver

a.k.a. The Bicycle
Heat Index: ★★★★★
Benefits: You can enjoy the view of your penis thrusting.

Stand at the edge of a bed or desk while she lies back and raises her legs to her chest. Her knees are bent as if she's doing a "bicycling" exercise. Grab her ankles and enter her. Thrust slowly as the deep penetration may be painful for her.
Now try this: Have her place her heels on your shoulders, which will open her hips so her labia press against you.

Butter Churner

a.k.a. Squat Thruster
Heat Index: ★★★★★
Benefits: An extra rush of blood to her head to increase her ecstacy.

Have your partner lie on her back with her legs raised over her head. This is *not* a plain Jane position! Squat over her and dip your penis in and out of her. Be extra careful to thrust lightly to avoid stressing her neck.
Now try this: By removing yourself fully, you'll give her the extremely pleasurable feeling of you first entering her over and over again.

Hot Tip —Ours

Novelty ignites passion by increasing your brain's levels of dopamine, a neurotransmitter linked to romance and sex drive, says biological anthropologist Helen Fisher, PhD. The Butter Churner qualifies for novelty, but you don't need to go to such extremes to sustain romance. Anything that's new and different will do the trick.

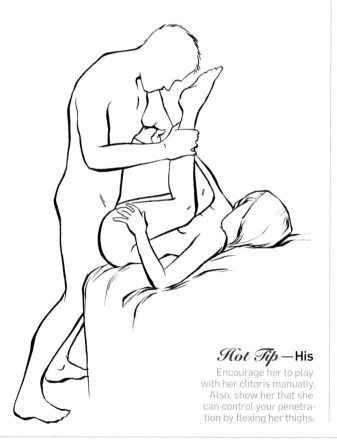

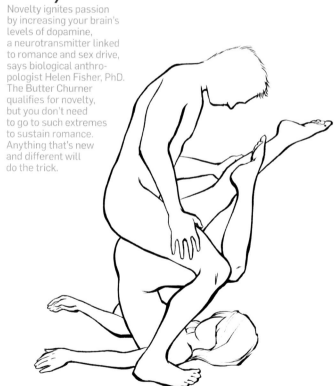

Hot Tip —His

Encourage her to play with her clitoris manually. Also, show her that she can control your penetration by flexing her thighs.

Kneeling

The Flatiron

a.k.a. Downward Dog, The Belly Flop
Heat Index: ★★★★★
Benefits: Intensifies vaginal pleasure.

She lies face down on the bed, knees slightly bent and hips slightly raised. For comfort, and to increase the angle of her hips, she can place a pillow under her lower abs. You enter her from behind and keep your weight off of her by propping yourself up with your arms. This position creates a snug fit, making you feel larger to her.
Now try this: You'll last longer in this position if you switch to shallower thrusts and begin deep breathing.

Hot Tip —His

Less friction means less stimulation—and can help you last longer. Try using a very slippery silicon-based lubricant like Durex Play More, which may allow you to thrust longer before reaching orgasm.

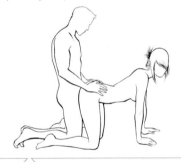

YOUR NEXT MOVE

Man's Best Friend

Entering her from behind, you'll be able to thrust deep so the tip of your penis touches her cervix, an often-neglected pleasure zone. But you should do this slowly and gently. Some women find it painful.

Hot Tip —Hers

You may be able to increase the intensity of your orgasm by pushing your pelvic floor muscles outward, as if you are trying to squeeze something out of your vagina. This causes your vaginal walls to lower, making your G-spot more accessible.

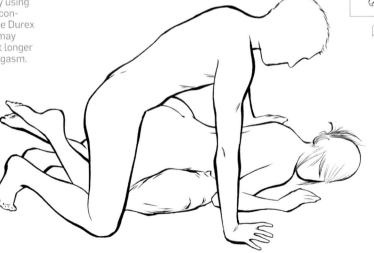

The G-Whiz

a.k.a. The Shoulder Holder, The Anvil
Heat Index: ★★★★
Benefits: Allows deep penetration and targeting the G-spot.

She lies on her back. You kneel between her legs and raise them, resting her calves over your shoulders. Rock her in a side-to-side and up-and-down motion to bring the head and shaft of your penis in direct contact with the front wall of her vagina. Because this angle allows for deep penetration, thrust slowly at first avoid causing her discomfort.

Now try this: Bring her legs down and have her place her feet on your chest in front of your shoulders. This allows her to control the tempo and depth of thrusts.

Hot Tip —His

Notice her nearing orgasm. You do that by listening for her breath to become short and shallow. Flushed skin and slightly engorged breasts also indicate she's nearing the peak of her arousal.

The Pretzel

a.k.a. The Pretzel Dip, The Camel Ride
Heat Index: ★★★★
Benefits: The deep penetration of doggy-style while face to face.

Kneel and straddle her left leg while she is lying on her left side. She will bend her right leg around the right side of your waist, which will give you access to enter her vagina. For many women, rear entry hurts their backs. This position allows her to lounge comfortably while enjoying deep penetration.

Now try this: Manually stimulate her using your fingers. Or withdraw your penis and, holding the shaft with your left hand, rub the head against her clitoris to bring her to the brink of orgasm then you can reinsert when she wants you inside her.

Hot Tip —His

Be gentle with her clitoris. It's more sensitive than your penis, so touch lightly at first. Some women even prefer gentle pressure around it rather than direct stimulation. Go soft, then increase speed and pressure. And ask her to direct you, faster, slower, lighter, harder.

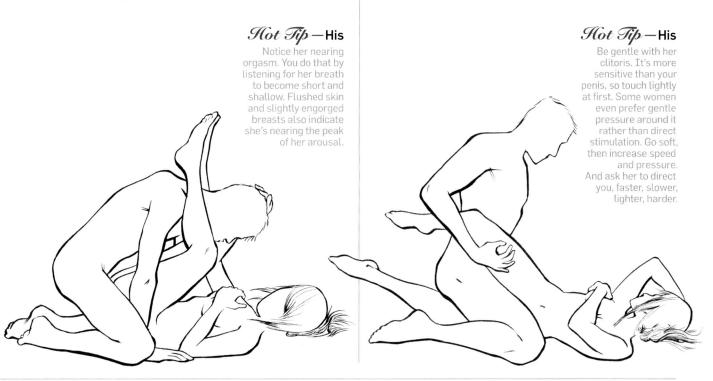

Oral

One Up

a.k.a. Over Your Shoulder, The Hamstring Stretch
Heat Index: ★★★
Benefits: This position is ideal for women who are particularly sensitive along one side of the clitoris.

Kneel on the floor with her lying on the edge of the bed. Raise one of her legs and ask her to support the leg by wrapping her hands around her hamstring just below the knee. With one hip raised, she'll be able to add some movement to aid in your stroking or to help move you to the perfect spot.

Now try this: Encourage her to wriggle a little to help you get the rhythm right.

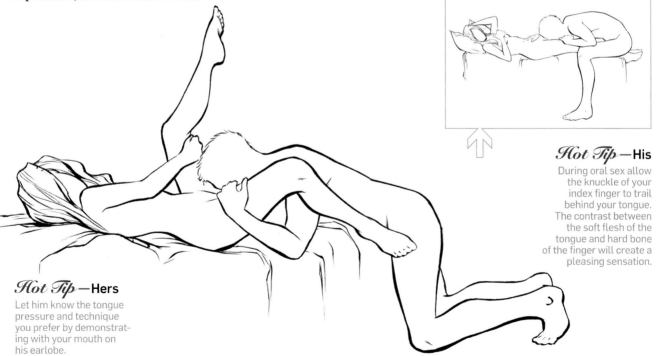

YOUR NEXT MOVE

Closed for Business

Some women find direct clitoral stimulation uncomfortable. Having her close her legs during oral sex may help. Place your hand above her public mound applying light pressure, then rub your firm tongue on the area around the clitoris to add indirect stimulation.

Hot Tip **—His**
During oral sex allow the knuckle of your index finger to trail behind your tongue. The contrast between the soft flesh of the tongue and hard bone of the finger will create a pleasing sensation.

Hot Tip **—Hers**
Let him know the tongue pressure and technique you prefer by demonstrating with your mouth on his earlobe.

Heir to the Throne

a.k.a. Lazy Girl
Heat Index: ★★★★
Benefits: The ultimate position for oral on the go, use this to get her in the mood and help her cut loose.

Have your partner sit on a chair with her legs wide open. You take it from there. This is a good position for either beginning the slow build-up with loose, broad, strokes, or ending with strong suction. Your partner is able to easily guide you, and she's able to get a full view of you between her legs, which is a turn-on for many women.
Now try this: Switch to a swivel chair and turn it left and right as you hold your tongue stationary.

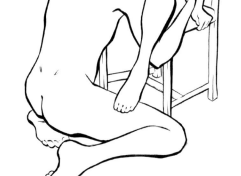

Hot Tip —His

Insert your index and ring fingers and stroke in a "come hither" motion to wake up her G-spot. With either your tongue or other hand, apply pressure to her pubic bone. This dual stimulation executed just right will send her over the edge.

David Copperfield

a.k.a. Trick & Treat
Heat Index: ★★★
Benefits: This position is the pièce de résistance for women who prefer a strong, upward stroking motion.

Hot Tip —His

Let your tongue rest firmly and flat against the full length of her vaginal entrance, then have her move and grind against your tongue.

Place a pillow under her hips to tilt her pelvis up. Bend her knees so she can place her feet on your shoulder blades.
Now try this: Amplify your oral efforts with a simple sleight-of-hand trick:

While you lap away, try using your hands to push gently upward on her abdomen, stretching her skin away from her pubic bone, and helping to coax the head of her clitoris out from beneath the hood.

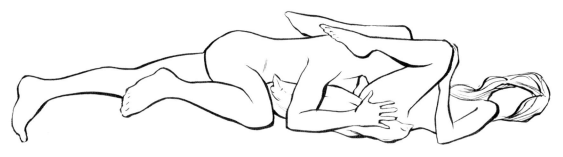

His Favorite Positions

Size, shape, and flexibility all play a role in which sex positions rock your world. Your lucky task is to experiment for best fit. These 15 positions, detailed on the following pages, should keep you busy.

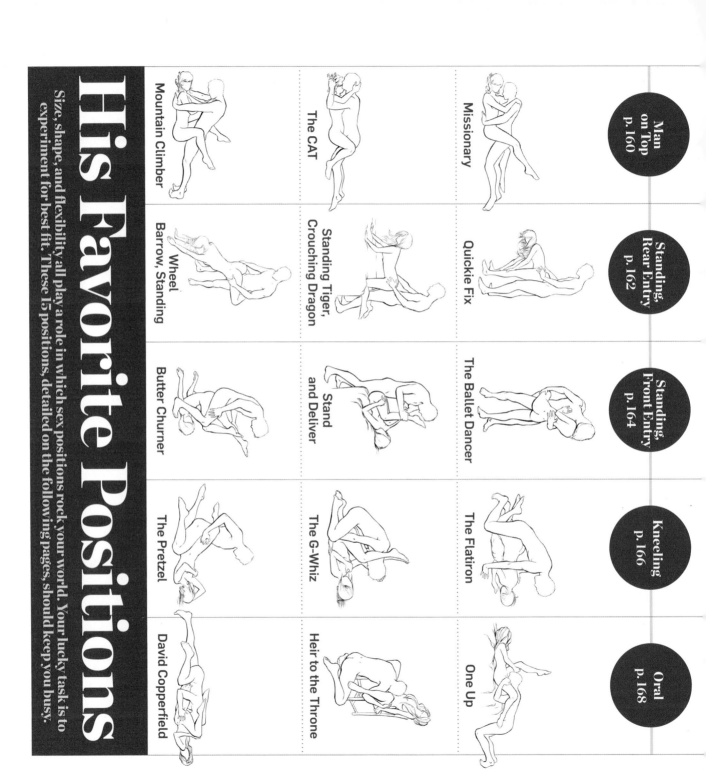

Man on Top p. 160	Standing, Rear Entry p. 162	Standing, Front Entry p. 164	Kneeling p. 166	Oral p. 168
Missionary	Quickie Fix	The Ballet Dancer	The Flatiron	One Up
The CAT	Standing Tiger, Crouching Dragon	Stand and Deliver	The G-Whiz	Heir to the Throne
Mountain Climber	Wheel Barrow, Standing	Butter Churner	The Pretzel	David Copperfield